PEDIATRIC CARDIOLOGY

A Problem Oriented Approach

PEDIATRIC CARDIOLOGY

A Problem Oriented Approach

Ira H. Gessner, M.D.

G.L. Schiebler Eminent Scholar
Department of Pediatrics
Division of Cardiology
University of Florida
College of Medicine
Gainesville, Florida

Benjamin E. Victorica, M.D.

Virginia Root Sutherland Professor
Department of Pediatrics
Division of Cardiology
University of Florida
College of Medicine
Gainesville, Florida

W.B. SAUNDERS COMPANY
A Division of Harcourt Brace & Company
Philadelphia / London / Toronto / Montreal / Sydney / Tokyo

W. B. SAUNDERS COMPANY

A Division of
Harcourt Brace & Company
The Curtis Center
Independence Square West
Philadelphia, Pennsylvania 19106

Library of Congress Cataloging-in-Publication Data

Pediatric cardiology: a problem oriented approach / [edited by] Ira
H. Gessner, Benjamin E. Victorica.
    p. cm.
    ISBN 0 – 7216 – 4564 – X
    1. Pediatric cardiology — Case studies. 2. Pediatric cardiology —
Examinations, questions, etc. I. Gessner, Ira H. II. Victorica,
Benjamin E.
    [DNLM: 1. Cardiovascular Diseases — in infancy & childhood — case
studies. WS 290 P3712 1993]
RJ421.P423   1993
618.92′ 1209 — dc20
DNLM/DLC   92 – 48475

Pediatric Cardiology: A Problem Oriented Approach   ISBN 0-7216-4564-X

Printed in Mexico.

Last digit is the print number: 9   8   7   6   5   4   3   2   1

This book is dedicated to many people, all of whom have been important to us throughout our careers in Pediatric Cardiology. Our patients, who number in the thousands, have given us invaluable experience from which we believe that we continue to learn daily. Students of medicine, both undergraduate and postgraduate, have provided stimulation and motivation. Most importantly, we include in this dedication our wives, Gerri Gessner and Blanca Victorica, and our children who have given us love, understanding, support, and continuity.

Contributors

JAMES A. ALEXANDER, M.D.
Professor of Surgery, Chief, Thoracic and Cardiovascular Surgery, University of Florida College of Medicine, Gainesville, Florida
Cardiovascular Surgery

HUGH D. ALLEN, M.D.
Professor of Pediatrics and Medicine, Vice-Chairman of Pediatrics, Director, Division of Pediatric Cardiology, Ohio State University, Columbus, Ohio
Life Style Issues

ELIA M. AYOUB, M.D.
Professor of Pediatrics, Chief, Division of Infectious Diseases, University of Florida College of Medicine, Gainesville, Florida
Rheumatic Fever

DAVID BAUM, M.D.
Professor of Pediatrics, Chief, Division of Pediatric Cardiology, Stanford University Medical Center, Palo Alto, California
Heart and Lung Transplantation in Children

CARROLL G. BENNETT, D.D.S., M.S.
Professor of Pediatric Dentistry, College of Dentistry, University of Florida, Gainesville, Florida
Dental Issues for the Primary Care Physician

DANIEL BERNSTEIN, M.D.
Assistant Professor of Pediatrics, Division of Pediatric Cardiology, Stanford University Medical Center, Palo Alto, California
Heart and Lung Transplantation in Children

FREDRICK Z. BIERMAN, M.D.
Professor of Pediatrics, Chief, Pediatric Cardiology, Schneider Children's Hospital of Long Island Jewish Medical Center, Albert Einstein College of Medicine, New Hyde Park, New York
Echocardiography

ADNAN S. DAJANI, M.D.
Professor of Pediatrics, Wayne State University School of Medicine; Chief, Division of Infectious Diseases, Children's Hospital of Michigan, Detroit, Michigan
Endocarditis

RICHARD J. DECKELBAUM, M.D.
Professor of Pediatrics, Director, Division of Gastroenterology and Nutrition, Director, Institute of Human Nutrition, Columbia University College of Physicians and Surgeons, New York, New York
Integrated Cardiovascular Health Promotion in Childhood

MICHAEL L. EPSTEIN, M.D.
Associate Professor of Pediatrics, Chief, Division of Cardiology, University of Florida College of Medicine, Gainesville, Florida
Disturbances of Cardiac Rhythm

WAYNE H. FRANKLIN, M.D.
Assistant Professor of Clinical Pediatrics and Internal Medicine, Ohio State University College of Medicine, Columbus, Ohio
Life Style Issues

JAIME L. FRIAS, M.D.
Professor and Chairman, Department of Pediatrics, University of South Florida College of Medicine, Tampa, Florida
Genetic Issues of Congenital Heart Defects

WELTON M. GERSONY, M.D.
Professor of Pediatrics, College of Physicians and Surgeons of Columbia University, Pediatric Cardiology, Babies Hospital South, New York, New York
The Older Child and Adolescent with Chest Pain, Mitral Valve Prolapse, Syncope

IRA H. GESSNER, M.D.
G.L. Schiebler Eminent Scholar, Department of Pediatrics, Division of Cardiology, University of Florida College of Medicine, Gainesville, Florida
Physical Examination; Congestive Heart Failure; Evaluation of the Infant and Child with a Heart Murmur

SAMUEL S. GIDDING, M.D.
Associate Professor of Pediatrics, Northwestern University Medical School, Chicago, Illinois
Integrated Cardiovascular Health Promotion in Childhood

RAE-ELLEN W. KAVEY, M.D.
Associate Professor of Pediatrics, Division of Pediatric Cardiology, SUNY Health Sciences Center, Syracuse, New York
Integrated Cardiovascular Health Promotion in Childhood

DANIEL G. KNAUF, M.D.
Associate Professor of Surgery, Division of Thoracic and Cardiovascular Surgery, University of Florida College of Medicine, Gainesville, Florida
Cardiovascular Surgery

DANIEL J. O'BRIEN, Ph.D., R.N.
Assistant Professor, College of Nursing; and Division of Thoracic and Cardiovascular Surgery, University of Florida, Gainesville, Florida
Cardiovascular Surgery

CHERYL L. PERRY, Ph.D.
Professor, Division of Epidemiology, School of Public Health, University of Minnesota, Minneapolis, Minnesota
Integrated Cardiovascular Health Promotion in Childhood

ROBERT E. PRIMOSCH, D.D.S., M.S., M.E.R.
Professor of Pediatric Dentistry, University of Florida College of Dentistry, Gainesville, Florida
Dental Issues for the Primary Care Physician

ANNE H. ROWLEY, M.D.
Assistant Professor of Pediatrics, Northwestern University Medical School, The Children's Memorial Hospital, Chicago, Illinois
Kawasaki Syndrome

STANFORD T. SHULMAN, M.D.
Professor of Pediatrics, Northwestern University Medical School; Chief, Division of Infectious Diseases, The Children's Memorial Hospital, Chicago, Illinois
Kawasaki Syndrome

WILLIAM B. STRONG, M.D.
Leon Henri Charbonnier Professor of Pediatrics, Chief, Section of Pediatric Cardiology, Medical College of Georgia, Augusta, Georgia
Integrated Cardiovascular Health Promotion in Childhood

BENJAMIN E. VICTORICA, M.D.
Virginia Root Sutherland Professor, Department of Pediatrics, Division of Cardiology, University of Florida College of Medicine, Gainesville, Florida
How to Read a Chest Radiograph; Electrocardiogram Interpretation and Diagnostic Value; Cyanotic Newborns; Newborns with Low Systemic Output; Cardiomyopathy

REGINALD WASHINGTON, M.D.
Associate Clinical Professor of Pediatric Cardiology, University of Colorado School of Medicine, Denver, Colorado
Integrated Cardiovascular Health Promotion in Childhood

JACK H. WILMORE, Ph.D.
Professor of Kinesiology and Health Education, University of Texas at Austin, Austin, Texas
Integrated Cardiovascular Health Promotion in Childhood

Acknowledgments

Many individuals have influenced both directly and indirectly our education as Pediatric Cardiologists. Of all those from whom we have learned over the past 30 years we would like to particularly acknowledge two; Richard T. Smith, M.D., first Chairman of the Department of Pediatrics at the University of Florida College of Medicine, who brought us to this institution; and Gerold L. Schiebler, M.D., first Chief of Pediatric Cardiology and second Chairman of the Department of Pediatrics at the University of Florida College of Medicine, whose outstanding qualities as a teacher and as a leader have been so important to us. Each of these fine human beings has enriched our lives in many ways.

We would like to acknowledge our co-authors who have contributed their time and talent to this project. We hope that the end result meets with their approval.

We acknowledge with great appreciation and gratitude the superb editorial assistance of Ms. Laura Monday who typed, managed, and organized each chapter through many revisions. Her contributions were essential. Ms. Debbie Floyd, Office Manager in the Division of Pediatric Cardiology helped considerably both directly and by her skillful management of our office thereby allowing the workload generated by this book to be assimilated. Finally we wish to acknowledge the interest and support of W.B. Saunders Company, particularly as expressed by Mr. Richard Zorab, Senior Medical Editor. His help has been invaluable.

Ira H. Gessner
Benjamin E. Victorica

Preface

Heart disease in infants and children often challenges the primary care pediatric physician both in regard to recognition and management particularly because heart disease can present as acute illness, sometimes life-threatening, especially in the newborn. Furthermore, the field becomes more complex as one delves into it; pediatric cardiology can seem to be an enormous array of bizarre and complicated anomalies. We believe, however, that it is not necessary for the practitioner to be able to identify specifically all congenital heart defects together with their various combinations; but it is important to be able to recognize the possibility or probability that cardiac disease is present. From this perspective, cardiac disease in infants and children becomes simpler. Cyanosis, heart failure, or both, account for most symptomatic disease. An asymptomatic heart murmur is the most common observation prompting outpatient evaluation of a child. Chest pain is a frequent complaint of the older child and adolescent, and concerns about diet, cholesterol, and blood pressure are prevalent.

Most textbooks of pediatric cardiology, whether written for the sub-specialist or for the non-cardiologist, present this subject lesion by lesion. We believe that it is more useful for the primary care physician to approach pediatric cardiology from the standpoint of the clinical setting in which the patient is first seen. A newborn with cyanosis requires evaluation of possible causes; for the cardiovascular system that means a physical examination, chest x-ray, electrocardiogram, and a few blood tests. If heart disease is present or likely, stabilization, acute therapy as needed, and transportation to a pediatric cardiology center are indicated. A child with an asymptomatic heart murmur should be evaluated primarily from the standpoint of a yes/no decision. Is there heart disease, or a likelihood of such, or not? The practitioner should be able to make that judgment on the basis of history and physical examination, sometimes supplemented by an electrocardiogram and chest x-ray. If the answer is yes, referral may be indicated.

The objective of this book is to provide the primary care pediatric physician with an opportunity to read about pediatric aged patients with documented or suspected heart disease from the standpoint of the patient's presenting problem which is, after all, the reality of the initial encounter. Each of the major problems in pediatric cardiology is addressed in this way. One can read about tetralogy of Fallot from the standpoint of a cyanotic newborn or an infant with a heart murmur but there is not a chapter on tetralogy of Fallot. Similarly, an infant with a large ventricular septal defect may present because of heart failure while a child with a small ventricular septal defect has only a heart murmur; the former appears in the chapter on heart failure and the latter in the chapter on asymptomatic heart murmur.

The book is divided into three sections. Section one describes basic diagnostic skills emphasizing physical diagnosis and simple laboratory tests. The second section presents common general clinical problems in pediatric cardiology as they present to the primary care physician. The third section reviews some specific clinical problems and management issues.

It is our hope that by focusing elsewhere than on specific anatomic diagnosis, the reader will be able to use this book as a guide to recognition, evaluation and management of the patient's problem; as a source of instruction in fundamental diagnostic skills; and as a reference for specific information. Our goal is to help the primary care physician provide more accurate, timely, efficient and cost effective care for infants and children with cardiovascular abnormalities.

Ira H. Gessner
Benjamin E. Victorica

Contents

Part I
BASIC DIAGNOSTIC SKILLS

1

PHYSICAL EXAMINATION

Ira H. Gessner

Physical examination remains the cornerstone of cardiac diagnosis. This principle is as true for the primary care physician as it is for the cardiologist, as most patients with a cardiovascular abnormality are referred to a cardiologist by a primary physician. Initial recognition or suspicion of pathology may be based entirely on physical findings. Just as it is important to be able to recognize abnormal physical findings, it is also important to be able to accurately and confidently characterize normal findings.

It is not possible to learn how to examine a patient's heart by reading about it in a book. Technical skills are learned best by performing them repetitively. It is possible, however, to acquire an understanding of facts, principles, and concepts that form the foundation and framework for skill acquisition. The rest is up to the individual. One becomes good at cardiac physical diagnosis in the same way as one becomes skilled in playing the piano. As the saying goes, the answer to How do you get to Carnegie Hall? is Practice, practice, practice.

This chapter presents the foundation and framework for cardiovascular physical examination. Cardiac anatomy, including surface anatomy, is reviewed. Mechanical events of the cardiac cycle are discussed because they are essential to understanding what is happening in the heart during each phase of the cardiac cycle. Concepts of heart sound and murmur generation are presented; and finally, conduct of a complete cardiovascular physical examination is reviewed.

CARDIAC ANATOMY

It is not the purpose of this section to review cardiac anatomy in detail. Textbooks of

anatomy, as well as other major works, present the subject in great detail, making use of color drawings and diagrams. It is important to have the fundamentals of cardiac anatomy firmly in mind because it makes certain features of cardiac physical examination more easily understood. In large part, cardiology is a logical discipline. There is a displacement pump with one-way valves, and there are pipes. What goes wrong can be considered to be a plumbing problem. Knowledge of how the system is constructed is essential for determining how the system is functioning or malfunctioning.

Gross Anatomy

The heart lies in the chest, with most of the cardiac mass located to the left of midline. The two sides of the heart are designated right and left, although the right side actually is anterior to the left side. Consideration of the borders of the cardiac silhouette viewed in the anteroposterior position should make this positioning apparent (see Fig. 2–11).

Knowledge of the internal structure of the ventricles and particularly of the position and interrelations of the four cardiac valves is important to understanding why sounds generated within the heart are heard where they are. The right ventricle is somewhat tubular, or U shaped (Fig. 1–1). The tricuspid valve consists of three cusps and several papillary muscles from which chordae tendineae attach to the leaflets. It is oriented more or less vertically, with its orifice directed to the left and slightly anteriorly. Its superior edge is separated from the pulmonic valve by the crista supraventricularis. Its inferior rim leads to the right ventricular inflow portion, characteristically heavily trabeculated particularly at the apex of the

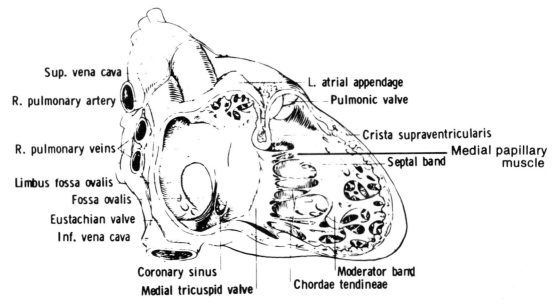

FIGURE 1–1. Anatomy of the opened right side of the heart, illustrating the right atrium and the right ventricle. Inf = inferior; L = left; R = right; Sup = superior. (From Krovetz LJ, Gessner IH, Schiebler GL: Handbook of Pediatric Cardiology. 2nd Ed. Baltimore, University Park Press, 1979. By permission.)

right ventricle. The inflow portion of the right ventricle leads into the vertically directed outflow portion, with the circular division between the two, called the os infundibulum, formed by the parietal, moderator, and septal muscular bands. The right ventricular outflow tract is smooth-walled and ends at the pulmonic valve located at the upper left border of the heart. The pulmonic trunk runs superiorly and posteriorly, bifurcating in such a way that the left pulmonary artery seems to be the continuation of the pulmonic trunk, whereas the right pulmonary artery turns sharply to the right.

The left ventricle is shaped like a cone, with its tip forming the cardiac apex (Fig. 1–2). The aortic and mitral valves, which abut each other, form the base of the cone. The mitral valve consists of two major leaflets and is oriented so its orifice is directed to the left and slightly anteriorly toward the left ventricular apex. Two papillary muscles, anterior and posterior, give rise to chordae tendineae, which attach to each leaflet.

The ventricular septum bulges toward the right ventricle, making the left ventricle rather circular in shape while flattening the right ventricle somewhat. The septum is primarily muscular with a small membranous portion located just below the juncture of the right and posterior (noncoronary) aortic cusps viewed from the left ventricle and just below the crista supraventricularis, behind the juncture of the medial and anterior tricuspid valve leaflets, viewed from the right ventricle (Fig. 1–3). The muscular septum is a curvilinear structure, so it does not lie in any single plane.

The left ventricle does not have a true outflow tract, although inclination of the ventricular septum slightly toward the right creates the illusion of one. The aortic and pulmonic valves are in continuity, as they are derived from the same embryonic vessel, the truncus arteriosus. Keep in mind that the aortic valve is located inferiorly, posteriorly, and to the right of the pulmonic valve. The aortic valve is inclined obliquely, with its orifice facing to the left and inferiorly toward the left ventricle and to the right and superiorly toward the ascending aorta. The ascending aorta rises superiorly and slightly to the right before giving off the innominate artery and turning posteriorly, coursing to the left of the trachea and esophagus.

Surface Anatomy

Surface anatomy refers to projection of internal structures onto the surface of the body. The subject is particularly important to cardiology because of sound generation, which forms the basis of auscultation. Where cardiac chambers and valves are located in relation to the body surface determines the areas designated the primary listening areas.

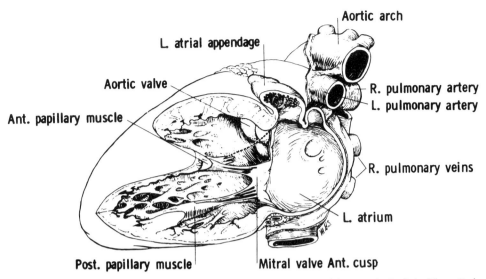

FIGURE 1−2. View of the opened left side of the heart. A portion of the anterior leaflet of the mitral valve has been cut away (dotted line) to view the aortic valve. Ant = anterior; L = left; Post = posterior; R = right. (From Krovetz LJ, Gessner IH, Schiebler GL: Handbook of Pediatric Cardiology. 2nd Ed. Baltimore, University Park Press, 1979. By permission.)

Anatomic designations used here are in a supine patient.

The tricuspid valve lies underneath the sternum at about the level of the fourth intercostal space (Fig. 1–4). Depending on body build, it may be closer to the left sternal edge (tall, thin individual) or to the right sternal edge (stocky individual). The right ventricle projects onto the surface along the left sternal edge from the fifth intercostal space almost to the second intercostal space, extending to the left just medial to the nipple line (Fig. 1–5). The pulmonic valve lies underneath the third costosternal junction a bit to the left of the left sternal edge.

The left atrium lies posteriorly, reaching superiorly to the left pulmonary artery. It projects posteriorly just to the left of the

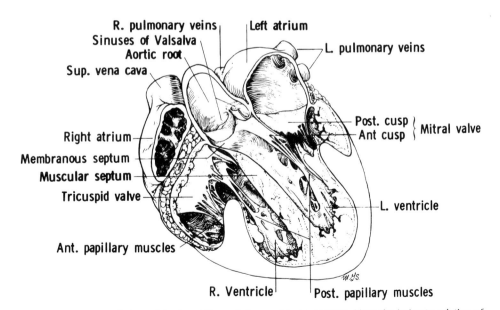

FIGURE 1−3. Frontal view of the heart through the ventricular septum. Note the intimate relation of the mitral and aortic valve. See Figures 1–1 and 1–2 for abbreviations. (From Krovetz LJ, Gessner IH, Schiebler GL: Handbook of Pediatric Cardiology. 2nd Ed. Baltimore, University Park Press, 1979. By permission.)

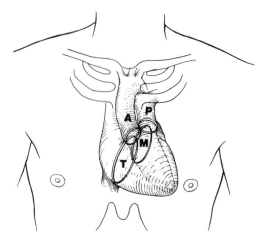

FIGURE 1–4. Transparent drawing of the heart indicating the location of the four cardiac valves in reference to the anterior chest wall. The drawing is stylized to permit display of all valves. A = aorta; M = mitral valve; P = pulmonic trunk; T = tricuspid valve.

spine underneath the scapula. The left ventricle projects onto the surface from the third intercostal space at the sternal border to the apex of the heart in the fifth intercostal space, the midclavicular line (Fig. 1–5). The aortic valve lies under the third intercostal space at the sternal edge, just below and to the right of the pulmonic valve. It leads into the ascending aorta, which projects under the sternum, reaching the right sternal edge in the second intercostal space. The mitral valve lies underneath the fourth rib just to the left of the left sternal edge. Its projection onto the anterior body surface, like that of

the aortic valve, is covered by the right ventricle (Fig. 1–4).

Several implications of these anatomic features are important from the standpoint of cardiac auscultation. (1) Sound generated in the right ventricle may project toward the right lower sternal edge via the tricuspid valve or vertically along the left sternal edge toward the pulmonic valve (Fig. 1–5). (2) Sound generated at the pulmonic valve can project downward along the left sternal border, or it may be carried along the pulmonary arteries, more so toward the left pulmonary artery because it is a direct continuation of the pulmonic trunk whereas sound must turn a corner to follow the right pulmonary artery. (3) Sound generated at the mitral valve may project to the left and inferiorly toward the left ventricular apex, posteriorly to the left of the spine, or superiorly toward the left pulmonary artery. (4) Sound generated in the left ventricle or aortic valve projects along a diagonal line running from the apex of the left ventricle to the third left intercostal space at the sternal edge and then to the second right intercostal space (Fig. 1–5).

What does this mean in practical terms? It means, for example, that the murmur of left ventricular outflow tract obstruction may be loudest at the third left intercostal space at the sternal edge but projects along the diagonal line just described toward the left ventricular apex and the second right intercostal space. In contrast, the murmur of right ventricular outflow tract obstruction, which also may be loudest in the third left intercostal space at the sternal edge, projects vertically along the left sternal border, down into the right ventricle and up into the pulmonic trunk.

MECHANICAL EVENTS OF THE CARDIAC CYCLE

The events depicted in Figure 1–6 are the foundation on which cardiac auscultation is built.[1] It is essential to know what is happening during each phase of the cardiac cycle and to know how the various events relate to each other if the examiner is to appreciate the logic and orderliness of cardiac physical diagnosis. Accomplishing this task invariably leads to a satisfying and accurate assessment of the patient. There is little doubt that it is rewarding to the practitioner to be able to use one's personal skills to ac-

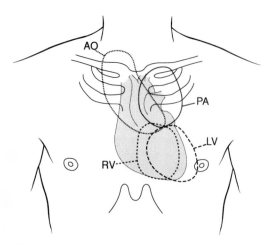

FIGURE 1–5. Projection of ventricles and great arteries onto the anterior chest wall indicating their areas of sound distribution. AO = aorta; LV = left ventricle; PA = pulmonary artery; RV = right ventricle.

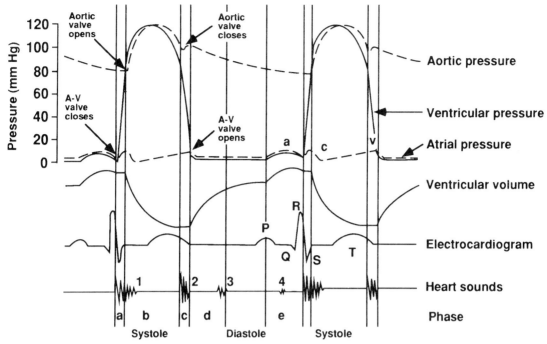

FIGURE 1–6. Mechanical events of the cardiac cycle, illustrating these events in the left heart. A-V valve = mitral valve. Atrial pressure curve: a = atrial contraction; c = ventricular contraction; v = atrial filling. Phase: a = isovolumetric contraction; b = ventricular ejection; c = isovolumetric relaxation; d = rapid ventricular filling; e = atrial contraction. Note that a and b comprise systole, and diastole includes c, d, and e. (Redrawn from several sources, primarily ref. 1.)

complish both an anatomic and a hemodynamic evaluation of a cardiac abnormality. This exercise is possible in most patients seen, including infants.

The cardiac cycle can be considered to begin with the onset of ventricular systole. Electrical systole starts with ventricular depolarization marked by the QRS complex on the electrocardiogram. Mechanical systole begins shortly thereafter with the onset of ventricular contraction. Figure 1–6 depicts left heart events. This discussion focuses on the left heart for the purpose of simplicity. A similar diagram and discussion could be presented for the right heart. The first phase of systole is marked by a rise in ventricular pressure. As it exceeds atrial pressure, the mitral valve closes. Until ventricular pressure exceeds aortic pressure, the aortic valve remains closed. Thus both the inlet and outlet valves of the left ventricle are closed and blood neither enters nor leaves it. This phase therefore is called *isovolumetric contraction*. Ventricular pressure continues to rise, exceeding aortic pressure, and the aortic valve opens allowing left *ventricular ejection*. Most of the blood that leaves the

ventricle does so during the early part of systole, producing the steep descent of the ventricular volume curve shown in Figure 1–6. The ventricle does not empty completely, at rest delivering approximately 65 per cent of its volume into the aorta[1]; this proportion, called the *ejection fraction*, is an important measure of systolic ventricular function. Ventricular emptying continues at a slower rate as its pressure falls just below aortic pressure. This situation is possible because of the momentum (inertiance) that ventricular contraction has imparted to the ejection volume. Some of the energy of ventricular contraction is transferred to the elastic wall of the ascending aorta, causing it to stretch. As left ventricular contraction ends and pressure begins to fall away from aortic pressure, the aortic wall recoils, pushing its volume downstream thereby maintaining a significant pressure throughout diastole.[1] Aortic recoil also pushes its blood volume back toward the ventricle and by doing so fills the aortic cusps, causing the valve to close. This reverse movement of blood coincides with the incisura of the aortic pressure curve and the point at which the aortic valve closes. This point marks the end of ventricular systole and the onset of ventricular diastole.

The first phase of ventricular diastole is *isovolumetric relaxation*. Ventricular pressure is falling but still exceeds atrial pressure; therefore both the aortic and mitral valves are closed, and ventricular volume is constant. Atrial pressure has been rising during ventricular systole as the left atrium continues to receive blood from the lungs. This action distends the atrium, raising its pressure and producing the atrial v wave. The mitral valve opens when falling ventricular pressure crosses the v wave. Flow into the ventricle therefore is passive; that is, it does not require active atrial contraction. This initial phase of flow into the ventricle also is rapid, hence the designation *rapid ventricular filling* phase. It can be seen readily on the ventricular volume curve. Ordinarily about 75 per cent of ventricular filling occurs during this phase.[1] Active ventricular relaxation is an important component of ventricular filling. The rate and amount of ventricular filling are influenced by diastolic ventricular function. The rapid filling phase ends with *atrial contraction* immediately following the P wave on the electrocardiogram. This contraction produces the atrial a wave. It also produces an analogous small wave at the end of ventricular diastole. Pressure in the left ventricle at the end of this wave is designated left ventricular end-diastolic pressure, an important measure of left ventricular diastolic function. Diastole ends with the onset of ventricular contraction.

GENERATION OF HEART SOUNDS AND MURMURS

Now is an appropriate point to discuss heart sounds. Figure 1–6 indicates the position of the four heart sounds. Remember that the fourth heart sound is not heard in a normal individual.

What produces these sounds? We associate the first and second heart sounds with closure of the atrioventricular valves and semilunar valves, respectively. It is not, however, the apposition of the valve leaflets or cusps themselves that produces these heart sounds.

The *first heart sound* (S_1) is a complex high-frequency event that is loudest at the cardiac apex, although it can be heard in all of the usual listening areas on the chest. It occurs at the onset of ventricular systole and is synchronous with mitral valve closure. Mitral valve papillary muscles contract, tensing the chordae, and blood flow into the ventricle decelerates. Vibrations occur in the mitral valves, in the myocardium and in the ventricular blood volume accounting for the complexity of S_1. The first sound is loudest when left ventricular systole begins with the mitral valve wide open as occurs with a more rapid heart rate or a short PR interval. It is also accentuated by particularly vigorous ventricular contraction, as may occur in children under conditions that increase cardiac output such as anemia, fever, or exercise. S_1 intensity is directly related to the peak rate of rise of the left ventricular pressure. The first sound is reduced in intensity by a long PR interval, left ventricular failure, and mitral regurgitation. Table 1–1 expands the list of conditions that affect the intensity of S_1. These observations suggest that the energy of ventricular contraction, perhaps in particular papillary muscle contraction, contributes most to S_1 generation.

The right ventricle also contributes to S_1 with the result that S_1 may have two audible components. The right ventricular component, however, is audible only over the right ventricle (i.e., at the lower left sternal edge). The interval between the two components is fixed because it is a function of the time of onset of the contraction of each ventricle, which is determined electrically by the depolarization sequence. This interval is not affected by respiration, ventricular filling, or outlet resistance. Splitting of S_1 can be confused with a single S_1 that is accompanied by either an ejection sound or a fourth heart sound (S_4). One can usually make the distinction based on the quality of the sounds and remembering that a split S_1 is heard only over the right ventricle, a location where neither an ejection sound nor an S_4 is likely to be isolated.

The *second heart sound* (S_2) marks clo-

TABLE 1–1. FIRST HEART SOUND

Loud	Soft
Short PR interval	Long PR interval
Tachycardia	Left ventricular failure
Anemia	Mitral regurgitation
Fever	Aortic regurgitation
Exercise	Left bundle branch block
Anxiety	
Mitral stenosis	

sure of the semilunar valves and the end of ventricular systole. It is the most important single feature of cardiac auscultation in the infant and child because it can tell the listener much about cardiac anatomy and physiology. One cannot become expert at cardiac physical diagnosis without being able to assess and interpret S_2.

The second heart sound is actually two sounds, as analogous events at the closure of each semilunar valve produce a sound. We consider, therefore, an aortic component and a pulmonic component of S_2, which may be designated A_2 and P_2. The sound is generated at the time blood flow reverses in the great arteries, filling the semilunar valve cusps and closing the valve orifice, thereby stopping this reversed flow. It is the sudden stopping of this reversed flow that creates the sound. Consider a hollow pipe, closed at each end, half filled with water. The pipe, held upright, is then suddenly inverted, sending the water to the opposite end of the pipe. The water has energy consistent with its velocity and the energy used to thrust the pipe downward. When the water reaches the opposite end of the pipe it stops suddenly, and its energy is transferred to the walls of the pipe, producing a sound. How loud is this sound? Suppose one inverts the pipe slowly and gently so the water reaches the opposite end of the pipe less rapidly and less energetically. It is evident that the sound is then softer than if the pipe were rapidly and vigorously inverted. In physiologic terms, the higher the pressure in the great artery driving blood backward toward its semilunar valve (i.e., diastolic great vessel pressure), the louder is that component of S_2.

Aortic diastolic pressure normally is much higher than pulmonic diastolic pressure; hence A_2 normally is louder than P_2. A_2 is heard in all listening areas but maximally at the apex and the upper right sternal edge. Normally P_2 is heard only in the second left intercostal space, where it might be as loud as A_2 at that location.

Two observations should help amplify this explanation for the generation of S_2. First, patients with truncus arteriosus have only one semilunar valve that leads into a common trunk, which immediately divides into a large aorta and usually a smaller common pulmonic trunk. Despite a single semilunar valve, S_2 commonly has two components.[2] Reversal of flow in the aorta and pulmonic trunk is not synchronous because impedance of the pulmonary vascular bed ordinarily is less than systemic impedance; thus flow downstream into the pulmonary arteries continues slightly longer than it does in the aorta. It is this asynchronous reversal of flow, and therefore asynchronous stopping of flow, in the two great arteries that allows the sound generated in each vessel to be audible. Second, patients with a mechanical prosthetic aortic valve have opening and closing sounds generated by the mechanical valve itself. These sounds are clearly identifiable as artificial sounds. In addition to the mechanical valve closure sound at the end of systole, one can also hear the usual aortic component of the second sound. The only source for the sound is the aortic wall.

The intensity of each component of S_2 is directly related to the diastolic pressure in the respective vessel. A_2 is increased by systemic hypertension and is decreased by aortic stenosis and significant aortic regurgitation. P_2 is increased by pulmonary hypertension and is decreased by severe pulmonic valve stenosis. P_2 may be absent with significant pulmonic regurgitation or with a combination of right ventricular outflow tract obstruction and pulmonic valve stenosis, as occurs commonly in patients with tetralogy of Fallot.

The relation of the two components of S_2 can provide both anatomic and physiologic information. A_2 occurs before P_2 because left ventricular mechanical events precede those in the right ventricle. The time interval between the two sounds varies, primarily due to respiration. Inspiration delays P_2, widening the interval for two reasons. The first, and more traditional, explanation is increased right ventricular filling, lengthening right ventricular ejection time. With inspiration, intrathoracic pressure decreases, tending to create a suction effect on the great veins, particularly the superior vena cava. More importantly, with inspiration the diaphragm descends, compressing the liver and thereby pushing blood into the thorax. The result of these events is an increase in right atrial filling during inspiration. The second, more important reason has to do with what is called hangout.[3] Simultaneous right ventricular and pulmonic artery pressure curves show a more gradual downslope of the pulmonic artery curve, so the two curves are separated at the time of the dicrotic notch. The time interval between the two curves is called the *hangout interval* (Fig. 1–7). The duration of this interval is inversely propor-

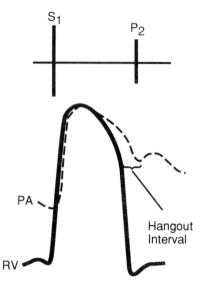

FIGURE 1–7. Concept of "hangout." Low impedance in the pulmonary arterial bed causes pulmonary artery pressure to fall more gradually than right ventricular pressure during late systole, resulting in separation of the two pressure curves. PA = pulmonary artery; RV = right ventricle. (Modified from Ronan JA: Heart Disease and Stroke. 1: 113–116, 1992.)

tional to the impedance of the pulmonary arterial system. Inspiration decreases impedance of the pulmonary arterial vascular bed, increasing the hangout interval.

The time between the two components of S_2 may be 25 to 30 ms during expiration, an interval that is just detectable by an experienced observer. The interval increases to 40 to 45 ms during quiet inspiration, an interval that makes the two sounds easily heard as independent events. The presence of two components of S_2 indicates that there are two great arteries, although for reasons just described it does not establish that there are two semilunar valves. Location of the pulmonic component of S_2 in an abnormal site can be a clue to the presence of an abnormality of cardiac position. For example, in situs inversus, splitting of S_2 is heard in the second right intercostal space.

Narrow splitting of S_2 can be caused by delay in A_2 (e.g., aortic stenosis) or by earlier occurrence of P_2 (e.g., pulmonary hypertension). Wide splitting of S_2 can be caused by increased right ventricular ejection volume (e.g., atrial septal defect), right ventricular outflow obstruction (e.g., pulmonic valve stenosis), or delayed activation of the right ventricle (e.g., right bundle branch block). Figure 1–8 illustrates the effect of respira-

tion on the auscultation of S_2 at the pulmonic listening area in various conditions.

The *third heart sound* (S_3) is a low-frequency event that occurs toward the end of rapid ventricular filling. It is caused by sudden limitation of rapid ventricular expansion, which in turn suddenly decelerates blood flow entering the ventricle, transferring its energy to the ventricular wall and creating the sound. S_3 therefore is related specifically to ventricular wall vibrations during rapid filling.[4] The ability of the left ventricle to expand rapidly is characteristic of a healthy, compliant ventricle, and therefore S_3 is heard normally in children and young adults. Disappearance of S_3 later in life, conversely, represents some deteriora-

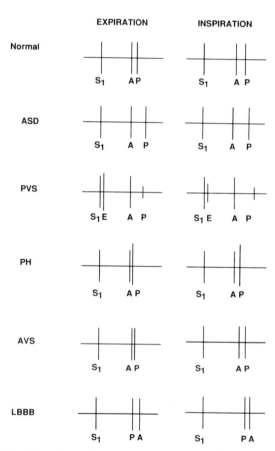

FIGURE 1–8. Effect of respiration on auscultation of S_1 and S_2 (A and P) at the pulmonic listening area in various conditions. See the text in this chapter and in Chapter 8 for details. Height of vertical lines representing heart sounds suggest relative intensity of these sounds. Note paradoxical splitting of S_2 in left bundle branch block. A = aortic component of S_2; ASD = atrial septal defect; AVS = aortic valve stenosis; E = ejection sound; LBBB = left bundle branch block; P = pulmonic component of S_2; PH = pulmonary hypertension; PVS = pulmonic valve stenosis; S_1 = first heart sound.

tion in left ventricular function. Furthermore, decreased ventricular compliance at any age can cause a pathologic S_3. The context in which this sound is heard is critical to its correct interpretation.

Left ventricular S_3 is located at the apex, and it is seldom as loud as S_1 or S_2 at that site. It should be apparent that S_3 can be generated in either ventricle, although a right ventricular S_3 is less often recognized. S_3 in the right ventricle is located at the lower left sternal edge and increases during inspiration owing to augmented right ventricular filling. An abnormal S_3, uncommon in the pediatric age group, almost always appears in conjunction with other abnormal auscultatory findings. When S_3 is pathologic, it is usually caused by either an increase in myocardial stiffness (decreased ventricular compliance) or a significant increase in the rate and volume of ventricular inflow during rapid ventricular filling.[4] In the latter instance S_3 is accentuated, although the principles of its generation remain normal.

An audible *fourth heart sound* (S_4) always should be considered abnormal in the young. S_4 occurs in response to atrial contraction, driving an additional quantity of blood into the ventricle. Its cause is similar to that of S_3, but its implication is different. A ventricle that is not capable of expanding normally during the rapid ventricular filling phase of mid-diastole causes an excessive volume of blood to remain in the atrium. Contraction of the atrium forces further expansion of the ventricle, causing low-frequency vibrations of the ventricular wall. S_4 therefore indicates poor ventricular compliance, which may come about because of significant ventricular hypertrophy or by heart (pump) failure.[5] Either ventricle may produce an S_4. The location of the sound is the same as an S_3.

It is apparent that some individuals demonstrate both S_3 and S_4. Left heart failure together with left heart volume overload, as may occur in an infant with severe coarctation of the aorta and mitral regurgitation, is one example. The ability to hear both of these sounds, however, depends on their separation by sufficient time for recognition, which is unlikely in the infant example just mentioned, as the heart rate would be rapid and diastole therefore shortened. As a result, the events that create S_3 and S_4 (i.e., rapid ventricular filling followed by atrial contraction) may occur so close together that one hears only a single, prominent diastolic sound. This sound can be called an S_3-S_4 *summation sound*.[6] It is heard often in infants and young children with significant heart disease, particularly in the presence of heart failure. Prolongation of the PR interval also may create an S_3-S_4 summation sound by causing atrial contraction to occur at about the same time as rapid ventricular filling. In this case the sound really is an augmented S_3, as there may be no reason for an S_4 to have occurred in and of itself.

Additional Heart Sounds

Other abnormal heart sounds can be heard during either systole or diastole. *Systolic ejection sounds* (also called systolic ejection clicks) are high-frequency, clicking sounds of short duration that occur early during systole in association with opening of a semilunar valve and the onset of ventricular ejection. Two pathophysiologic mechanisms explain an ejection sound. First, a stenotic, but mobile, semilunar valve may literally snap open, producing this sound. It takes little obstruction to cause an ejection sound. In fact, an ejection sound may be heard with only a bicuspid aortic or pulmonic valve. Second, either a large ejection volume or a normal volume ejected under high velocity and pressure can cause sudden augmented distension of the great vessel wall, producing an ejection sound with acoustic properties similar to those generated by a stenotic valve.

Both right- and left-sided ejection sounds occur. They do have certain distinguishing characteristics, however. A *pulmonic ejection sound* is heard best in the second and third left intercostal space and seldom outside that area. If caused by pulmonic valve stenosis, the click has distinct respiratory variation, becoming softer during inspiration (Fig. 1–8). This softening occurs for two reasons. First, inspiration results in increased right atrial filling, leading to more forceful atrial contraction and producing a larger a wave. This a wave is transmitted into the right ventricle, moving the pulmonic valve toward the open position before the onset of ventricular contraction. Excursion of the pulmonic valve therefore is reduced, and the sound diminishes. Second, inspiration decreases pulmonary impedance, reducing the energy needed to open the pulmonic valve. The pulmonic ejection sound is one of the few right heart acoustic events that is diminished by inspiration. Almost all right heart sounds and murmurs either are louder or more easily heard during inspiration.

An *aortic ejection sound* is produced by a mobile bicuspid or stenotic aortic valve. It is maximal at the apex and second right intercostal space. In the presence of aortic valve stenosis, the ejection sound is more easily heard at the apex because the murmur of aortic stenosis is loudest in the second right intercostal space and tends to obscure the ejection sound in that location. The ejection sound, being high frequency, radiates better to the apex than does the lower-frequency murmur. An aortic ejection sound is not affected by respiration.

An aortic ejection sound also can be caused by a large volume ejection into a dilated aorta, as may occur with tetralogy of Fallot in which the aorta receives all of the left ventricular ejection volume plus some from the right ventricle. In that condition the aorta also is more anterior in location, making its sound easier to hear.

Mid- (and late) systolic sounds usually are caused by mitral valve prolapse. In this case the term *mid-systolic click* is preferred. This sound (or sounds, as multiple clicks may occur) is of short duration and high frequency, and it is best heard at the apex. It is generated by tensing of the chordae tendineae of the mitral valve as a mitral leaflet billows toward the left atrium. The mid-systolic click of mitral valve prolapse is variable. Moving from supine to standing position causes the click to occur earlier during systole, as does the Valsalva maneuver, because of a momentary decrease in left ventricular volume. Conversely, squatting or sustained hand grip exercise (maintaining respiration to avoid an involuntary Valsalva) delays the click by increasing the left ventricular volume. In some patients a click is not heard at all with the patient supine. The cardiac examination therefore should include apical auscultation with the patient sitting or standing.

Additional diastolic sounds also occur. One that is described regularly is an *opening snap*, which is a high-frequency sound produced by energetic but limited opening of a stenotic atrioventricular valve as in mitral stenosis secondary to rheumatic heart disease. The opening snap in this instance is analogous to the aortic ejection sound. Rheumatic mitral stenosis seldom is en-

countered in the pediatric population in the United States; therefore hearing an opening snap in a child is a rare event. An opening snap is not produced by a congenitally stenotic mitral valve, the pathology of which is different.

A mid-diastolic sound can be heard at the lower left sternal border in a patient with constrictive pericarditis. The sound is produced during rapid and forceful right ventricular filling from a high-pressure right atrium. Sudden restriction of right ventricular distension by the rigid pericardium produces the sound that has been called a *pericardial knock*. It has a striking quality, simulating knocking on a wood door with one's knuckle.

Mechanical prosthetic valves produce sounds as they open and close. These sounds are readily identifiable as artificial because they sound so different from any naturally occurring event, normal or abnormal. Opening of a prosthetic aortic valve simulates an aortic ejection sound; its closing is simultaneous with the normal S_2, as discussed earlier. Opening of a prosthetic mitral valve simulates an opening snap; its closure is simultaneous with the left ventricular component of S_1, which may be soft because the mitral valve papillary muscles have been surgically removed. Listening to artificial valve sounds is good practice for timing the analogous events. It also is important to recognize that the sounds are normally clear and sharp; otherwise valve malfunction might be suspected.

Murmurs

The word *murmur* derives from the Latin word *murmur*. Perloff[7] called attention to Pepper's[8] suggestion that murmur has an onomatopoeic origin.

A heart murmur is a series of audible sounds whose duration is sufficiently long to exceed that which one could call a sound. The distinction between a sound and a murmur seldom is difficult, as most murmurs are sufficiently long for clarity. Murmurs that may be difficult to recognize as such are mid-diastolic right and left ventricular filling murmurs, particularly when heard in the infant with a rapid heart rate. These murmurs may be short enough that some observers would label them S_3.

Murmurs have been attributed to turbulent movement of blood, which need not be marked to cause vibrations that are audible.[9]

An alternative explanation suggests Aeolian phenomena or vortex shedding distal to an obstruction.[10]

There are at least 11 characteristics that can be described regarding each heart murmur. This information should not be intimidating to the examiner, as learning to describe a murmur in a complete and orderly manner is logical and not difficult. Discussion of each of these characteristics follows.

1. *Location.* Each murmur should be evaluated carefully for the location on the body (usually on the chest) where the murmur is loudest. It may require listening in nontraditional areas, particularly in a child with congenital heart disease whose heart and its component parts may not be located in normal position.

2. *Timing.* Murmurs are either systolic, diastolic, or continuous. Keep in mind that systolic and diastolic are ventricle-specific. A long systolic murmur originating in the right ventricle may extend beyond the aortic component of S_2 (i.e., beyond the end of left ventricular systole).

   a. *Systolic murmurs* also must be timed within systole. An early systolic murmur begins immediately with S_1 occupying isovolumetric contraction. A mid-systolic murmur begins after S_1 and cannot start until the semilunar valve opens. It ends just before the semilunar valve closes. A late systolic murmur begins during mid-systole to late systole and continues to the end of ventricular contraction. Figure 1–9 illustrates these murmurs.

   b. *Diastolic murmurs* also must be timed. An early diastolic murmur begins immediately with its respective component of S_2 occupying isovolumetric relaxation. A mid-diastolic murmur begins just after the atrioventricular valve opens, and it is synchronous with rapid ventricular filling. A late diastolic murmur occurs after atrial contraction and may last until S_1 (Fig. 1–10). Exactness of timing is important and is emphasized later in regard to specific murmurs.

   c. *Continuous murmurs* begin during systole and continue through S_2 into diastole. It is not necessary that the murmur be present throughout systole and diastole. There are no murmurs that begin during diastole and continue through S_1 into systole. With one rare exception, all continuous murmurs are generated within blood vessels (Fig. 1–11).

3. *Intensity (loudness).* Murmurs are graded on a scale of 1 to 6.[11] The major dividing line is between grades 3 and 4. If a thrill is felt, the murmur is grade 4 or more; and if no thrill is present, the murmur is grade 3 or less. Distinction

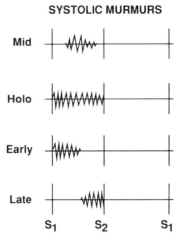

SYSTOLIC MURMURS

Mid

Holo

Early

Late

S_1 S_2 S_1

FIGURE 1–9. Timing of systolic murmurs. S_1 = first heart sound; S_2 = second heart sound.

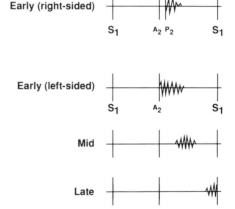

DIASTOLIC MURMURS

Early (right-sided)

S_1 A_2 P_2 S_1

Early (left-sided)

S_1 A_2 S_1

Mid

Late

FIGURE 1–10. Specific timing of diastolic murmurs. An early diastolic murmur must begin with the respective component of S_2. L = left; R = right; S_1 = first heart sound; S_2 = second heart sound; A_2 = aortic component of S_2; P_2 = pulmonary component of S_2.

CONTINUOUS MURMURS

AORTO-PULMONARY
(patent ductus arteriosus)

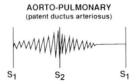

S₁   S₂   S₁

ARTERIAL

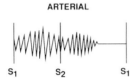

S₁   S₂   S₁

VENOUS

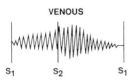

S₁   S₂   S₁

FIGURE 1–11. Continuous murmurs characterized by etiology. A continuous murmur begins during systole and ends during diastole. Note that the murmur of PDA peaks at S₂, the murmur of an AVM has two peaks, and the murmur of a venous hum peaks during diastole. S₁ = first heart sound; S₂ = second heart sound.

within grades 1 to 3 and grades 4 to 6 is somewhat arbitrary and depends to some extent on observer subjectivity despite criteria that have been described (Table 1–2). It is not particularly important that observers agree completely on whether a murmur is, for example, grade 2 or grade 3. It is valuable for each observer to be consistent, so the murmur is graded identically from one examination to the next.

TABLE 1–2. GRADING OF MURMURS

Grade 1:	Murmur is heard with effort or special attention.
Grade 2:	Murmur is readily heard but is not loud.
Grade 3:	Murmur is apparent immediately upon listening and seems loud, but no thrill is felt.
Grade 4:	Thrill is present, and a murmur is heard with the stethoscope fully in contact with the chest wall.
Grade 5:	Thrill is present, and a murmur can be heard with the stethoscope lifted so only one edge is in contact with the chest wall.
Grade 6:	Thrill is present, and a murmur can be heard with the stethoscope completely off the chest wall.

Consistency is important for recognizing change.

4. *Duration.* A murmur that begins with S₁ and ends with S₂ is said to be holosystolic. A murmur that begins with S₂ and ends with S₁ could be called holodiastolic. For the most part, the duration is the observer's estimation of the amount of systole, diastole, or both that is occupied by a murmur. One might note that a systolic murmur begins just after S₁ and lasts midway through systole or that a murmur is confined to mid-diastole. Time of onset of the murmur is more important than how long the murmur lasts.

5. *Frequency (pitch).* Frequency refers to a rough estimate of dominant sound range. Murmurs are described as either of low, middle, or high frequency. These terms are in relation to all murmurs and are not meant to imply a specific Hertz designation.

6. *Shape.* A murmur can begin softly and increase in intensity. Its shape is called crescendo. A murmur that is loud at the beginning and then decreases in intensity has a decrescendo shape. A murmur that rises and falls is said to be crescendo-decrescendo, or diamond-shaped. A murmur that is of constant intensity is said to be plateau-shaped.

7. *Quality (timbre).* Quality is a term used to describe how noisy a murmur sounds. All murmurs are noise, but some are noisier than others. In a musical sense timbre is the characteristic that allows one to identify two instruments playing the same musical note. For example, a clarinet and saxophone may each play middle C whose dominant frequency is 256 Hz. The listener would know which instrument is being played, though, without seeing them because they sound different: The instruments are not producing a pure tone as would a tuning fork. There are many overtones that, added onto the dominant frequency, give each instrument its particular quality. In a musical instrument these overtones are harmonic and the note sounds pleasant. In the heart the overtones are discordant, and noise results. Various terms are applied to describe murmurs, such as harsh, coarse, rough, blowing, vibra-

tory, and musical. These descriptions are in large part arbitrary, and each observer should try to establish a framework that can be used as a reference for murmur characterization

8. *Radiation.* Murmurs have a direction of spread from their point of maximal intensity. It is determined by site of murmur generation, by murmur intensity, and by direction of blood flow from the site of origin of the murmur. For example, the systolic murmur of aortic stenosis radiates to the upper right sternal edge because that is the direction of the turbulent blood flow as it leaves the aortic valve and ascends in the aorta.

9. *Transmission.* A murmur may have a secondary point of loudness. For example, the murmur of mitral regurgitation is loudest at the apex, but if the regurgitant jet is directed anterosuperiorly the murmur also may be prominent at the upper left sternal edge in the pulmonic area without being well heard between these two locations.

10. *Effect of normal respiration.* Some murmurs, particularly those generated in the right heart, vary with the respiratory phase. For example, the diastolic murmur of pulmonic regurgitation and the systolic murmur of tricuspid regurgitation both increase during inspiration.

11. *Response to intervention.* Several simple maneuvers can be accomplished during routine cardiac auscultation that can affect murmur characteristics. Change in body position from supine to sitting, squatting, sustained hand grip exercise, and Valsalva maneuver can influence features of some murmurs.

Etiology of Heart Murmurs

It is possible to classify heart murmurs in such a way as to reduce to a manageable level what may seem to be an enormous number of possible causes. This section attempts to do that. After reviewing this material the reader may want to look at Chapter 8, which illustrates how fundamental concepts are applied to clinical problem solving.

Systolic Murmurs. There are only four causes of systolic murmurs: (1) atrioventric-

ular valve regurgitation; (2) ventricular outflow obstruction; (3) ventricular septal defect; (4) innocent. Every systolic murmur must be due to one of these four etiologies. This statement may seem an oversimplification, but it is not. The primary care physician is concerned with one fundamental decision. Is the murmur pathologic? Determining whether a murmur is subvalvar aortic stenosis or valvar aortic stenosis is not as important as identifying that there is a murmur of left ventricular outflow tract obstruction.

Each category of systolic murmur is discussed in detail in Chapter 8, so murmur evaluation can be placed in the context of total patient assessment. At this point only a brief description is presented for the purpose of providing continuity and clarity.

ATRIOVENTRICULAR VALVE REGURGITATION. The murmur of atrioventricular valve regurgitation usually begins with S_1, thus occupying isovolumetric contraction, and it is classified as early systolic. If it persists throughout systole, it can be classified as holosystolic. Some forms of atrioventricular valve regurgitation begin during midsystole, but in children mid-systolic to late systolic atrioventricular valve regurgitation is caused only by mitral regurgitation due to mitral valve prolapse. Mitral regurgitation is much more common than tricuspid regurgitation, particularly in the context of a child not previously known to have a cardiac abnormality.

VENTRICULAR OUTFLOW OBSTRUCTION. For any form of ventricular outflow obstruction to produce a murmur, blood must be flowing through an open semilunar valve. This murmur cannot begin until isovolumetric contraction is complete and therefore must be separated from S_1. It is classified as mid-systolic. Cardiac output and myocardial function can influence this murmur substantially. If there is no flow, there is no murmur. That statement sounds absurd, but it serves to emphasize the point that low-flow states (e.g., congestive heart failure) reduce murmur intensity.

VENTRICULAR SEPTAL DEFECT. The murmur of a ventricular septal defect (VSD) occupies isovolumetric contraction as flow begins with the onset of left ventricular contraction prior to opening of the aortic valve. It is therefore classified as early systolic.

A VSD causes a murmur because turbulence is produced by flow through the defect. Turbulence occurs with small to moderate-size defects because a significant systolic pressure difference exists between the two ventricles, generating high velocity flow across the defect, which produces a high-frequency murmur. A large VSD, on the other hand, allows blood to flow freely across it, producing little or no turbulence—hence little or no murmur. For example, the VSD in tetralogy of Fallot is by definition large. It causes no murmur, regardless of the magnitude and direction of shunt flow. More is said about that situation later.

INNOCENT CAUSE. The innocent murmur is by far the most common heart murmur, occurring in almost all children. The term innocent means that the murmur has been determined to be due to normal blood flow in a normal cardiovascular system. Only flow out of the ventricle can initiate these murmurs; therefore the murmur cannot occupy isovolumetric contraction, and it is classified as mid-systolic.

It should be apparent that only one mechanical cardiac event occurs that is relevant to systolic murmur generation, and that event is ventricular contraction. All systolic murmurs, innocent and pathologic, are initiated by ventricular contraction. Diastolic murmurs, on the other hand, are created by several mechanical events.

Diastolic Murmurs. There are three distinct phases of diastole as previously discussed. There are therefore three specific types of diastolic murmur: (1) early; (2) mid; (3) late. All diastolic murmurs should be considered abnormal. Specific pathologic conditions causing these murmurs are discussed in Chapter 8.

EARLY DIASTOLIC MURMUR. An early diastolic murmur begins synchronously with closure of the semilunar valve, thereby occupying isovolumetric relaxation. Only semilunar valve regurgitation can cause this murmur.

MID-DIASTOLIC MURMUR. A mid-diastolic murmur is generated by rapid ventricular filling. The atrioventricular valve must open for this murmur to occur. Isovolumetric relaxation is silent; therefore a distinct interval exists between S_2 and the onset of this murmur. There are two mechanisms of sound generation. First, a stenotic atrioventricular valve creates turbulence in a manner analogous to a stenotic semilunar valve. The concerned atrium is dilated and its pressure abnormally high. Ventricular pressure falls

through the phase of isovolumetric relaxation, reaching atrial pressure, and the stenotic valve opens. The distended, tense atrium forces blood through the restricted orifice, creating the mid-diastolic murmur. Atrial contraction is not required. Second, a mismatch can occur between the volume of blood entering the ventricle during rapid ventricular filling and ventricular compliance. This situation generates sound from the distending ventricular walls. It can be thought of as an extended S_3—hence the difficulty at times when deciding whether one is hearing only an S_3 or a short diastolic murmur. If the atrium is significantly overfilled during ventricular systole, the large volume of flow entering the ventricle can create this murmur in an otherwise normal ventricle. If ventricular compliance is decreased, however, a normal volume of blood entering this ventricle during rapid ventricular filling also can cause the murmur.

LATE DIASTOLIC MURMUR. A late diastolic murmur is one that occurs in response to active atrial contraction following the P wave on the electrocardiogram. It may continue until S_1. The most common mechanism is turbulent flow across a stenotic atrioventricular valve which restricts the rapid phase of ventricular filling, leaving a larger than normal volume of blood in the atrium. Atrial contraction drives this volume through the stenotic valve, producing a murmur analogous with that just described for mid-diastole. Mitral stenosis due to rheumatic heart disease is the classic example of this type of late diastolic murmur.

Left atrial contraction also can cause a late diastolic murmur in the absence of mitral valve pathology. This murmur, first described by Austin Flint in 1862 in patients with severe aortic regurgitation,[12] has been explained in several ways. Flint proposed that partial closure of the mitral valve during mid-diastole by the dilated left ventricle results in mitral valve vibrations with subsequent atrial contraction. One study presented evidence that this murmur is caused by vibration of the ventricular wall and that its presence correlates with the severity of aortic regurgitation.[13]

Continuous Murmurs. Blood flow is not continuous anywhere within cardiac chambers; therefore it should be apparent that continuous murmurs must be generated in blood vessels. (There is one rare exception to this requirement: the presence of a small atrial septal defect together with mitral atresia or severe stenosis can cause continuous high-velocity flow across the atrial septal defect secondary to markedly increased left atrial pressure. A continuous murmur may result.) These murmurs can be the result of: (1) patent ductus arteriosus; (2) arteriovenous malformation; (3) coronary artery–cardiac chamber fistula; (4) altered arterial flow; (5) altered venous flow.

The mechanism of murmur production is continuous turbulence as blood flows through the particular abnormality. One innocent continuous murmur exists, the venous hum; and it is by far the most common continuous murmur. A venous hum can be heard in almost every child placed in the sitting position. It is located at the right sternoclavicular junction and is produced by turbulence in the jugular vein due to partial compression of the vessel. The murmur is usually soft in quality and of medium frequency, with accentuation during mid-diastole when the tricuspid valve opens. Turning the patient's head or compressing the jugular vein obliterates the murmur.

Pericardial Rubs. A pericardial friction rub, strictly speaking, is not a murmur, as it is not caused by blood flow. It is generated by inflamed visceral and parietal pericardial surfaces rubbing against each other. Each of the three major phases of the cardiac cycle can produce a rub: ventricular systole, rapid ventricular filling, and atrial contraction. If all three are present, there is a major systolic component and two diastolic components. Rubs are heard in patients with acute pericarditis and now are heard most commonly during the first few days after open heart surgery.

COMPLETE CARDIOVASCULAR PHYSICAL EXAMINATION

Examination of an infant or child for the presence of a cardiovascular abnormality includes techniques common to all clinical situations. Some features of the cardiac examination are specific, and this section is designed to help the reader develop a logical, orderly approach to this skill.

Aspects of the examination that are reviewed here are: (1) environment and equipment; (2) appearance of the patient; (3) respiration; (4) abdominal examination; (5) cardiovascular examination. The latter includes evaluation of venous waves, arterial pulses and blood pressure, precordial palpation, and auscultation.

Environment and Equipment

There is no substitute for a calm, quiet patient in a quiet room. Achieving that goal, or even coming close, can be a challenge, especially with an infant or toddler. Anyone who conducts physical examinations in this age group is aware of these difficulties and no doubt has developed a method to manage them.

Newborns and young infants are seldom a problem, as they do not cry or struggle unless uncomfortable. The older infant and toddler, however, may not be a willing participant. There is no doubt that it helps to spend a few minutes in the examining room talking with the family, thereby allowing the patient to get used to your presence. This interval is a good time to assess the patient's appearance and respiration. The toddler's behavior at this point can tell you whether the hands-on evaluation will be difficult. The patient should be supine for cardiac examination. An infant or young child who seems unlikely to remain calm in this position may require that you allow the patient to sit in the mother's lap. By the time you conduct the examination in that manner, the child may be willing to lie down next to the mother or across her lap so a supine position is achievable.

The examiner must have a good stethoscope. There are differences of opinion regarding which type is preferable. The Sprague-Rappaport design by Hewlett-Packard is a fine instrument, comfortable to use, and durable. Its component parts are replaceable so it can be maintained easily. It is designed for the pediatric patient, as it has two diaphragms and three bells of varying size. The only disadvantage is its short tubing length, which is necessary to achieve outstanding sound transmission. I have evaluated many stethoscopes, and this one is the only one I recommend. The investment is not great; after 30 years I am now on my third instrument.

Proper-size blood pressure cuffs must be available, and a mercury manometer is preferred. Automated equipment is satisfactory for screening purposes but not if an accurate blood pressure measure is needed. Blood pressure cuff width should measure approximately three fourths of the limb section to which it is applied (i.e., arm or calf). The cuff bladder should be long enough to exceed arm circumference by 20 to 25 per cent. This fit can be a problem with an obese child and sometimes a chubby infant. A cuff that is too narrow or one whose bladder is too short results in falsely high blood pressure measurements.

Appearance of the Patient

Take a moment to look at the patient. Some syndromes (e.g., Down syndrome) may be readily apparent; others are not. Is body build unusual? Height and weight should be recorded and plotted on a standard growth chart. Is the patient's color normal? Cyanosis may be obvious or subtle or, in a black patient, obscure. Is the patient pale or jaundiced?

Take a moment to decide whether the patient is ill. This point is particularly important for an infant. Recognizing that a patient is distressed is not difficult for anyone who has reasonable experience, but one does have to be aware of the possibility.

Respiration

Before attempting to examine the patient physically, observe the patient's respiratory rate and pattern. If there is tachypnea, is there also laboring? Hyperpnea may be present in the chronically hypoxemic patient. Look for nasal flare, tracheal tug, and intercostal retractions. Look at the chest cage for abnormal shape or deformity, such as pectus excavatum or carinatum.

Abdominal Examination

The abdomen is examined primarily to assess liver size and structure because it is crucial to the evaluation of congestive heart failure. Palpate the spleen and for other masses to be complete. The liver edge should be palpated gently so the examiner can evaluate its contour and consistency as well as identify its location. If the liver is displaced downward by hyperinflated lungs, the edge remains sharp and the consistency firm. One can easily push this liver up into the chest. A liver that is enlarged because of congestive heart failure has a soft, rounded edge, and it cannot be pushed into the chest to any extent. Measure the distance the liver edge extends below the right costal margin in the midclavicular line. Each physician carries a convenient measuring device—the index

finger. The distance from the proximal interphalangeal joint to the tip of the index finger in an adult is close enough to 5 cm to allow one to make a relatively accurate assessment. If the liver edge cannot be felt, it may be possible to detect it by listening over the liver with the stethoscope bell while gently scratching the abdomen, starting low and gradually moving cephalad. As the liver edge is crossed, the scratching sound suddenly intensifies.

Cardiovascular Examination

Venous Waves

Venous waves are difficult to assess in infants and toddlers because these patients often have short, chubby necks. The heart rate often is too fast to allow accurate visual identification of these waves. In the older child and adolescent useful information can be obtained. Are the veins distended? Is pressure obviously abnormal based on persistent distension despite elevation of the head (or arm) above the right atrial level? Are the waves regular, suggesting sinus rhythm? Is there an excessively large a or v wave? Each of these observations may be useful when interpreting subsequent auscultatory observations.

Arterial Pulses and Blood Pressure

Assess pulse rate amplitude and quality at each examination. Compare both right and left brachial artery pulses with those in the feet. Learn to assess the posterior tibial artery or dorsalis pedis artery pulses (or both) instead of the femoral artery pulses for all age patients. In the infant it is easier to do, as one need not disturb the infant by hyperabducting the leg; and it is safer for the examiner because the diaper need not be removed. The older child squirms if you attempt to feel femoral pulses. More importantly, a normal pulse in the feet is more meaningful. Be careful not to press too firmly, particularly in an infant, as the peripheral arterial pulse is easily obliterated. If pulses are decreased in amplitude in all four extremities, check the carotid artery or temporal artery.

While palpating pulses, also evaluate peripheral perfusion. It is particularly important in a sick infant. Evaluate capillary refill time: Are the color and temperature of the hands and feet appropriate?

It is also a convenient time to look for clubbing in a hypoxic patient. Clubbing is swelling of the distal phalanx of the fingers and toes. It is most easily detected by noting obliteration of the obtuse angle at the base of the fingernail or toenail.

If you do not measure the blood pressure yourself, be sure the person who does so is properly trained. The stethoscope diaphragm should be used to auscultate the Korotkoff sounds. Systole is easily determined, as it is the point at which sound is first heard as the pressure in the cuff is slowly released. Discussion continues as to whether diastolic blood pressure correlates best with sound muffling (phase 4) or sound disappearance (phase 5) as the cuff is gradually deflated at a rate of a few millimeters of mercury per heart beat. The observer should record both points if phase 4 and phase 5 differ by more than a few millimeters.[14] Be careful not to press on the diaphragm as you listen to the sounds. Doing so may partially compress the artery with the result that Korotkoff sounds continue to a much lower level.

If a pulse amplitude differential seems to be present between the arms and legs or the patient has elevated systolic blood pressure in the arm, it is essential that blood pressure is measured in the feet. It is done most easily using Doppler equipment to measure systolic pressure. Blood pressure should be measured in both arms and at least one foot. An adequately sized cuff is placed on the arms and then on the calf, and the Doppler signal is recorded at the brachial artery and posterior tibial or dorsalis pedis artery. It should be measured in both feet if there is a palpable difference between them or if there is a significant difference between the arm and the first leg measured.

Precordial Palpation

Develop a method for placing your hand on the chest that allows you to palpate comfortably and accurately. Palpation includes search for a thrill, evaluation of the apical impulse, and assessment of the right ventricle.

A *thrill* is the tactile equivalent of a murmur. If the vibrations producing the audible noise are sufficiently strong, they are transmitted to the surface. Learn to distinguish between a thrill, which has duration, and a forceful impulse, which is discrete. A thrill may be systolic or diastolic, although the lat-

ter is rare, as diastolic murmurs seldom are that loud. Use either the palm at the base of the fingers or the tips of the fingers to feel the thrill. For many observers the fingertips are not as sensitive as the hand. One can place the distal palm anywhere on the chest, even on the chest of a premature infant, by spreading the fingers on either side of the neck. It is necessary to use the fingertips to detect a thrill in the suprasternal notch. This observation is important, as it is almost diagnostic of an abnormal, usually stenotic, aortic valve.

Assess the apical impulse for size, duration, and quality. A vigorous hyperactive, healthy left ventricle may cause a forceful systolic impulse, or lift. An apical impulse displaced to the left indicates cardiomegaly. A slow, sustained systolic impulse, called a heave, indicates poor left ventricular contractile force.

Palpate along the left sternal border for increased right ventricular activity. A hyperdynamic right ventricle causes a short, forceful lift against your hand during early systole. A more prolonged systolic impulse, or heave, indicates an hypertrophied right ventricle whose function may be abnormal.

Pulmonary hypertension may cause a systolic impulse in the second left intercostal space owing to forceful expansion of the pulmonic trunk.

Auscultation

The technique of auscultation is not complicated, but training and repetition are required to attain a skill level that allows the observer to develop confidence. Learn the skills of auscultation while listening with a proper stethoscope to a cooperative child who is lying supine in a quiet room. Do not try to master this skill while examining a fussy infant with a heart rate of 150 beats/ minute. That skill will evolve, but the basics must be learned first.

Start by listening with the bell at the second right intercostal space. (A few seconds spent warming the chest piece, especially the diaphragm, by rubbing it against your palm is appreciated by the older patient and may keep the infant or toddler from crying.) Many instructors suggest starting auscultation at the apex, but it is easier to start where there is less likelihood of hearing anything other than a single S_1 and S_2. This method allows you to become comfortable with rhythm and rate and to identify systole and diastole. At this location you hear the left heart components of S_1 and S_2. The right heart components of S_1 and S_2 normally are not heard in the second right intercostal space; and murmurs, both innocent and pathologic, are uncommon. There should be little difficulty identifying S_1 and S_2, regardless of rate. S_1 is somewhat broad and soft. S_2 is of high frequency, narrow, and louder. It is essential to recognize S_1 and S_2 because it allows you to identify systole and diastole. A slow heart rate helps with the timing because systole is noticeably shorter than diastole. Once the rate exceeds 100 beats/minute or so, this aid is lost. Therefore you must learn to recognize S_1 and S_2 by how they sound. They are different. Establishing the pattern of S_1 and S_2 (i.e., the heart rhythm) is analogous to listening to the rhythm section of a musical group. The drum and bass are there in the background; you may not pay direct attention to them, but they are vital to setting the framework for the other instruments—additional heart sounds and murmurs, if you will. Musical aptitude and ability are helpful during cardiac auscultation. There are many similarities.

Move to the second left intercostal space and evaluate S_2. You should be able to hear both components and to assess their response to respiration. It may be easier to hear both components by using the diaphragm. Determine if the distance between the two components (S_2 splitting) is of normal duration and that splitting varies with breathing (increasing with inspiration and decreasing with expiration). If splitting cannot be heard, try augmenting the right ventricular filling by compressing the abdomen with your hand during each inspiration. Evaluate the intensity of the pulmonic component of S_2. Listen for a specific pulmonic flow murmur and concentrate on S_1 to determine if a pulmonic ejection sound is present. Remember that it is loudest during expiration. Sometimes recognizing that a low-intensity click is present is based entirely on phasic changes in the quality of S_1 that have no other explanation.

Move to the lower left sternal border and listen for a split S_1. Both components should be of similar quality and intensity, and their interval does not vary with respiration. Note any systolic or diastolic murmurs (or both).

Move to the apex. S_1 and S_2 should be single. Listen for an ejection sound or a midsystolic click. Note the presence of S_3, remembering that this finding is normal in children and adolescents. Note any murmurs.

Now evaluate what you have heard during this systematic once-over examination of the four major listening areas (Fig. 1–12). If no abnormalities have been detected, you may be through. If you have listened only with the bell chest piece, you may want to go back over the four areas using the diaphragm. The bell provides the maximal intensity of all sounds. The diaphragm distinguishes high-frequency sounds by damping the low-frequency sounds. The high-frequency sounds are not louder, just easier to hear.

If you detected a murmur, you should return to it and assess it in detail according to the scheme presented earlier in the chapter. At this point you should make a simple yes/no decision. Is the murmur pathologic or innocent? If you are satisfied that it is innocent, the examination is complete. If you believe that it is pathologic or possibly so, you should evaluate the possible causes and assess whether additional cardiac findings are present that would support this impression and that may not have been heard during the initial review. For example, if you hear a murmur that you believe may represent aortic stenosis, listen more carefully at the apex with the diaphragm for an aortic ejection sound.

How long does it take to accomplish thorough cardiac auscultation? It takes less time than it does to read about it. An experienced pediatric cardiologist can accomplish all but the most complex examinations in 5 minutes or less. Be honest with yourself. How often have you spent 5 minutes performing cardiac auscultation? You cannot develop this skill to your potential if you do not make a reasonable effort.

There are some tricks to accomplishing cardiac auscultation that are particularly useful in infants. Many learners are discouraged by the infant in congestive failure with a heart rate of 150 beats/minute. Such an infant, with a large ventricular septal defect, has at least two murmurs—S_1 and both components of S_2—each of which must be evaluated. Thus there are five sound events per cardiac cycle; at a rate of 150 beats/minute, there are then 12.5 sound events per second in a relatively simple, straightforward cardiac examination for an infant with heart disease. Do not be discouraged by these numbers. The examination is easier than it seems. One of the first methods you should

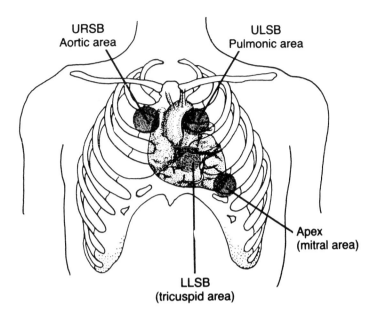

FIGURE 1—12. Traditional listening areas and cardiac outline in relation to the anterior chest. LLSB = lower left sternal border; ULSB = upper left sternal border; URSB = upper right sternal border. (From Lehrer S: Understanding Pediatric Heart Sounds. Philadelphia, WB Saunders, 1992. By permission.)

develop to manage auscultation of a patient with a rapid heart rate is the ability to listen selectively: You must evaluate each sound event independently, concentrating on it during each cardiac cycle. It is not difficult. You probably do it often, as whenever you listen to a musical group; many instruments may be playing simultaneously, but you can pick out the bass, the lead, the piano, and so on and concentrate on it. It need not be the loudest instrument. Practice this skill the next time you go to a concert or play a record. It is easier to do it during cardiac auscultation because for the most part sound events from the heart are consecutive, not simultaneous, and they are repetitive.

It is difficult to begin cardiac auscultation in an unknown patient by listening to low-intensity sounds, particularly when there is a loud murmur demanding your attention. In this case it may be wise to modify the order in which you gather information. You must first identify the rhythm of systole and diastole but then go ahead and assess the loud murmur. Characterize it in your mind and satisfy yourself that you have done all that is required to evaluate it. You can then tune it out and listen to other sounds and quieter murmurs. Selective listening ability is an essential skill. Fortunately, it is not difficult to learn in regard to cardiac auscultation, as most of us accomplish it frequently in other contexts.

Another useful aid to auscultation, especially with fast heart rates and multiple sound events, is "inching" of the stetho-scope. With this technique the auscultation starts in an area at which sounds are clear, and then gradually the stethoscope is moved to another area where they are uncertain. As you listen, staying in tune with the basic rhythm, additional sound events gradually fade in, and their place in the cardiac cycle becomes clear.

There are occasions when auscultation in nontraditional listening areas is indicated. For example, the presence of heart failure in a newborn raises the possibility of a cerebral arteriovenous malformation. This abnormality is almost always readily audible by listening to the head. It is a rare lesion, and if you do not think about it you may not diagnose it. This is not to say that routine examination of every newborn should include auscultation of the head, abdomen, and anywhere else an arteriovenous malformation may occur. It does suggest that observation of one abnormality, in this example heart failure, should direct further evaluation.

REFERENCES

1. Guyton AC: Textbook of Medical Physiology. 8th Ed. Philadelphia, WB Saunders, 1991.
2. Victorica BE, Gessner IH, Schiebler GL: Phonocardiographic findings in persistent truncus arteriosus. Br Heart J *30*:812–816, 1968.
3. Curtiss EI, Matthews RG, Shaver JA: Mechanism of normal splitting of the second heart sound. Circulation *51*:157–164, 1975.
4. Glower DD, Murrah RL, Olsen CO, et al: Mechanical correlates of the third heart sound. J Am Coll Cardiol *19*:450–457, 1992.

5. Jordon MD, Taylor CR, Nyhuis AW, Tavel ME: Audibility of the fourth heart sound: relationship to presence of disease and examiner experience. Arch Intern Med *147*:721–726, 1987.

6. Grayzel J: Gallop rhythm of the heart: II. Quadruple rhythm and its relation to summation and augmented gallops. Circulation *20*:1053–1062, 1959.

7. Perloff JK: Heart sounds and murmurs: physiological mechanisms. *In* Braunwald E (ed): Heart Disease. 4th Ed. Philadelphia, WB Saunders, 1992.

8. Pepper OHP: Medical Etymology. Philadelphia, WB Saunders, 1949.

9. Sabbah HN, Stein PD: Turbulent blood flow in humans: its primary role in the production of ejection murmurs. Circ Res *38*:513–525, 1976.

10. Bruns DL: A general theory of the causes of murmurs. Am J Med *27*:360–374, 1959.

11. Freeman AR, Levin SA: The clinical significance of the systolic murmur: a study of 1000 consecutive "non-cardiac" cases. Ann Intern Med *6*: 1371–1385, 1933.

12. Flint A: On cardiac murmurs. Am J Med Sci *44*: 29–54, 1862.

13. Landzberg JS, Pflugfelder PW, Cassidy MM, et al: Etiology of the Austin Flint murmur. J Am Coll Cardiol *20*:408–413, 1992.

14. Report of the Second Task Force on Blood Pressure Control in Children—1987. Task Force on Blood Pressure Control in Children: National Heart, Lung, and Blood Institute. Pediatrics *79*: 1–25, 1987.

2

HOW TO READ A CHEST RADIOGRAPH

Benjamin E. Victorica

The routine chest radiograph continues to be of diagnostic value for heart disease despite newer and more sophisticated imaging techniques. Upright posteroanterior and lateral chest radiographs, with or without barium in the esophagus, can suggest the presence of structural cardiovascular abnormalities and can also estimate their hemodynamic significance. The procedure is simple, readily available, and by far the least expensive imaging technique. The primary care physician should be able to perform basic chest radiography interpretation and correlate the findings with other clinical data to arrive at a preliminary diagnosis. It does not mean that chest radiography is required for routine patient evaluation. Specific indications for the procedure should exist.

Proper evaluation of a chest radiograph requires a systematic approach so important diagnostic information is not overlooked or misinterpreted. Combining information on heart size, heart shape, and pulmonary vascularity is important for determining the cardiac diagnosis and hemodynamic status.

TECHNICAL ASPECTS

The first step in chest radiograph analysis is to determine if the films are technically adequate for proper interpretation (Fig. 2–1). Chest radiography should be done with the patient upright and the arms elevated, in a straight posteroanterior view and, if possible, during inspiration. Proper position and film penetration are essential particularly for evaluation of pulmonary vascularity.

INTERPRETATION

Chest radiograph interpretation should be accomplished in an orderly, stepwise fashion to include the following:

1. Extracardiac structures
   a. Abnormalities of the thoracic skeleton
   b. Diaphragms and lungs
   c. Lung parenchyma
2. Cardiovascular structures
   a. Organ position: heart, stomach, liver
   b. Cardiac size and shape
   c. Aortic arch anomalies
3. Pulmonary vascularity

Extracardiac Structures

Abnormalities of the Thoracic Skeleton

Congenital skeletal anomalies occur in association with congenital heart defects. Hemivertebrae and rib anomalies are often present in patients with tetralogy of Fallot or truncus arteriosus. They are also a manifestation of the VACTERL syndrome (vertebral anomalies, anal atresia, cardiac defects, tracheoesophageal fistula, renal and limb anomalies). Down syndrome frequently is marked by the presence of 11 ribs (Fig. 2–2). Skeletal chest deformities (scoliosis, pectus excavatum, straight back syndrome, narrow posteroanterior diameter of the chest) may be seen in conditions such as Marfan syndrome and are often present in patients with mitral valve prolapse (Fig. 2–3).

Bilateral rib notching can be seen in older children with coarctation of the aorta (Fig. 2–4). Unilateral rib notching is uncommon

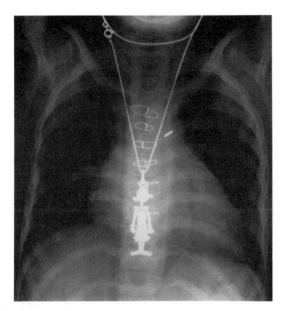

FIGURE 2–1. Technically inadequate radiograph: superiorly angulated view with the clavicles seen from above. This particular view, associated with a poor inspiratory effort, results in a triangular heart and gives a false impression of cardiomegaly. Presence of the child's necklace also does not help.

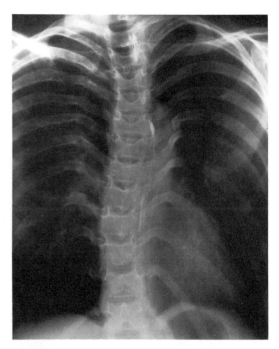

FIGURE 2–3. Young girl with mitral valve prolapse showing scoliosis and left displacement of the heart due to a narrow anteroposterior diameter of the chest.

but may be present on the same side as a Blalock-Taussig shunt.

Radiographic evidence of previous chest surgery can be useful when evaluating car-

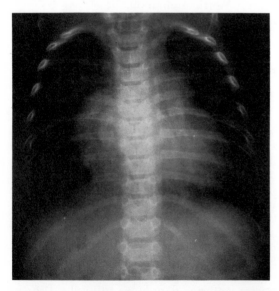

FIGURE 2–2. Infant with an endocardial cushion defect resulting in a hemodynamically significant left-to-right shunt. Note the presence of 11 ribs bilaterally, consistent with Down syndrome. The film is overexposed, making skeletal structures clear but obscuring pulmonary vascular markings.

diac patients. A lateral thoracotomy can be suspected by comparing the outline of the thoracic cage on both sides. A deformed rib and indented rib margin or narrow intercostal space indicate the side and level of previous surgery (Fig. 2–5). Sternal deformity or sternal wires indicate a previous midline thoracotomy. Metallic clips, artificial valves, or pacemaker wires are easily detectable (Fig. 2–6). The site of previous surgery reflects the type of operation accomplished (Table 2–1).

Diaphragm and Lungs

Elevation of a hemidiaphragm due to its paralysis can affect interpretation of cardiac size and pulmonary vascularity. Diaphragmatic hernia can result in shift of the cardiac structures; for example, a left hernia can displace the heart into the right chest, resulting in cardiac dextroposition. Right chest and lung hypoplasia also can result in cardiac dextroposition. In this situation one must consider the possibility of associated partial anomalous drainage of the right lung pulmonary veins into the inferior vena cava. The dilated vein directed toward the inferior vena cava junction may resemble a curved

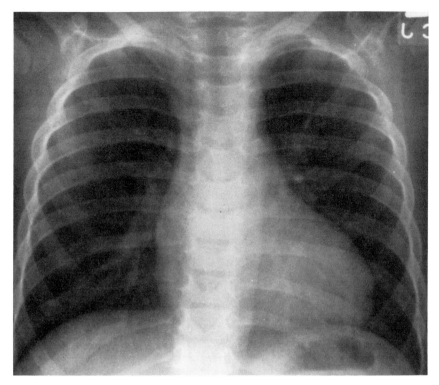

FIGURE 2–4. Child with coarctation of the aorta. There is periosteal thickening and notching of the inferior aspect of ribs 4, 5, and 6 secondary to prominent collateral circulation.

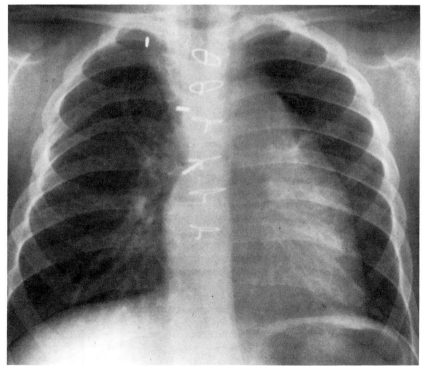

FIGURE 2–5. Postoperative patient with sternal wires indicating midline thoracotomy. The narrow intercostal space between the deformed right 4th and 5th ribs denotes a right thoracotomy.

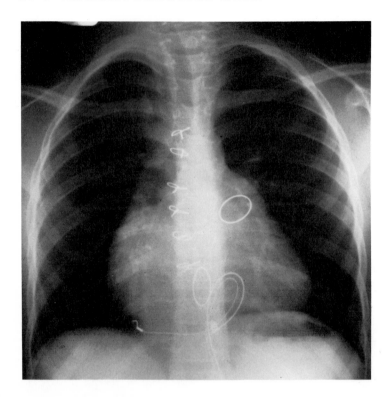

FIGURE 2–6. Patient after Hancock valve replacements of the pulmonary and tricuspid valves and placement of a sequential artificial pacemaker with epicardial leads on the right atrium and ventricle.

sword—thus the name scimitar syndrome (Fig. 2–7).

Left lower lobe atelectasis can result from bronchial compression by an enlarged left atrium. It also may occur following cardiac surgery.

Lung Parenchyma

Lung disease may be present in many patients with cardiac abnormalities. The subject is beyond the scope of this book.

Cardiovascular Structures

Organ Position: Heart, Stomach, Liver

The usual patient has a left-sided cardiac apex and stomach bubble indicating that the internal organs have normal position and relation (situs solitus). A right-sided cardiac apex and stomach bubble would indicate the presence of mirror-image dextrocardia (situs inversus) with complete reversal of internal organ positions (Fig. 2–8). In this particular situation one can simply flip the frontal film over and interpret the film in the usual way.

Interpretation is more difficult when there is discordance between the position of the cardiac apex and the stomach bubble (e.g., stomach bubble on the left side with cardiac apex on the right). In this case the patient may have situs solitus and cardiac dextroversion as if the cardiac apex had been rotated toward the right side (Fig. 2–9). Patients with dextroversion have a higher incidence of cardiac defects than do those with situs inversus. When the stomach bubble is close to the midline, the possibility of asplenia should be suspected (isomerism) (Fig. 2–10).

TABLE 2–1. SITE OF CARDIAC VASCULAR SURGERY

Right Thoracotomy	Midline Sternotomy	Left Thoracotomy
Blalock-Taussig shunt	Pulmonary valvotomy (closed heart)	Blalock-Taussig shunt
Glenn anastomosis	Central shunts	Patent ductus arteriosus
	Hemi-Fontan	Coarctation of the aorta
	Open heart	Pulmonary artery banding

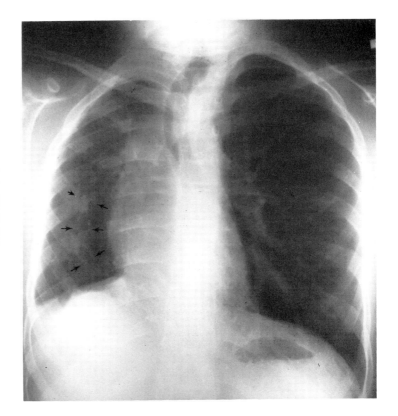

FIGURE 2–7. Cardiac dextroposition secondary to right lung hypoplasia. The left lung is hyperexpanded, and the trachea is deviated toward the right. Arrows indicate the curved right lower pulmonary veins draining anomalously toward the inferior vena cava (scimitar syndrome).

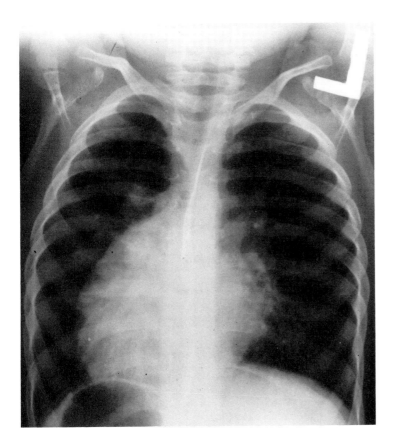

FIGURE 2–8. Situs inversus and mirror-image dextrocardia. Note the stomach bubble and the cardiac apex on the right side.

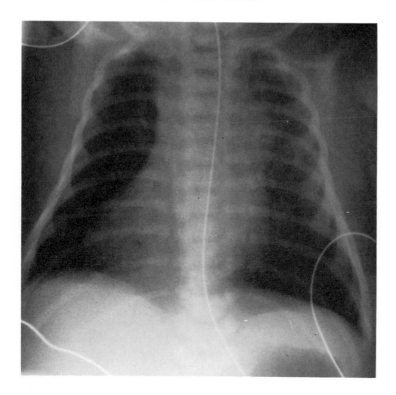

FIGURE 2–9. Newborn with situs solitus (stomach bubble on the left side) and cardiac dextroversion.

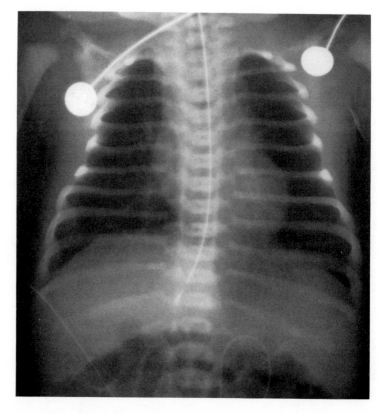

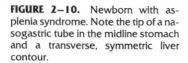**FIGURE 2–10.** Newborn with asplenia syndrome. Note the tip of a nasogastric tube in the midline stomach and a transverse, symmetric liver contour.

Cardiac Size and Shape

Traditionally the cardiothoracic (CT) ratio has been used to estimate heart size. It is obtained by comparing the transverse diameter of the heart with the maximal transverse diameter of the chest. A CT ratio of more than 50 per cent is considered abnormal, representing cardiomegaly. This ratio is almost impossible to apply to an infant chest radiograph because usually there is some degree of rotation and often inadequate inspiration. The presence of a large thymus also can affect the measurements.

Isolated pressure overload lesions, such as aortic or pulmonic valve stenosis, do not enlarge heart size. Volume overload lesions, such as a significant left-to-right shunt or atrioventricular valve regurgitation, cause cardiac chamber dilation, which enlarges the cardiac silhouette on chest radiograph. Congestive heart failure, severe anemia, and myocardial dysfunction cause cardiomegaly. It is difficult to entertain the clinical diagnosis of congestive heart failure in the presence of normal heart size.

A chest radiograph demonstrating normal heart shape is shown in Figure 2–11. The right heart border is formed superiorly by the straight lateral wall of the superior vena cava (SVC) and inferiorly by the right lateral wall of the right atrium. The left heart border is formed superiorly by the aortic knob, which continues with the proximal descending aorta. The convexity below that represents the pulmonic trunk, whose identification in normal position is important as it indicates the presence of normally related great arteries. Below the pulmonic trunk, the remainder of the convexity of the left

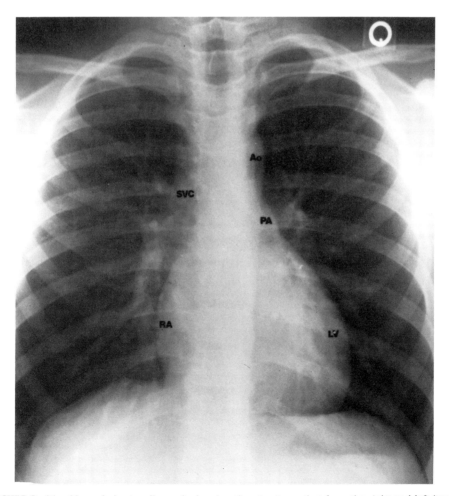

FIGURE 2–11. Normal chest radiograph showing the structures that form the right and left heart borders. SVC = superior vena cava; RA = right atrium; Ao = aortic knob and first of the descending aorta; PA = main pulmonary artery (pulmonic trunk); LV = left ventricle. The right ventricle and left atrium do not participate in the cardiac silhouette.

heart border is formed by the anterolateral wall of the left ventricle. In the normal heart there is a concavity between the pulmonic trunk and the left ventricular contour.

Displacement of the SVC to the right is seen in the presence of a right aortic arch, which also produces an indentation on the right side of the trachea just above the carina. A right aortic arch is present in approximately 25 per cent of patients with tetralogy of Fallot and 25 per cent of patients with truncus arteriosus (Fig. 2–12). The SVC also can be displaced to the right by a dilated ascending aorta as a result of aortic valve stenosis (Fig. 2–13). A dilated SVC suggests the presence of anomalous systemic or pulmonary venous drainage into this vein. A prominent right atrial contour suggests right atrial enlargement, which is seen with right heart volume overload lesions such as an atrial septal defect. A large right atrium may be present with Ebstein anomaly of the tricuspid valve (Fig. 2–14), causing marked tricuspid valve regurgitation.

An indentation in the descending aorta suggests the presence of a localized aortic coarctation. It results in the characteristic "3 sign," which is formed by the aortic knob, indentation at the site of coarctation, and poststenotic dilatation of the descending aorta (Fig. 2–15).

Dilation of the pulmonic trunk is seen with pulmonic valve stenosis (Fig. 2–16), idiopathic dilation of the pulmonary artery, and pulmonary hypertension. A localized convexity between the aortic knob and pulmonary artery is typical of a patent ductus arteriosus (Fig. 2–17).

Protrusion of a density occupying the normal concavity between the pulmonic trunk and the superior left ventricular border represents dilation of a left atrial appendage. This picture is almost diagnostic of chronic rheumatic heart disease (Fig. 2–18).

Young infants can have a broad upper mediastinum due to the presence of a large thymus. The lateral edges of the thymus are usually irregular (thymic wave) with indentations caused by the anterior ribs. One may also see the characteristic "sail sign," partic-

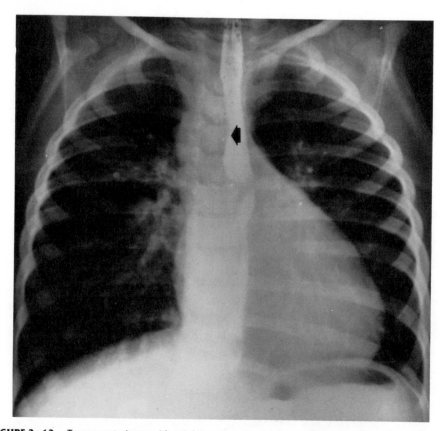

FIGURE 2–12. Truncus arteriosus with a right aortic arch and descending aorta. The right arch causes the esophagus and trachea to be displaced to the left of midline. The right arch also indents the right side of the barium-filled esophagus (arrow).

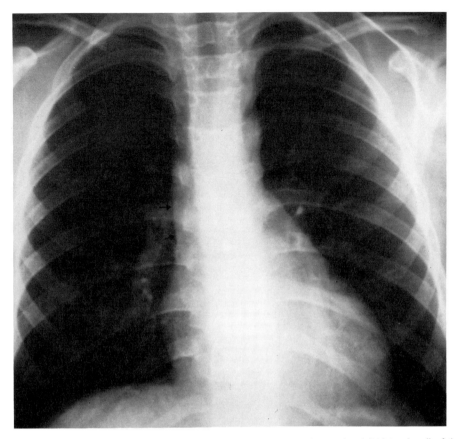

FIGURE 2–13. Teenage boy with aortic valve stenosis. Arrows point to the right lateral wall of the SVC displaced by a dilated ascending aorta.

ularly if the heart is rotated slightly to one side or the other.

A "figure of eight," or "snowman," configuration is highly suggestive of supracardiac total anomalous pulmonary venous return. The upper part is formed by the dilated left vertical vein (usually the left superior vena cava) on the left and the dilated superior vena cava on the right. The lower part is formed by the large right atrium and the ventricular mass (Fig. 2–19).

Right ventricular hypertrophy is suggested by an upturned apex. If this sign is combined with a concave pulmonary trunk segment, tetralogy of Fallot (Fig. 2–20) is likely to be present. A "left ventricular" configuration caused by left and downward displacement of the cardiac apex is seen in the presence of chronic left ventricular dilation (Fig. 2–21). A dilated left atrium can elevate the left main stem bronchus and can cause double density behind the right atrium. It also produces an anterior indentation on the lower third of the barium-filled esophagus (Fig. 2–22).

Aortic Arch Anomalies

Posteroanterior and lateral chest radiographs with barium-filled esophagus are needed to diagnose these abnormalities. An aberrant subclavian artery originates from the descending aorta rather than from the innominate artery. The anomalous vessel courses upward and behind the esophagus toward the arm opposite the side of the aortic arch (Fig. 2–23A). The aberrant vessel causes a discrete posterior indentation on the upper barium-filled esophagus (Fig. 2–23B).

A vascular ring can result in compression of the trachea and esophagus. The most common type, fortunately creating a loose ring that is seldom symptomatic, is produced by the combination of a right aortic arch and an aberrant left subclavian artery associated with a left-sided ductus ligamentum. In this case the posterior indentation in the esophagus is larger than with an isolated aberrant

text continues on page 36

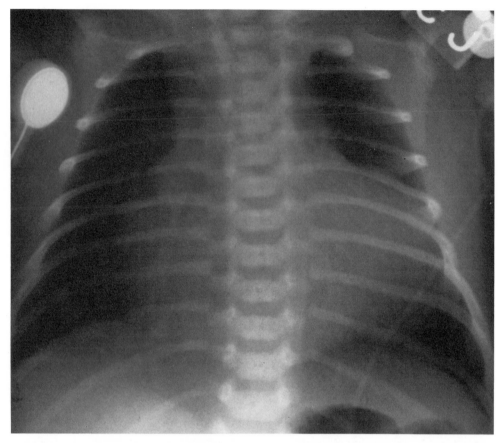

FIGURE 2–14. Cyanotic newborn with Ebstein anomaly of the tricuspid valve. There is cardiomegaly, an enlarged right atrium, and diminished pulmonary arterial vascularity.

FIGURE 2–15. Child with coarctation of the aorta. Note the "3 sign" formed by the aortic knob, the indentation at the site of coarctation, and the post-stenotic dilatation of the descending aorta.

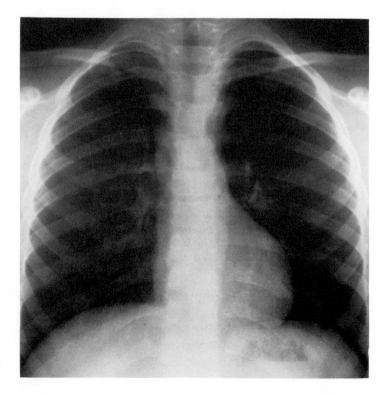

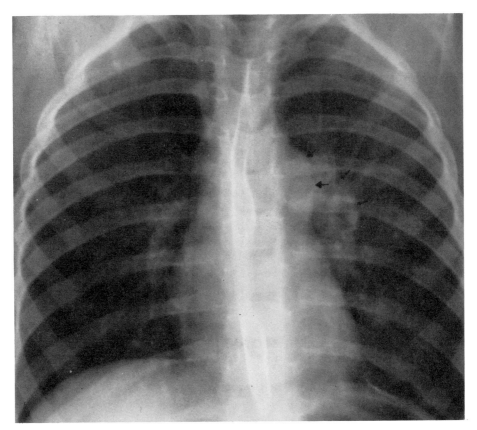

FIGURE 2–16. Child with pulmonic valve stenosis showing poststenotic dilation of the pulmonic trunk (large arrows) and left (small arrows) pulmonary artery.

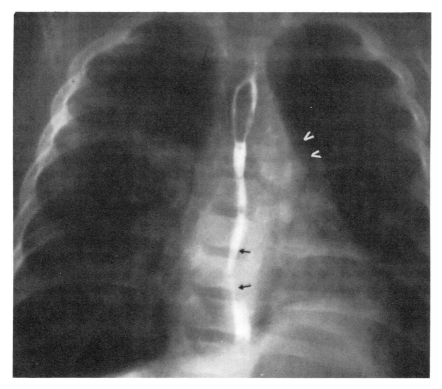

FIGURE 2–17. Infant with a large patent ductus arteriosus and lung disease. The dilated ductus forms a convexity (arrowheads) between the aortic knob and the pulmonic trunk. Left atrial enlargement is indicated by displacement of the esophagus to the right (arrows) and by elevation of the left main stem bronchus so its convexity is directed superiorly.

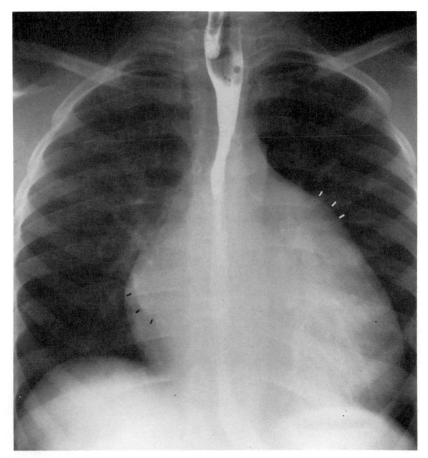

FIGURE 2–18. Patient with chronic rheumatic heart disease. The white bars show the almost pathognomonic sign of a dilated left atrial appendage bulging between the pulmonic trunk and the left ventricular convexity. The black bars indicate the right edge of a markedly dilated left atrium. Note the cardiomegaly and evidence of pulmonary venous obstruction with dilated pulmonary veins in both upper lung lobes.

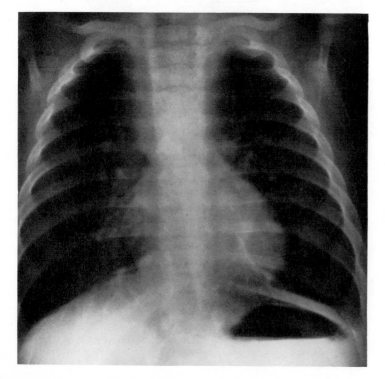

FIGURE 2–19. Infant with supracardiac total anomalous pulmonary venous return. Note the "figure of eight," or "snowman," formed superiorly by the dilated left vertical vein and the right superior vena cava and inferiorly by the atrioventricular mass.

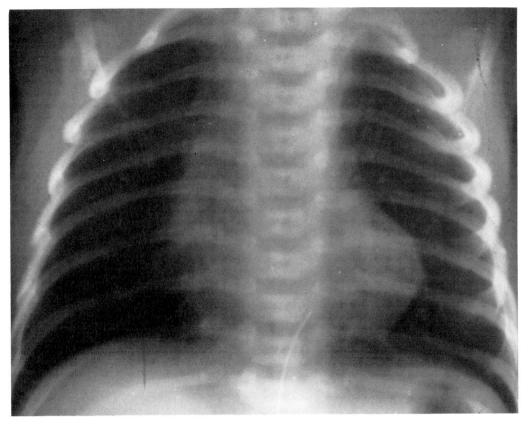

FIGURE 2–20. Newborn with tetralogy of Fallot. There is a "right ventricular configuration" with an upturned apex and a concave right ventricular outflow tract-pulmonary trunk area. Heart size is normal; the shape is not.

FIGURE 2–21. Child with chronic rheumatic mitral valve regurgitation. The heart shows a left ventricular configuration with left and downward displacement of the apex. The arrowheads point to the diagnostic dilated left atrial appendage.

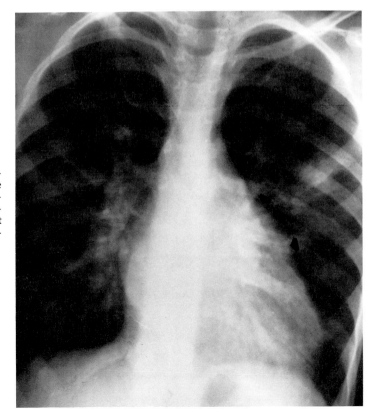

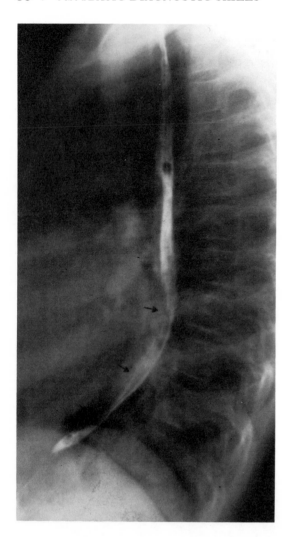

FIGURE 2–22. Chest radiograph of the same child shown in Figure 2–21 illustrating that left atrial dilation causes anterior indentation and posterior displacement of the barium-filled esophagus (arrows).

Normal Pulmonary Vascularity

Normal pulmonary vascular markings rule out the presence of a hemodynamically significant left-to-right shunt, pulmonary venous congestion, or inadequate pulmonary blood flow (Fig. 2–25).

Increased Pulmonary Vascularity

Increased pulmonary vascularity is always an abnormal finding. Once this observation has been made, it is necessary to differentiate between the presence of increased arterial vascularity due to a left-to-right shunt and increased pulmonary venous vascularity due to pulmonary venous obstruction.

Left-to-Right Shunt Vascularity

Enlarged pulmonary arteries indicate the presence of increased pulmonary blood flow as a result of a significant left-to-right shunt (e.g., an atrial or ventricular septal defect). Pulmonary arteries may be dilated and tortuous centrally and distally throughout both lung fields (Fig. 2–26A). This type of vascularity also is suggested by the presence of prominent hilar vessels on the lateral film (Fig. 2–26B). Once evidence of left-to-right shunt has been detected, the next step is to determine the presence of left atrial enlargement. Increased pulmonary arterial vascularity without left atrial enlargement would indicate the presence of an atrial level left-to-right shunt (Fig. 2–27). As increased pulmonary blood flow returns to the left atrium, it can either enter the left ventricle or cross the atrial septal defect thereby avoiding dilation of the left atrium itself. If the atrial septum is intact, however, the only outlet is the mitral valve. In this situation, as pro-

subclavian artery. A double aortic arch, on the other hand, is a vascular ring that commonly produces symptomatic obstruction of the trachea and esophagus. The frontal chest radiograph (Fig. 2–24A) shows bilateral indentation of the barium-filled esophagus with the right-sided indentation larger and higher than that on the left. The lateral film shows a large posterior indentation (Fig. 2–24B). Narrowing of the trachea just above the carina may be apparent. Angiography illustrates the vascular anatomy (Fig. 2–24C).

Pulmonary Vascularity

Adequate interpretation of pulmonary arterial and venous vascularity is an essential step when assessing the hemodynamic status of the patient.

text continues on page 44

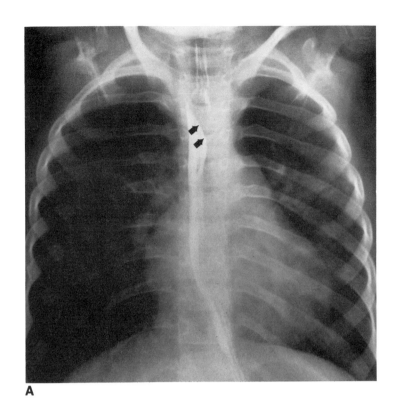

A

FIGURE 2–23. (A) Posteroanterior radiograph showing the presence of a left aortic arch and an aberrant right subclavian artery producing an oblique indentation (arrows) on the upper third of the barium-filled esophagus. (B) On the lateral film the aberrant artery is seen to cause a small posterior indentation (arrow) of the upper barium-filled esophagus.

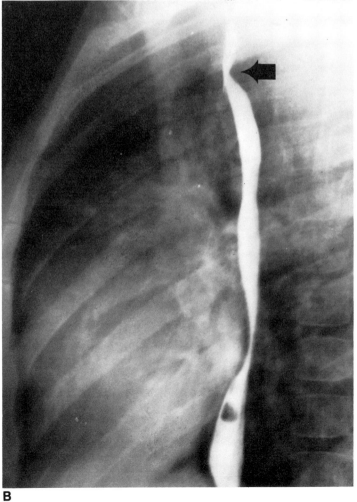

B

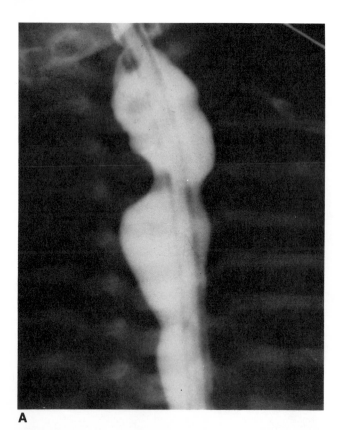

A

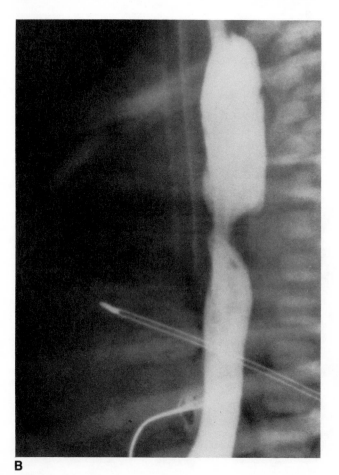

B

FIGURE 2–24. Barium swallow in an infant with signs and symptoms of significant upper airway obstruction. (*A*) Frontal view shows bilateral, right larger than left, indentation of the barium-filled esophagus. (*B*) Lateral film shows a large posterior indentation of the esophagus. (*C*) Aortogram clearly demonstrates the presence of a double aortic arch.

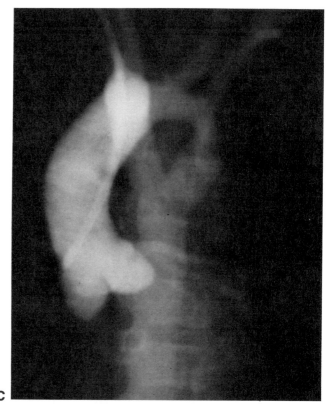

FIGURE 2–24. (*continued*)

C

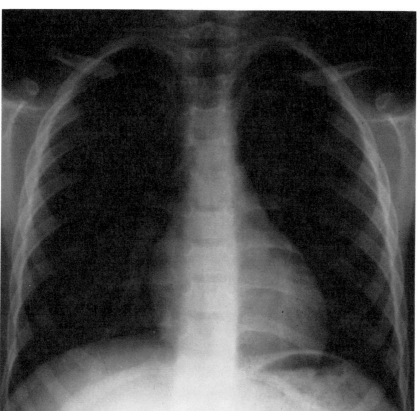

FIGURE 2–25.   Technically excellent chest radiograph showing normal heart size and configuration. The pulmonary vascularity is normal and equally distributed throughout both lung fields.

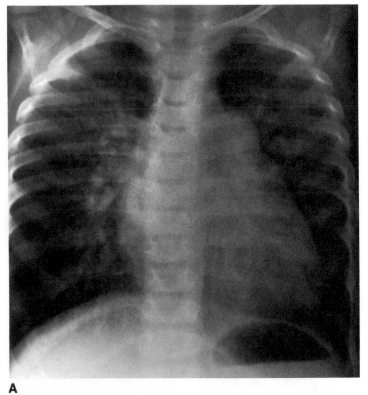

A

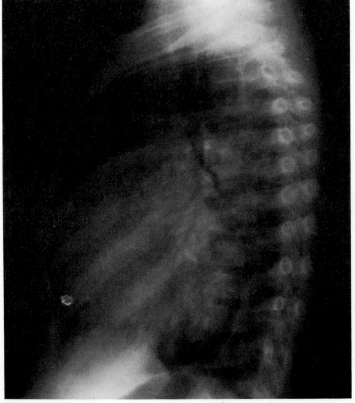

B

FIGURE 2–26. (*A*) Child with a hemodynamically large ventricular septal defect producing a large left-to-right shunt. There is prominent pulmonary arterial vascularity with dilated and tortuous pulmonary arteries throughout both lung fields. (*B*) Lateral view confirms the presence of shunt vascularity with prominent, dilated hilar vessels.

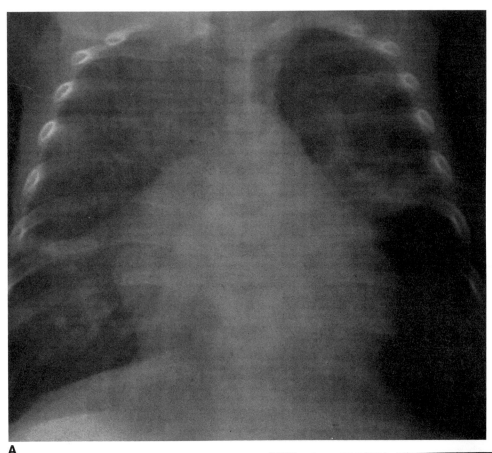

A

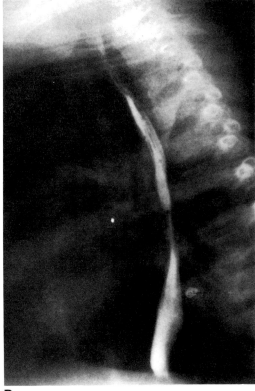

B

FIGURE 2–27. Infant with an endocardial cushion defect. (*A*) Frontal view shows increased pulmonary venous and arterial vascularity, lung atelectasis, and lung infiltrates. (*B*) Lateral view with barium shows no evidence of left atrial enlargement, consistent with the presence of an atrial level left-to-right shunt. It does not, however, rule out an additional ventricular level shunt.

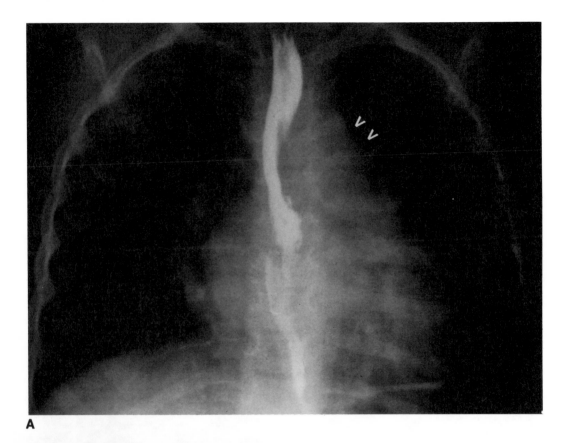

A

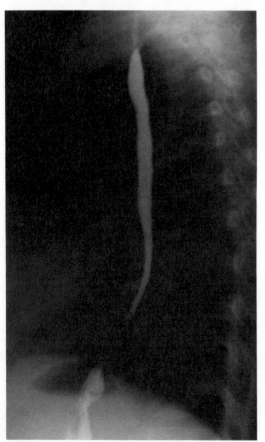

B

FIGURE 2–28. (*A*) Infant with a large patent ductus arteriosus. Note the prominent pulmonary vascularity of the shunt type. Convex density between the aortic knob and pulmonic trunk (arrowheads) is caused by the ductus itself. (*B*) Presence of a dilated left atrium indenting the lower barium-filled esophagus indicates that the left-to-right shunt is distal to the atrioventricular valve.

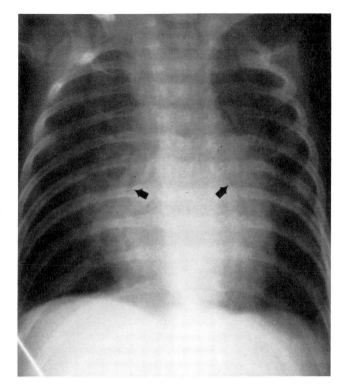

FIGURE 2–29. Infant with severe congenital mitral valve stenosis. The heart is of normal size, but there is evidence of pulmonary venous obstruction and congestion. Note the redistribution of pulmonary blood flow toward the upper lobes with dilated and indistinct pulmonary veins. Spread of the right and left main stem bronchi (arrows) indicates left atrial dilation.

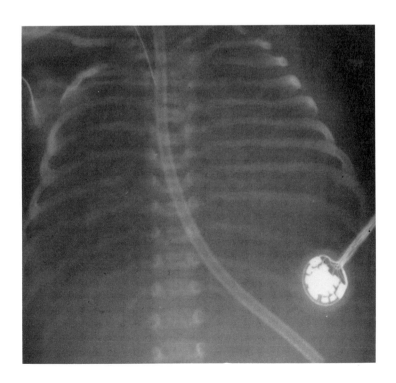

FIGURE 2–30. Pattern of severe pulmonary venous obstruction in a newborn infant with infradiaphragmatic total anomalous pulmonary venous return.

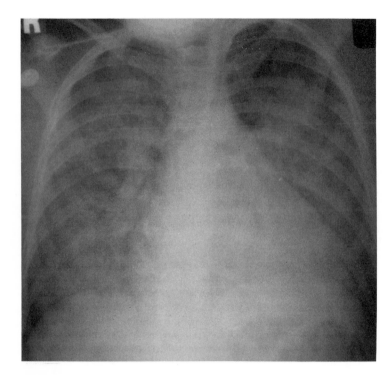

FIGURE 2–31. Patient with florid pulmonary edema. There is marked cardiomegaly, and "fluffy" infiltrates are present in both lung fields.

duced by a ventricular septal defect or patent ductus arteriosus, the left atrium is dilated. In the posteroanterior projection, left atrial dilation often is manifested by elevation of the left main stem bronchus (Fig. 2–28A). On a normal chest radiograph the left main stem bronchus has its convexity di- rected downward. The left atrium lies directly underneath the left main stem bronchus. If the left atrium dilates, it elevates the left main stem bronchus initially causing it to be straight; with greater enlargement, it causes it to have a convexity directed upward. Left atrial dilation also is indicated by

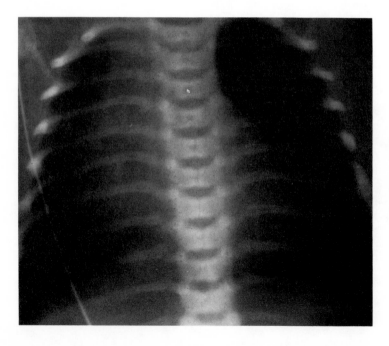

FIGURE 2–32. Cyanotic newborn with pulmonary valve atresia and an intact ventricular septum. Pulmonary vascularity appears markedly diminished with black lung fields, indicating diminished pulmonary arterial blood flow.

posterior displacement of the lower barium-filled esophagus viewed in lateral position (Fig. 2–28B).

Pulmonary Venous Obstruction

Pulmonary venous obstruction (PVO) is characterized by redistribution of pulmonary arterial blood flow toward the upper lobes of both lungs, resulting in prominence of the upper lobe pulmonary veins. In contrast, the lower lobes show somewhat diminished vascularity (Fig. 2–18). This type of pulmonary vascularity, often unrecognized, is seen in the presence of obstructive left heart lesions such as aortic stenosis. A more significant degree of PVO causes pulmonary congestion, again particularly in the upper lobes (Fig. 2–29). A severe form of PVO is seen in newborn infants with infradiaphrag-matic total anomalous pulmonary venous return. The obstructive venous pattern is so severe the film resembles hyaline membrane disease (Fig. 2–30). An extreme form of PVO results in pulmonary edema with diffuse and changing fluffy infiltrates in both lung fields (Fig. 2–31).

Decreased Pulmonary Arterial Vascularity

Diminished arterial vascularity with small arterial vessels is seen in patients with pulmonic valve stenosis or atresia associated with an intracardiac right-to-left shunt. This combination of defects results in decreased pulmonary arterial blood flow (Fig. 2–32). Pulmonic valve stenosis does not cause decreased pulmonary arterial blood flow unless a right-to-left shunt is present.

3

ELECTROCARDIOGRAM INTERPRETATION AND DIAGNOSTIC VALUE

Benjamin E. Victorica

The 12-lead electrocardiogram continues to be an important diagnostic tool in cardiology. Most physicians have an understanding of the principles of electrocardiography. Reading electrocardiograms, however, can be a difficult and stressful task, particularly for those not routinely involved in their interpretation. Reading electrocardiograms is much like other skills. The ability is developed and maintained by doing it on a regular basis.

Pediatricians and other physicians caring for infants and children should not assume that routine reading of electrocardiograms in their hospital or community is as accurate as it should be or as accurate as can be done by a knowledgeable children's physician. In many hospitals electrocardiographic interpretation is provided only by cardiologists trained in the care of adults. Adult cardiologists are concerned primarily with acquired heart disease and for the most part have little experience with congenital heart disease, particularly in the newborn and infant. It is our belief, based on experience with numerous individuals, that a physician interested in childrens' heart disease can become a valuable community resource by acquiring the ability to interpret pediatric electrocardiograms.

In many hospitals electrocardiograms are now provided with an interpretation generated by a computer program. This reading may be satisfactory for the older child and adolescent, but these programs are limited in usefulness when applied to infants and young children. Computerized pediatric reading programs are available, but all have

limitations and none can be relied on without experienced physician review.

It is important for primary pediatric physicians to be able to distinguish between normal and abnormal electrocardiograms. Subtleties in interpretation and specific abnormalities may not be recognized, but major variations from normal should be identified.

BASIC CONCEPTS

One does not need to be a student of electrophysiology to learn to interpret electrocardiograms. This chapter therefore does not review the basic science of electrocardiography. Those interested in reading about this subject should consult standard textbooks of physiology, electrocardiography, or cardiology. Only some fundamentals are reviewed here.

The heart beats in response to an electrical signal that normally is generated in the sinus node located in the right atrium. (Chapter 11 reviews principles of impulse generation and spread.) This electrical signal depolarizes the atria and ventricles in succession, creating an impulse that can be recorded by electrodes applied to the skin. This recording is the electrocardiogram. The configuration of the signal depends on where on the body the electrodes are applied. These different positions are defined as specific ECG leads. The same electrical signal looks different depending on what lead is recorded.

By international standards an electrical impulse that is moving toward an electrode is recorded as an upward deflection from baseline on the recording paper, and an impulse moving away from the electrode writes a downward deflection. This principle applies to all electrocardiographic waves: P, QRS, and T.

The P wave represents depolarization of the atria. Right atrial depolarization precedes left atrial depolarization, but the time difference is so short that the P wave usually is smooth and one does not observe independent depolarization of the two atria. Atrial repolarization seldom is recorded on a standard electrocardiogram, as this small wave is lost in the much larger QRS. It is possible, however, for a large P to be followed by the so-called T of the P.

The QRS represents ventricular depolarization. It may begin as a negative deflection or a positive deflection. By convention, if the QRS begins with a negative deflection, that negative deflection is designated a Q wave. If the QRS begins with a positive deflection, that deflection is designated an R wave. The first negative deflection after an R wave is designated an S wave. A second positive deflection is designated R′ and a second negative deflection S′. The T wave represents ventricular repolarization. It may be biphasic (i.e., partially positive, partially negative) but still is considered as a unit.

Theoretically, there is no limit to the number of leads that can be obtained, although most instruments are designed to record 12 leads often in groups of three simultaneously. For the standard electrocardiogram, electrodes are placed on all four extremities. These electrodes record the bipolar standard leads designated I, II, and III, which represent electrode pairs as follows: lead I, right arm/left arm; lead II, right arm/left leg; and lead III, left arm/left leg. The limb electrodes also record the augmented limb leads aVR, aVL, and aVF. These leads represent unipolar electrodes on the right arm, left arm, and left leg, respectively. Six additional electrodes, placed across the chest, are designated unipolar precordial V leads. It is useful for the physician to know where the electrodes should be placed to record the V leads, as the skills of electrocardiographic technicians vary, particularly among part-time staff. Adult electrocardiograms and some pediatric electrocardiograms record precordial leads V_1 through V_6 positioned as follows:

V_1 = fourth intercostal space at right sternal edge
V_2 = fourth intercostal space at left sternal edge
V_3 = midway between V_2 and V_4
V_4 = fifth left intercostal space in the midclavicular line
V_5 = fifth left intercostal space in the anterior axillary line
V_6 = fifth left intercostal space in the midaxillary line

Many pediatric electrocardiograms are recorded substituting two other V leads that extend the chest recording farther to the right and to the left. Lead V_3R is placed on the right chest in a position analogous with V_3 on the left. Lead V_7 is placed in the fifth intercostal space in the posterior axillary line. Many electrocardiography machines allow only six V leads to be recorded, in which case leads V_3 and V_5 can be omitted to allow use of V_3R and V_7.

It is useful to think of these 12 leads in two groups of six. The limb leads and augmented limb leads can be considered to view the electrical activity of the heart from the front of the patient—hence the designation frontal plane. Direction of the electrical forces is either left or right and either superior or inferior.

The chest leads view electrical activity of the heart in the horizontal plane, that is, from above. Direction of electrical activity is therefore either left or right and either anterior or posterior. In most instances the right-sided V leads V_3R and V_1 best reflect right ventricular electrical forces, and the left-sided leads V_6 and V_7 best illustrate left ventricular electrical forces.

The electrocardiogram is usually recorded at a paper speed of 25 mm/second. It is essential that the tracing contain a calibration signal so the magnitude of the waves can be evaluated. Every electrocardiogram should be recorded at a calibration of 10 mm deflection equals 1 mV. If some electrocardiographic waves are too large, the tracing can be recorded also at one half sensitivity, or 5 mm deflection equals 1 mV. The appropriate calibration signal must be recorded in order to indicate this change in sensitivity during that portion of the recording.

ELECTROCARDIOGRAM READING

Interpretation of electrocardiograms requires an orderly step-by-step approach developed from good habits. These habits are best obtained by following a form that forces the reader to fill in all of the blank spaces, plot the QRS axis, and pay attention to specific details of each of the components. In this manner chances of overlooking significant findings are diminished. There are many types of reading forms. One adapted for pediatric interpretation is shown in Figure 3–1. Items 1 through 8 in Figure 3–1 are discussed in detail in this section.

The heading of the form should record patient identification data. One should thereafter proceed in an orderly fashion to analyze, measure, and record each component of the tracing.

Rhythm

Rhythm refers to the origin of the heartbeat and to its regularity. Most tracings demonstrate sinus rhythm manifested by the presence of a P wave in front of each QRS complex with normal mean P axis (positive P waves in leads I and aVF) and normal PR interval. Most rhythms are reasonably regular; that is, beats occur at approximately equal time intervals.

The P wave that is negative in lead I and positive in aVF should be considered abnormal. The most common cause for this abnormality is a technical error due to reversal of the left and right arm leads. In this case lead

PEDIATRIC ELECTROCARDIOGRAM

Name ———————————————————————— Date ——————————
Age ————— Medical Record# ———————————

1. Rhythm———————————————
2. Atrial rate————————————— bpm.
   Ventricular rate ————————— bpm.

3. Intervals
   a. PR——————— sec.
   b. QRS ————— sec.
   c. QTc ————— sec.

4. QRS axis

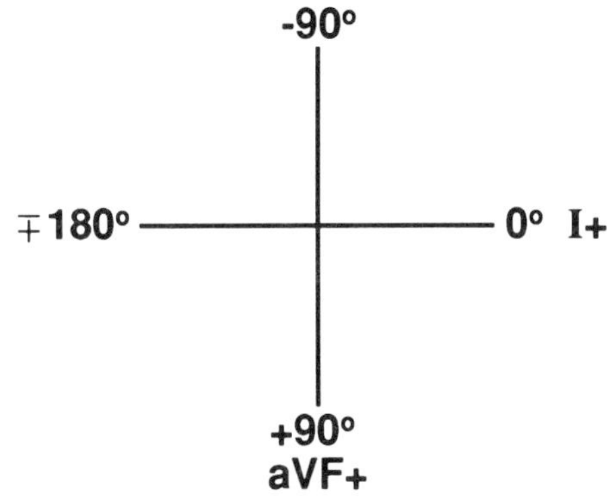

5. Atrial enlargement (P waves)————————————————————————
6. Septal forces (q waves)———————————————————————————
7. Ventricular hypertrophy (QRS complexes)————————————————
   ———————————————————————————————————————
   ———————————————————————————————————————

8. Ventricular repolarization (ST-T waves)
   ———————————————————————————————————————
   ———————————————————————————————————————
   ———————————————————————————————————————

Interpretation
   ———————————————————————————————————————
   ———————————————————————————————————————
   ———————————————————————————————————————

FIGURE 3–1. Working form for interpretation of pediatric electrocardiograms.

aVR is also reversed from normal. If lead placement is correct, one should consider the possibility of mirror-image situs inversus. The remainder of the tracing should supply supporting information if that is the case. If the supraventricular pacemaker is located elsewhere than the sinus node, the P wave generally reflects this abnormal origin. For example, negative P waves in leads II, III, and aVF indicate an ectopic atrial pacemaker. Absent P waves with normal QRS complexes may indicate the presence of junctional rhythm. Chapter 11 provides additional information on some of these conditions.

The most common cause for an irregular rhythm with no change in either the PR interval or the configuration of the P and QRS is respiratory sinus arrhythmia. Inspiration increases heart rate, and expiration decreases it. The electrocardiogram demonstrates, therefore, a regular slowing and speeding of the heart rate with the time necessary to complete a slowing–speeding cycle consistent with the patient's respiratory rate. If the patient is available for physical examination at the time the electrocardiogram is being recorded, this explanation can be easily confirmed. Sinus arrhythmia is a normal finding even if marked. Slowing of the heart rate during expiration may be sufficient to result in the appearance of a beat that either does not have a P wave or has a P wave just in front of the QRS with a distinctly short PR interval. This pattern denotes junctional escape during the bradycardiac phase of the respiratory sinus arrhythmia.

Heart Rate

A close estimate of heart rate can be determined by dividing 300 by the number of large squares on the electrocardiographic

TABLE 3–1. ESTIMATING HEART RATE[a]

No. of Large Squares on ECG Paper Between Two P Waves or QRS Complexes	Heart Rate (bpm)
1	300
2	150
3	100
4	75
5	60
6	50

[a] Divide 300 by the number of large squares on ECG paper between two P waves or two QRS complexes.

TABLE 3–2. CALCULATING VENTRICULAR RATE[a]

No. of Small Squares on ECG Paper Between Two QRS Complexes	Heart Rate (bpm)
5	300
10	150
15	100
20	75
25	60
30	50

[a] Divide 1500 by the number of small squares on ECG paper between two QRS complexes.

paper between two P waves or between two QRS complexes (Table 3–1). This method is adequate for routine electrocardiographic interpretation. If more accurate calculation of the ventricular rate is needed (e.g., in a patient with an artificial pacemaker) divide 1500 by the number of small squares on the electrocardiographic paper between two QRS complexes (Table 3–2).

Intervals

PR Interval

The PR interval (Fig. 3–2) represents atrial depolarization plus the time required for the impulse to travel through the atrioventricular specialized conduction tissue (atrioventricular node, bundle of His, bundle branch). It is measured from the beginning of the P wave to the beginning of the QRS complex regardless of whether the QRS complex begins with a Q wave or an R wave. The length of the PR interval is inversely related to heart rate and is affected by patient age. A useful guideline for the upper limits of normal at various ages (assuming normal heart rate for that age) is as follows:

Newborn 0.11 second
Child 0.14 second
Adolescent 0.16 second

Prolongation of the PR interval is defined as first degree heart block. This term is useful, although it does imply the presence of a conduction disturbance that may not, in fact, be present. Although a prolonged PR interval may be due to delayed conduction through the atrioventricular specialized conduction tissue, it also may be due to right atrial enlargement, especially dilation. Furthermore, prolongation of the PR interval may be caused by an inflammatory process

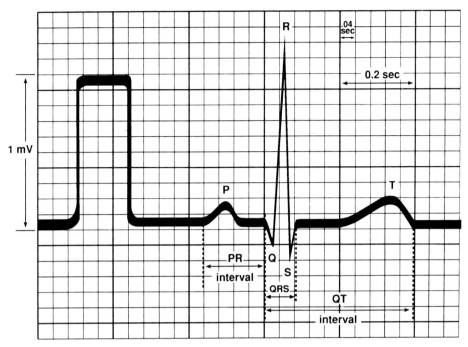

FIGURE 3–2. Waves and intervals in a P–QRS–T complex. Standard calibration is 1 mV = 10 mm; paper speed is 25 mm/second.

such as rheumatic fever, although this observation cannot be considered a criterion for diagnosis of carditis in rheumatic fever (see Chapter 10). Digitalis therapy prolongs the PR interval, as may the effects of open-heart surgery. Shortening of the PR interval with a normal P wave can be seen in preexcitation syndromes such as in Wolff-Parkinson-White syndrome (see Chapter 11) or glycogen storage disease (type II Pompe's disease). Shortening of the PR interval with an abnormally directed P wave suggests an ectopic supraventricular pacemaker.

QRS Interval

The QRS interval (Fig. 3–2) represents ventricular depolarization. It is measured from the beginning to the end of the QRS complex. The interval should be less than 0.10 second. Longer QRS duration suggests ventricular conduction delay. Right ventricular conduction delay causes slowing of the terminal portion of the QRS, with this portion directed toward the right ventricle so as to produce a large-voltage, wide R' in precordial leads V_3R and V_1. If the QRS has a similar configuration but the duration is 0.12 second or longer, one usually can label the problem right bundle branch block (RBBB). This pattern is seen frequently in post-cardiac surgery patients, especially after surgery involving the right ventricle. Left bundle branch block (LBBB) causes slowing of the middle portion of the QRS complex, resulting in a wide, moderately tall, 100 per cent R wave in precordial leads V_6 and V_7. True LBBB is rare in children. It may occur with left ventricular cardiomyopathy and after surgery in the left ventricular outflow tract; the LBBB pattern is simulated in patients with Wolff-Parkinson-White syndrome of the type in which there is early activation of the right ventricle; and it is produced by an artificial ventricular pacemaker implanted into the right ventricle.

QT Interval

The QT interval (Fig. 3–2), measured from the beginning of the QRS complex to the end of the T wave, is inversely proportional to the heart rate. Correction for heart rate should be done by dividing the measured QT interval by the square root of the preceding RR interval. This corrected measurement is referred to as the QT_c interval. Standard tables should be consulted for maximal and minimal QT_c interval durations in infants and children. Beyond the first month of life, however, the QT_c duration normally is not longer than 0.45 second.

Prolongation of the QT_c interval may be seen with some forms of active carditis, with hypocalcemia, or after quinidine administration. Prolongation of the QT_c interval also may be observed in some syndromes associated with sudden death, such as Romano-Ward and Lange and Jerveil-Nielson, discussed briefly in Chapter 17. In these patients the QT_c interval is markedly prolonged, and one is not faced with concerns over a few hundredths of a second. Shortening of the QT_c interval occurs following digitalis administration and in the presence of hypercalcemia.

QRS Axis

Electrical forces represented by the QRS have a mean magnitude and direction that can be drawn as a vector. When constructed from the six limb leads, this vector represents the mean QRS axis as seen in the frontal plane. Exact calculation of the mean QRS axis is a rather time-consuming task that is of little added value, as plotting the frontal

QRS axis by quadrant is more than adequate for clinical purposes. For this simple and practical approach, the R/S ratio in leads I and aVF is used (Fig. 3–3). Lead I records the electrical potential between the right arm and left arm with the left arm being designated the positive pole. In normal patients, therefore, a positive QRS complex in lead I (dominant R or R' wave) indicates that the axis is directed left of the vertical line. If the QRS complex is primarily negative in lead I (dominant S wave), on the other hand, the axis is oriented to the right of the vertical line. The R/S ratio in lead aVF designates whether the mean QRS axis is directed superiorly or inferiorly. This augmented, unipolar limb lead views the heart's electrical activity from the left leg, with impulse direction toward the leg considered positive. A positive QRS complex in aVF (dominant R wave) therefore designates the mean QRS axis as being inferior to the horizontal line, whereas a negative QRS complex (dominant S wave) in lead aVF indicates that the axis is directed superiorly to the horizontal line.

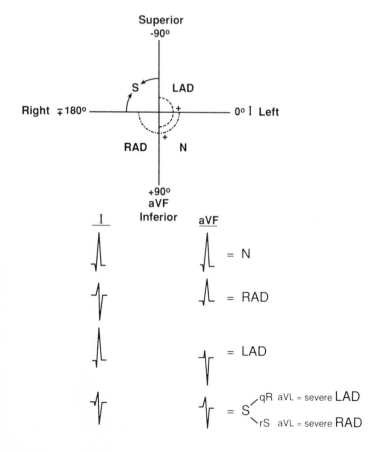

FIGURE 3–3. Plotting of the mean QRS axis by quadrant using the R/S ratio in leads I and aVF.

The frontal plane QRS axis normally is directed between 0 degrees and +90 degrees; that is, toward the left lower quadrant (Fig. 3–3). The electrocardiogram demonstrates predominantly positive QRS complexes in leads I and aVF (N). The term right axis deviation is applied when the QRS axis is directed between +90 degrees and +180 degrees (or more). The electrocardiogram demonstrates QRS complexes that are predominantly negative in lead I and positive in aVF. The mean QRS axis falls in the right lower quadrant, or right axis deviation (RAD). Right axis deviation may be seen in patients with cardiac lesions characterized by right ventricular hypertrophy as in tetralogy of Fallot, transposition of the great arteries, pulmonic stenosis, atrial septal defect, or lung disease (i.e., cor pulmonale). Keep in mind that RAD is a normal finding in the newborn and young infant because ventricular wall thicknesses are equal at birth. Occasionally a normal child or young adult has mild RAD.

Left axis deviation (LAD) indicates that the QRS axis is directed between 0 degrees and −90 degrees. QRS complexes are positive in lead I but negative in aVF, and the mean QRS axis is plotted in the left upper quadrant. This axis is seen typically in patients with either an endocardial cushion defect or tricuspid valve atresia. It is also characteristic of the conduction abnormality called left anterior hemiblock, which can occur after intracardiac surgery. In fact, explanation for this pattern in patients with an endocardial cushion defect probably is congenital absence or hypoplasia of the left anterior division of the left bundle branch, the congenital equivalent of acquired left anterior hemiblock. When the QRS complexes are negative in both leads I and aVF, the axis is directed toward the right upper quadrant (S) (i.e., between −90 degrees and ±180 degrees). An axis in this quadrant could be due either to severe right or severe left axis deviation. Distinguishing between these two possibilities usually is possible by looking at the QRS configuration in lead aVL. If the QRS complexes in aVL show an rS pattern, there is severe right axis deviation (> +180 degrees). This extreme right axis might be seen in newborns with severe right ventricular hypertrophy as, for example, in hypoplastic left heart syndrome. If the QRS complexes in aVL show a qR pattern, there is severe left axis deviation (> −90 degrees), as seen in patients with an endocardial cush-

ion defect, such as a complete atrioventricular canal with dominant right ventricular hypertrophy.

The terms severe LAD and RAD are used advisedly. The frontal axis must be either left or right and cannot truly be either more left than left or more right than right. What is meant by left or severe right axis deviation really is left and superior or right and superior axis deviations.

Certain dysmorphic syndromes (e.g., Noonan syndrome, postrubella embryopathy) may cause the QRS axis to be located in the right or left superior quadrants in the absence of a significant underlying anatomic abnormality of the heart. As always, clinical information should be available for the most effective interpretation of the electrocardiogram. It is important to obtain an electrocardiogram and to plot the QRS axis in a newborn with Down syndrome. If there is a distinctly superior QRS axis, one should be suspicious that the baby has an endocardial cushion defect.

Atrial Enlargement (P Waves)

The next step when reading an electrocardiogram is evaluation of specific chamber enlargement. Atrial depolarization starts at the superior vena cava–right atrial junction and spreads toward the inferior aspect of the right atrium and toward the left atrium. The P wave is the result of this electrical activity. The normal P wave is formed by summation of right and left atrial depolarization. Changes in P wave morphology can reflect atrial enlargement or dilatation (Fig. 3–4). Tall (> 2.5 mm) and peaked P waves indicate right atrial enlargement. This pattern is best seen in lead II and precordial level V$_2$. The definition of "peaked" is arbitrary. We have always taught that if the P looks as if you would not want to sit on it, it is peaked.

Prolonged, flat, or notched P waves, particularly in leads I, aVF, and V$_6$, reflect left atrial enlargement. One may also see a positive/negative P wave in precordial lead V$_1$. If the negative phase is a box wide (0.04 sec-

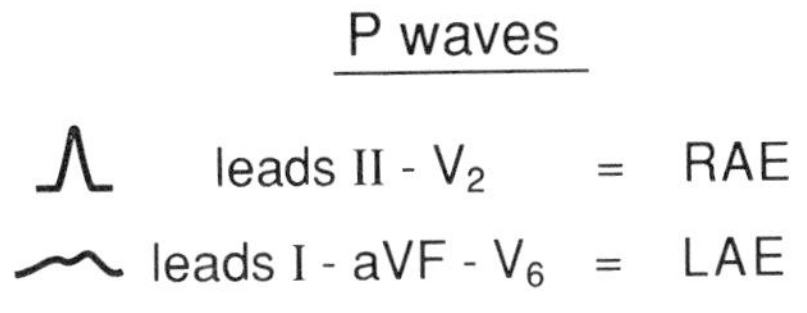

P waves

leads II - V$_2$ = RAE
leads I - aVF - V$_6$ = LAE

FIGURE 3–4. P wave configuration in atrial enlargement.

ond) and a box deep (1 mm), left atrial enlargement is present.

Septal Forces (Q Waves)

One of the most important differences between interpretation of pediatric and adult electrocardiograms is analysis of ventricular septal forces. These septal forces have particular significance in the pediatric age group. Once the electrical impulse travels through the atrioventricular specialized tissue and reaches the ventricles, the first area to be depolarized is the ventricular septum. Septal depolarization forms an electrical vector that originates on the left ventricular side of the septum and then is directed to the right and anteriorly toward the right ventricular surface of the septum. This vector, traveling away from the left ventricle, results in the inscription of a small negative deflection (q wave) in left precordial leads V_6 and V_7. A normal q wave in either one of these leads indicates the presence of the ventricular septum (and thus the presence of two functioning ventricles) and suggests normal ventricular position. This information is important particularly when interpreting the tracings from newborns. Unless there is a q wave in V_6 and V_7, one cannot accurately determine if there is a left ventricle or if the R waves in those leads actually represent left ventricular forces.

The presence of q waves in right precordial leads V_3R and V_1, on the other hand, suggests reversal of inscription of the septal forces. This finding is abnormal and represents either right ventricular hypertrophy or ventricular inversion.

Ventricular Hypertrophy (QRS Complexes)

Inscription of the septal forces is followed immediately by rapid depolarization of the ventricular free walls. The resultant electrical vectors from both ventricles travel in more or less opposite directions. Right ventricular vectors are directed right and anteriorly, whereas the normally stronger left ventricular vectors are directed left and posteriorly. These simultaneously competing electrical forces inscribe the remainder of the QRS complex, i.e., the major QRS forces. Precordial leads V_3R and V_1 are closest to the right ventricle and are the leads most likely to illustrate right ventricular en-

largement. Leads V_6 and V_7 are analogous for the left ventricle.

All of the precordial leads are "looking at" the same electrical force. How this force appears in any one lead depends on where that lead is placed. In a normal child, because the left ventricle is dominant, most of the QRS forces are directed away from the right precordial leads, resulting in a small r and dominant S pattern in V_3R and V_1, and toward the left ventricle, resulting in dominant R waves in V_6 and V_7. (The relative size of the R and S waves is indicated in the text by the use of lower case letters for the smaller wave and capital letters for the larger waves, e.g., rS or qRs.) The precordial leads normally show a more or less gradual progression from dominant S waves in V_3R and V_1 to dominant R waves in V_6 and V_7.

Changes in the normal relation between the ventricular forces are reflected in the precordial leads. It is important to evaluate configuration, extent, and direction of the QRS forces in all precordial leads before drawing conclusions. Voltage criteria alone may be misleading, as the size of precordial QRS complexes can be affected not only by the magnitude of the electrical forces but also by other factors such as the presence of pericardial effusion, chest wall thickness, electrode–skin contact, and equipment sensitivity.

Ventricular Hypertrophy

Right Ventricular Hypertrophy

See Figures 3–8 to 3–10, 3–14 to 3–16, 3–18, and 3–20 to 3–22, later in the chapter.

Precordial leads V_3R and V_1 "look" directly at the right ventricle and illustrate best the presence of right ventricular hypertrophy and dilation. It is, of course, necessary to know what is normal before one can identify abnormal. This point is true particularly in regard to the right ventricle because of the normal evolution of both the absolute and relative mass of the right ventricle that takes place over the first months of life. Prior to birth the ventricles are in parallel, both emptying into the aorta, the left ventricle directly and the right ventricle via the ductus arteriosus. Systolic pressure in the two ventricles therefore is identical and their wall thicknesses are approximately the same. At birth the right ventricle is dominant electrically because it is anterior to the left ventricle and therefore closer to the electrode

TABLE 3–3. NEWBORN ELECTROCARDIOGRAMS

Measurement	Normal	Abnormal
PR interval (second)	< 0.11	> 0.11
QRS axis (frontal) (degrees)	+45 to +180	0 to −90 (LAD) −90 to −180 (S)
V_3R and V_1	Rs R wave < 15 mm	qR 100% R rS R wave > 20 mm[a]
	Negative T waves > 3 days of age	Positive T waves > 3 days of age
V_6 and V_7	qrS	Rs

[a] R wave 15 to 20 mm can be normal but should heighten suspicion of abnormality.

placed on the chest wall. As a result, right precordial leads V_3R and V_1 demonstrate a dominant R wave, and left precordial leads V_6 and V_7 demonstrate a dominant S wave. Right ventricular hypertrophy is overdiagnosed in the newborn unless specific criteria are followed during interpretation of the tracing (Table 3–3).

In the normal newborn there is an Rs pattern in V_3R and V_1. The s wave is due to the presence of right and posterior terminal QRS forces that, in fact, are generated by depolarization of the right ventricular outflow tract. Both R and S waves are usually low voltage (< 10 mm). Right ventricular hypertrophy can be diagnosed when there is a "pure" (near 100 per cent) R or rR′ in V_3R and V_1. Right ventricular hypertrophy is also indicated when the R (or R′) is greater than 20 mm. A qR pattern in V_3R and V_1 is an indication of right ventricular hypertrophy. An rS pattern then should be present in V_6 and V_7 with no hint of a q wave (septal forces). On the other hand, when q waves apparently are present in V_3R and V_1 and in V_6 and V_7, septal forces are probably normal and the apparent qR pattern in $V_3 R$ and V_1 is likely an rsR′ with the initial r isoelectric and therefore not actually recorded, or so small in magnitude that it is not visible.

In the normal newborn the T wave is positive in V_3R and V_1. By the third day of life these T waves become biphasic and then fully negative by 7 days of age. Right ventricular hypertrophy is indicated when the T wave remains positive in V_3R and V_1 beyond 1 week of age, provided the T wave also is positive in V_6 and V_7.

Right ventricular hypertrophy also should be suspected if there is either right axis de-

viation greater than +180 degrees or severe right atrial enlargement. However, the latter is not valid if the patient has a primary tricuspid valve abnormality. It is useful to consider that there are some characteristic right ventricular hypertrophy patterns that can be associated with specific cardiac lesions. These patterns generally represent either ventricular volume or pressure overload (Fig. 3–5). Right ventricular hypertrophy of the volume overload type in a child is characterized by an rsR′ pattern in V_3R and V_1. The R′ is larger than the beginning r but usually is less than 15 mm. The R′ often is wide, simulating right ventricular conduction delay. This volume overload pattern is commonly present in patients with an atrial

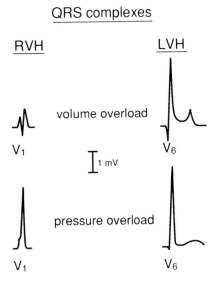

FIGURE 3–5. Ventricular hypertrophy patterns (volume and pressure overload) in precordial QRS complexes.

septal defect, a lesion that causes right ventricular dilation without an increase in right ventricular pressure and without substantial increase in right ventricular wall thickness. Typical right ventricular hypertrophy of the pressure overload type in a child is characterized by a tall R or R′ in V_3R and V_1. Generally, the taller the R wave, the greater is the hypertrophy. This pressure overload pattern usually is seen in patients with elevated right ventricular peak systolic pressure, as occurs in pulmonic valve stenosis. Severe pressure overload right ventricular hypertrophy may be represented by a qR pattern in V_3R and V_1. Hypoplasia of the left ventricle also results in a pattern of right ventricular hypertrophy.

Left Ventricular Hypertrophy

See Figures 3–11, 3–17, and 3–23 to 3–26, later in the chapter.

Left ventricular hypertrophy or dilation causes augmentation of the normally dominant left and posterior QRS forces. These changes are reflected in the electrocardiogram by the presence of deeper S waves in the right precordial leads (V_3R and V_1) and taller R waves in the left precordial leads (V_6 and V_7). Hypoplasia of the right ventricle also creates this pattern. With severe left ventricular hypertrophy the increased QRS forces may be directed even farther posteriorly. In those instances, the QRS complexes in V_6 and V_7 might not best reflect the severity of the hypertrophy, as the R waves may be only mildly increased. The diagnostic clue is the presence of deeper than normal S waves in V_1 or V_2 and a left shift of the transitional lead with an rS rather than an equiphasic RS pattern in V_4.

As with right ventricular hypertrophy, one can consider patterns of left ventricular hypertrophy to be associated with volume or pressure overload (Fig. 3–5). However, these patterns are less reliable in the presence of left ventricular hypertrophy. With left ventricular hypertrophy of the volume overload type, there usually are deep q waves (>3 mm) and tall R waves in V_6 and V_7. There may be mild ST segment elevation in V_6 and V_7 with a curved ST segment whose convexity is directed downward ("coving"). Tall, peaked T waves also suggest volume overload. These QRS and ST-T changes can be seen in a child with a large patent ductus arteriosus, a typical left ventricular volume overload lesion. Similar patterns can be seen with other left heart volume overload lesions. A distinct exception, however, is seen in patients with rheumatic heart disease manifested by mitral regurgitation, aortic regurgitation, or both, hemodynamic abnormalities that cause left ventricular dilation. In such patients, the q waves in V_6 and V_7 are small, the R wave is generally tall, and the T waves are of low voltage, a total pattern simulating left ventricular pressure overload. We believe that the difference derives from the fact that patients with rheumatic heart disease have significant myocardial involvement in addition to chamber dilation.

With left ventricular hypertrophy of the pressure overload type, the QRS pattern is characterized by small q waves and tall R waves in V_6 and V_7. The T waves are usually of lower amplitude than expected for the height of the R waves. These electrocardiographic findings are present, for example, in patients with aortic valve stenosis, a left ventricular pressure overload lesion. Two variations to this left ventricular pressure overload pattern should be noted. The first is in patients with hypertrophic cardiomyopathy. This condition, in which left ventricular outflow tract obstruction can occur, is uncommon in children. It is characterized by marked thickening of the ventricular septum. As a result, the electrocardiogram often reflects this anatomy by showing deep q waves (septal forces) in V_6 and V_7. These q waves are usually wider than those in patients with volume overload. The second variation is in children with coarctation of the aorta. In these patients, who have left ventricular pressure overload as a result of hypertension, the electrocardiogram often demonstrates an rSr′ in V_3R and V_1. Explanation for the r′ in this situation, indicating that terminal QRS forces are directed to the right, is unknown.

Biventricular Hypertrophy

See Figures 3–12, 3–18, and 3–27, later in the chapter.

There are few absolute criteria to diagnose biventricular hypertrophy, but it can be suspected in relative terms. For example, if an electrocardiogram shows definite criteria for right ventricular hypertrophy, one would expect to see dominant S waves or small R waves (or both) in V_6 and V_7. If, however, there are relatively tall or dominant R waves in V_6 and V_7, it may be considered evidence of additional left ventricular hypertrophy. Similarly, if there are definite criteria for left ventricular hypertrophy, larger than expected R waves in V_3R and V_1 suggest the presence of additional right ventricular hypertrophy. Biventricular hypertrophy can also be suspected when the midprecordial QRS complexes (V_2 and V_4) are of large amplitude (> 50 mm) with approximately equal-amplitude R and S waves. Voltage alone is a weak diagnostic criterion, as a normal patient with a thin chest wall also might have large midprecordial QRS complexes.

Ventricular Repolarization (ST Segment and T Waves)

Detailed analysis of the ST segment and the T wave can be of importance in the diagnosis of ventricular hypertrophy. Normal infants and children should have negative T waves in V_3R and V_1. At about 8 to 10 years of age these T waves become positive and remain so into adulthood. Positive T waves in V_3R and V_1 between the ages of 1 week and 8 to 10 years are indicative of right ventricular hypertrophy, provided the T wave is also positive in leads V_6 and V_7. If the patient has severe left ventricular hypertrophy, creating negative T waves in V_6 and V_7, the T wave may be "pushed" toward the right side, creating a positive T wave in leads V_3R and V_1. In this situation, it does not indicate right ventricular hypertrophy.

The T wave configuration in leads V_3R and V_1 also can be of help for evaluating the severity of right ventricular hypertrophy, particularly of the pressure overload type. In the presence of mild to moderate elevation of right ventricular pressure, these T waves are usually positive. In patients with peak right ventricular systolic pressure at the systemic level (equal to that in the left ventri-

cle), T waves in leads V_3R and V_1 become biphasic and of low amplitude. When right ventricular pressure is suprasystemic, there may be a depressed ST segment and negative T waves in leads V_3R and V_1. This pattern is referred to as right ventricular "strain," an ill-defined but reasonably meaningful term.

In patients with left ventricular hypertrophy, particularly those with pressure overload, it also is important to evaluate the ST-T configuration. A flat ST segment in V_6 and V_7, resulting in a sharper ST-T angle or a low-voltage, flatter negative T wave (or both) are signs of what can be called left ventricular "strain," which implies ventricular dysfunction; it probably represents a form of myocardial ischemia, relative or absolute.

CHARACTERISTIC ELECTROCARDIOGRAMS

A series of normal and abnormal electrocardiograms from newborns, infants, and children are depicted in this section. Rather than show the entire tracing, we focus on those leads that are most helpful in their interpretation. Frontal leads I and aVF are used to plot the mean QRS axis within a specific quadrant. Precordial leads V_3R and V_1 reflect primarily the right ventricular forces, and V_6 and V_7 reflect the left ventricular forces. The midprecordial lead V_4 shows the transitional forces between the right and left ventricles.

Figures 3–6 through 3–12 illustrate patterns in the newborn. Figures 3–13 through 3–18 are tracings from infants. Figures 3–19 through 3–28 were taken from electrocardiograms of children. The first tracing in each age group is normal.

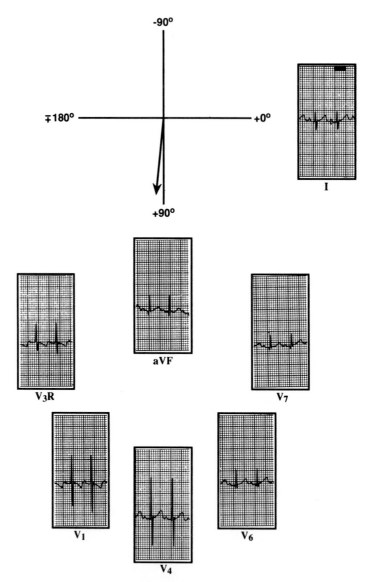

FIGURE 3–6. Newborn with a normal heart. The ECG shows an R/S pattern in V_3R and V_1 with negative T waves. Note the presence of a q wave (septal forces) in V_6 and V_7 indicating the presence of two functioning ventricles.

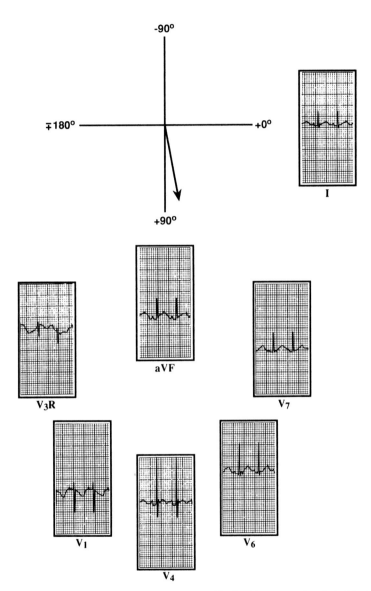

FIGURE 3–7. Premature newborn with a normal heart. The ECG in a premature infant typically shows a left ventricular dominant pattern with S waves in V_3R and V_1 and a qR pattern in V_6 and V_7. Right ventricular dominance on the newborn ECG develops late during gestation. There are nonspecific ST-T changes that are often seen in newborn tracings.

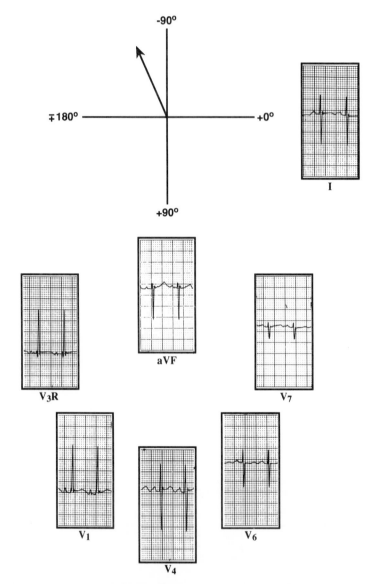

FIGURE 3—8. One-day-old neonate with Down syndrome. There is a superior QRS axis (negative QRS complexes in leads I and aVF). QRS complexes in V_3R and V_1 are almost totally positive, with tall R′ waves indicative of right ventricular hypertrophy. No q waves are seen in V_6 and V_7 but an rsR′ pattern in V_3R would indicate the presence of normally oriented septal forces.

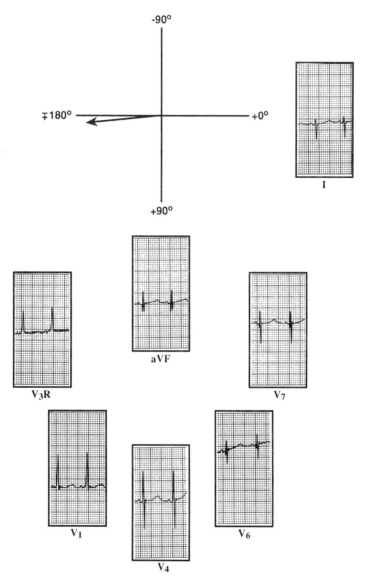

FIGURE 3–9. Five-day-old infant with tetralogy of Fallot. Dominant, 100% R waves in V₃R and V₁ with positive T waves at this age indicate right ventricular hypertrophy. The septal forces are normal, manifested by the presence of q waves in V₆ and V₇.

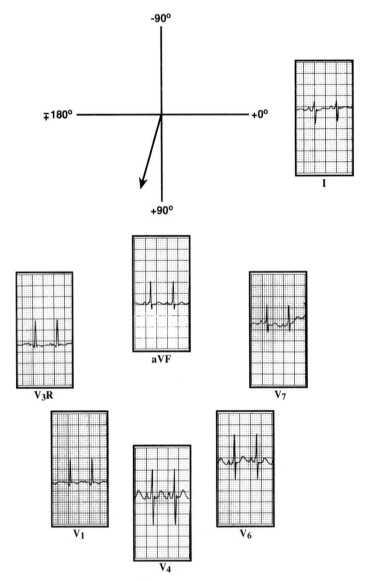

FIGURE 3–10. One-day-old baby with mitral valve atresia, transposition of the great arteries, and double-outlet right ventricle. The ECG shows severe right ventricular hypertrophy (qR pattern in V_3R and V_1).

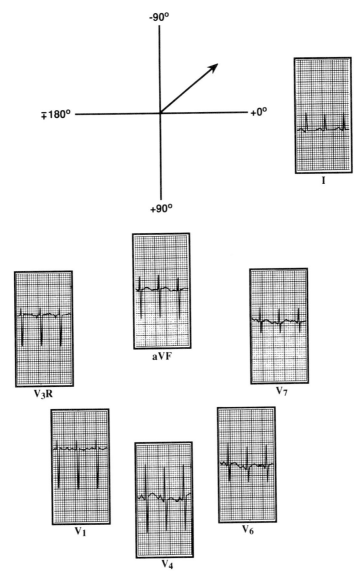

FIGURE 3—11. Two-day-old baby with tricuspid valve atresia. The ECG shows left superior axis deviation (positive QRS complexes in lead I but negative in aVF). Right ventricular forces are absent, reflecting the presence of a hypoplastic right ventricle (small r waves in V_3R and V_1). This pattern suggests left ventricular hypertrophy.

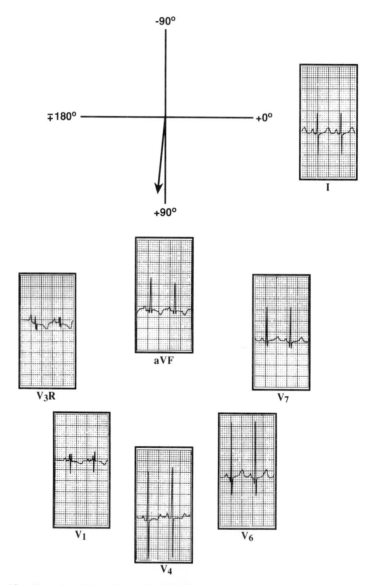

FIGURE 3–12. Nine-day-old newborn of a diabetic mother. The tracing shows left ventricular hypertrophy (dominant, tall R waves in V_6 and V_7), and suggests additional right ventricular hypertrophy (large voltage R/S in V_4 and rsr′ in V_3 and V_1).

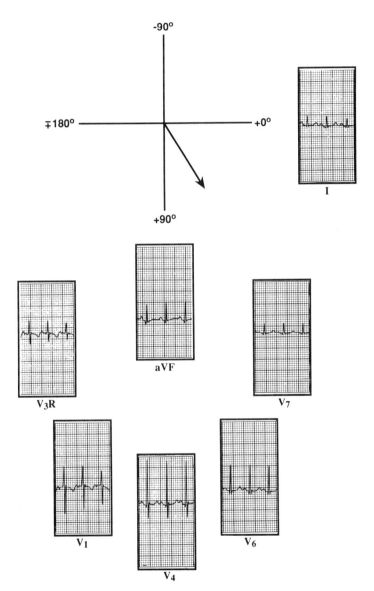

FIGURE 3–13. Three-month-old infant with a normal ECG.

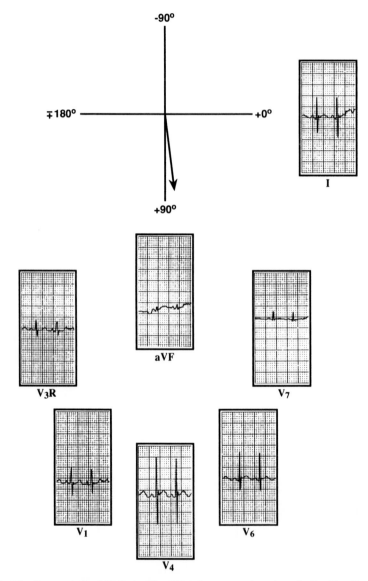

FIGURE 3–14. Four-month-old infant with mild pulmonary valve stenosis. Positive T waves in V_3R and V_1 are indicative of mild right ventricular hypertrophy.

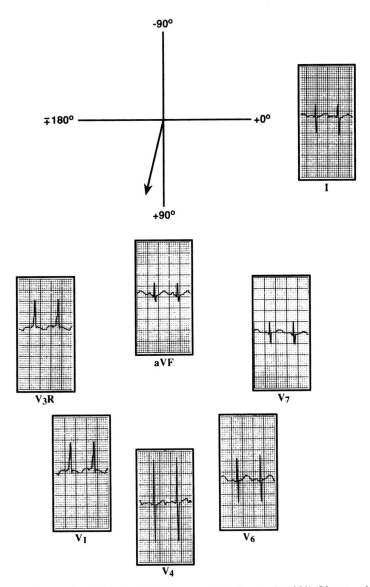

FIGURE 3–15. Six-month-old infant with tetralogy of Fallot. The nearly 100% rR′ pattern in leads V₃R and V₁ indicates right ventricular hypertrophy, pressure overload.

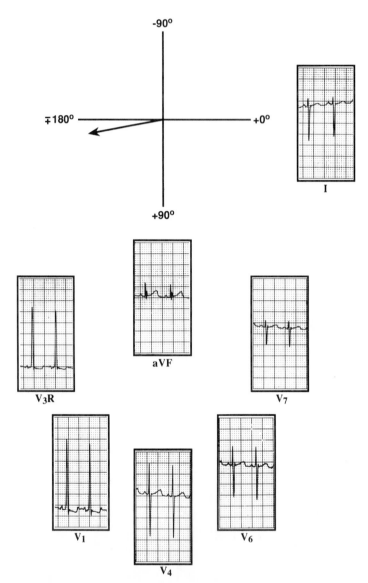

FIGURE 3–16. Six-month-old infant with severe pulmonary valve stenosis. The tracing shows right axis deviation and right ventricular hypertrophy, pressure overload (> 25 mm R waves in V_3R and V_1 with low voltage, biphasic T waves). ST and T wave abnormalities in V_3R and V_1 indicate right ventricular "strain."

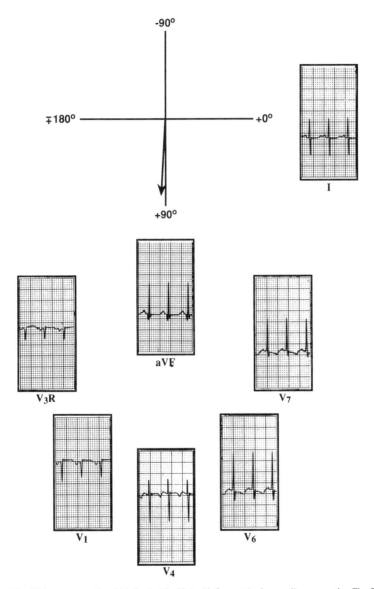

FIGURE 3–17. Thirteen-month-old infant with dilated left ventricular cardiomyopathy. The ECG shows significant left ventricular hypertrophy. Note the posterior shift of the QRS forces with large negative complexes not only in V_3R and V_1 but also in the midprecordial lead V_4. The negative T waves in V_6 and V_7 indicate an abnormality in left ventricular repolarization commonly referred to as "strain." (The resultant slightly positive T in V_3R and V_1 does not indicate additional right ventricular hypertrophy.)

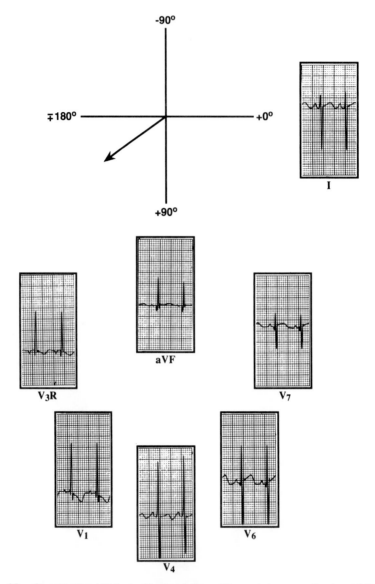

FIGURE 3–18. One-month-old infant with coarctation of the aorta in congestive heart failure. Dominant, tall R waves in V_3R and V_1 and deep S waves in V_6 and V_7 indicate right ventricular hypertrophy. In the presence of definite criteria for right ventricular hypertrophy, the R waves in V_6 suggest additional left ventricular hypertrophy. There are also some nonspecific ST-T changes in the tracing. Note that what seems to be a qR in V_3R is revealed in V_1 to be an rsR′. Normal q in V_6 and V_7 also confirms the presence of normal septal forces.

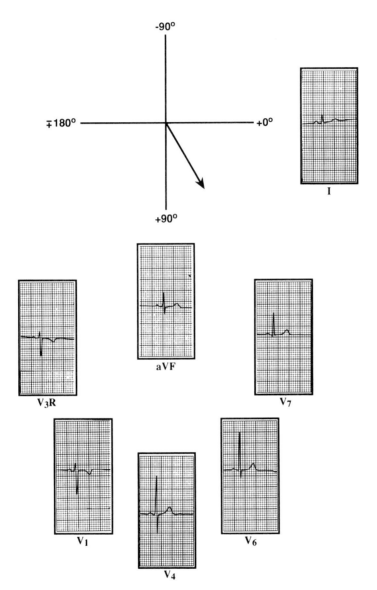

FIGURE 3–19. Ten-year-old girl with a functional murmur. The ECG is normal.

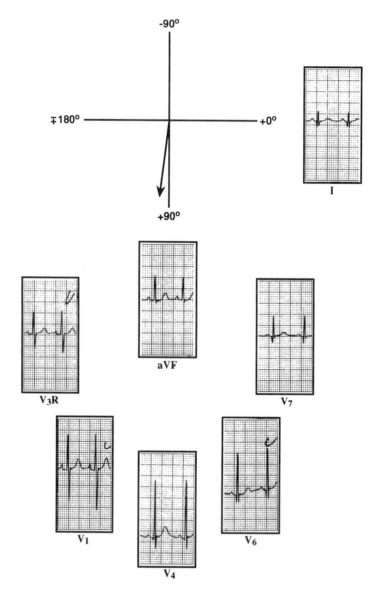

FIGURE 3—20. Five-year-old girl with mild pulmonary valve stenosis. The R/S ratio and positive T wave in V_3R and V_1 are signs of mild right ventricular hypertrophy.

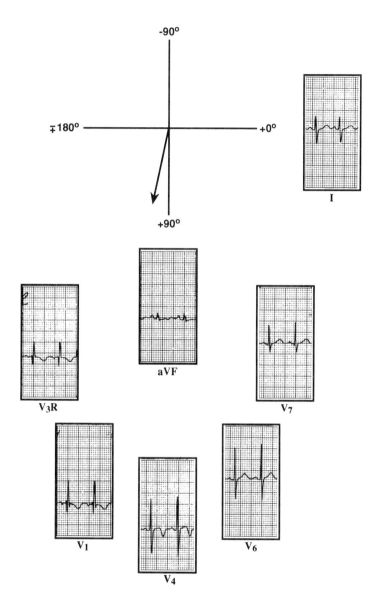

FIGURE 3–21. Three-year-old girl with an ostium secundum atrial septal defect. The ECG demonstrates mild right axis deviation and right ventricular hypertrophy, volume overload (rsR′ in V_3R and V_1).

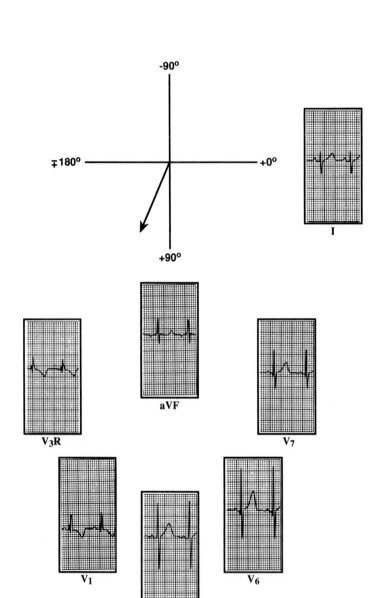

FIGURE 3–22. Four-year-old boy with a sinus venosus atrial septal defect. The tracing shows right axis deviation and right ventricular hypertrophy, volume overload (rsR′ in V$_3$R and V$_1$ and an R′ of less than 15 mm). Of interest is the presence of an ectopic atrial pacemaker with superior axis deviation of the P axis.

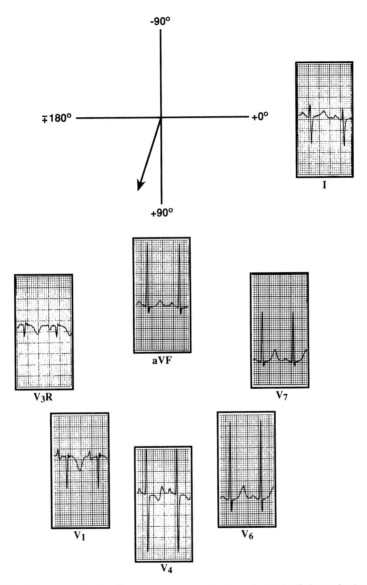

FIGURE 3–23. Five-year-old girl with pulmonary valve atresia and a markedly hypoplastic right ventricle. The ECG shows right axis deviation and biatrial enlargement (tall, peaked P waves in V_1 and V_4 and broad, notched P waves in leads I and V_6 and V_7). Right atrial enlargement is greater than left atrial enlargement. There is left ventricular hypertrophy (tall R waves in V_6) and absence of right ventricular forces (very small r waves in V_1).

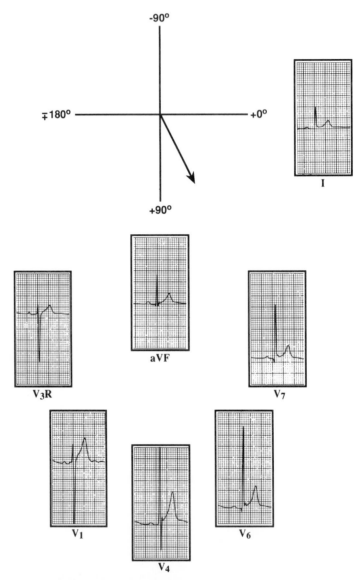

FIGURE 3–24. Six-year-old girl with a patent ductus arteriosus. The tracing shows left ventricular hypertrophy of the volume overload type. (Note the tall R and T waves in V_6 with "coving" of the ST segment.)

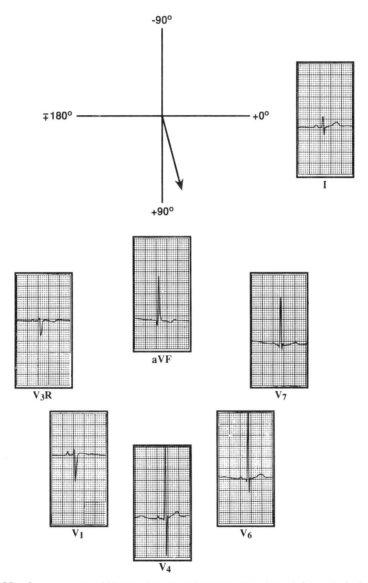

FIGURE 3–25. Fourteen-year-old boy with aortic valve stenosis. It shows left ventricular hypertrophy of the pressure overload type (small q waves, tall R waves, and low-voltage T waves in V_6 and V_7).

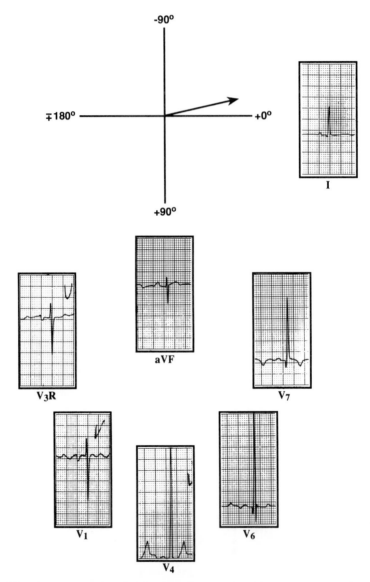

FIGURE 3–26. Thirteen-year-old girl with severe aortic stenosis. The tracing shows left axis deviation and left atrial enlargement (broad, notched P waves in V_6 and broad, negative P waves in V_3R and V_1). There is severe left ventricular hypertrophy with "strain" (tall R waves in V_6 and V_7 with negative T waves in V_7).

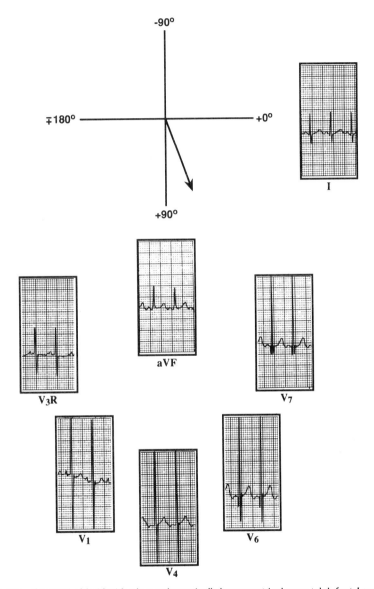

FIGURE 3–27. Six-year-old girl with a hemodynamically large ventricular septal defect. Large biphasic QRS complexes in midprecordial lead V_4 suggest biventricular hypertrophy. Deep q waves and tall R waves in V_6 indicate left ventricular volume overload. Tall R and positive T in V_1 indicates right ventricular hypertrophy.

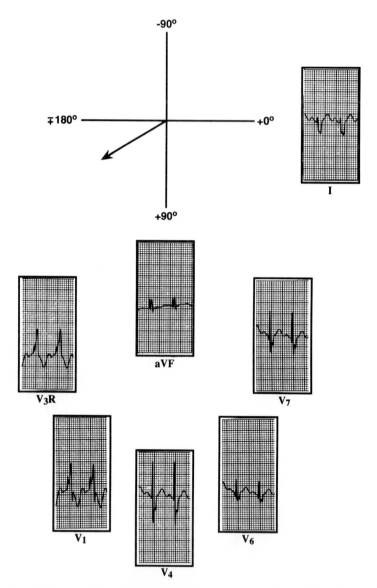

FIGURE 3–28. Eight-year-old boy who is status after repair of tetralogy of Fallot. The tracing shows sinus rhythm. Slow inscription of the terminal QRS forces resulting in QRS complexes of 0.12 second duration and prolonged R′ in V_3R and V_1 indicate right bundle branch block. This pattern is seen often after right ventriculotomy.

4

ECHOCARDIOGRAPHY

Fredrick Z. Bierman

Diagnosis and management of cardiovascular anomalies in the pediatric population requires integration of clinical and laboratory data. Historically, cardiac evaluation of the neonate, infant, child, or adolescent by the primary physician included the medical history, physical examination, electrocardiogram, and chest roentgenogram. The pediatric cardiologist was responsible for definitive diagnosis of the cardiovascular anomaly based on additional noninvasive or cardiac catheterization data.

During the 1980s cardiac ultrasonography evolved into a readily accessible laboratory procedure, allowing detailed evaluation of cardiovascular anatomy and function. In many tertiary care pediatric centers diagnostic information from echocardiography currently guides surgical intervention of many cardiovascular anomalies without additional invasive studies. General availability of cardiac ultrasonography warrants a practical understanding by the practitioner of the technology, the scope of its clinical applications, and its limitations. Initial evaluation by the primary care physician of an asymptomatic or stable symptomatic patient with suspected heart disease should not include echocardiography. Need for this study, and its performance, should be determined by the specialist. In some situations, such as a newborn with respiratory distress, primary evaluation may include echocardiography, provided appropriate support is available for recording and interpreting pediatric echocardiograms. Obtaining an echocardiogram should not delay referral to a tertiary center of a sick infant with probable heart disease determined by other clinical measurements.

FUNDAMENTALS OF CARDIAC ULTRASONOGRAPHY

Cardiac ultrasonography is an imaging technique using high-frequency sound waves or ultrasound—2.0 to 7.5 megahertz, or million cycles per second (MHz)—to display cardiac anatomy, function, and blood flow. Under this technical umbrella are included M-mode, two-dimensional, and Doppler echocardiography. Although an ultrasound signal is the basis for all these imaging methods, they differ in how the signal is transmitted, processed, and displayed.[1,2]

Production of an ultrasound signal is based on the mechanical or electrical response of ceramic crystal (i.e., piezoelectric property). When an electrical charge is applied, certain crystals oscillate producing an ultrasound signal with a predictable frequency. Acoustic lenses focus the signal at a target of interest, such as the heart. The reciprocal piezoelectric response of these crystals to mechanical compression is production of an electrical potential. A single crystal therefore functions as an acoustic transmitter when electrically stimulated and as a receiver when caused to oscillate by returning reflected sound waves.

Echocardiographic imaging is dependent on (1) the unique acoustic properties of fluid and soft tissue and (2) the propagation and reflection of an ultrasound signal at acoustic boundaries between contiguous tissues. Acoustic borders function as semipermeable mirrors that reflect a fraction of the ultrasound signal back to the piezoelectric crystal housed in the cardiac probe. The signal not reflected at the first acoustic border continues in a linear manner to the next acoustic boundary. Cardiac ultrasonography therefore involves reflection of some ultrasound signal at each tissue border with linear propagation of the nonreflected signal to deeper structures. Imaging depth is limited by the process of attenuation (i.e., absorption of the ultrasound signal as thermal energy by tissue and blood). Extensive use of cardiac ultrasonography in pediatric patients compared to adults is in part a consequence of the more favorable balance between subject size and signal attenuation. This balance allows imaging not only of intracardiac structures but also extracardiac structures typically not visualized in larger adult subjects.

Distinctive acoustic properties of connective tissue, muscle, fat, and blood permit echocardiographic display of internal as well as external organ architecture. Extreme differences in acoustic properties (e.g., muscle versus bone or biologic versus prosthetic material) compromises ultrasound imaging. Bone, cartilage, metals, or synthetic grafts reflect most of the ultrasound signal, creating an acoustic shadow that obscures adjacent soft tissue and deeper structures. Air in the lung or pleural or pericardial spaces, or air dissecting through a tissue plane, is the most common obstacle to cardiovascular ultrasonography. Air scatters the ultrasound signal, preventing its orderly propagation and reflection. The smaller residual lung volume in young subjects offers a large acoustic window for imaging cardiovascular structures from the surfaces of the chest, neck, and abdomen. It permits use of cardiac probes containing crystals that produce higher-frequency ultrasound signals (5.0 and 7.5 MHz) resulting in better resolution of cardiovascular anatomy. This technical advantage accounts for the more aggressive preoperative application of cardiac ultrasonography to the surgical management of congenital and acquired heart disease in the pediatric population.

M-MODE ECHOCARDIOGRAPHY

The time interval from transmission to return of an ultrasound signal is the practical basis of anatomic cardiac ultrasound imaging. M-mode echocardiography, using a signal generated by a single ceramic crystal, is the simplest application of this technology. This form of cardiac ultrasonography plots the changing distance of cardiac structures from the chest wall during the cardiac cycle. Figure 4–1 illustrates the M-mode presentations of the right ventricular outflow tract, aortic valve, left atrium, and mitral valve apparatus. The images are abstract displays of cardiac anatomy. The aortic valve is represented by the box-like tracing corresponding to systolic separation of the leaflets. Mitral valve motion has a biphasic configuration that corresponds to early passive and late atrial movements of the anterior and posterior leaflets during rapid ventricular filling and atrial contraction phases of ventricular diastole. Systolic closure of the mitral leaflets is identified by the diagonal line connecting one diastole with the next. Coving, or hammocking, of the systolic closure line is found with prolapse of the mitral valve apparatus. Although the latter is encountered with the mitral valve prolapse syndrome[3–5] and certain connective tissue disorders,[6–9] it may also be encountered as an isolated normal variant with no auscultatory or clinical evidence of mitral valve pathology.[10–12]

M-mode echocardiography is a limited imaging modality. When integrated with other cardiac ultrasound applications, however, it can offer a useful noninvasive index of left ventricular size and function.[13] When using M-mode echocardiography for serial follow-up of left ventricular size and function, one must recognize the pitfalls of the data (Fig. 4–2). The tracings in Figure 4–2 were obtained during a single examination of a patient at the same level of the left ventricle. Both recordings display the variation in left ventricular "diameter" corresponding to end-systole and end-diastole. Although recorded at the same long axis position of the ventricle (i.e., distance from the aortic valve and apex), the tracings differ in the position of the echo beam relative to the papillary muscles. The tracing in Figure 4–2B was recorded with the ultrasound signal equidistant to both left ventricular papillary muscles. In Figure 4–2C, the echo beam was closer to one papillary muscle. The resultant M-mode tracings differ in size and fractional shortening. This artifact due to beam orientation might obscure interval changes in ventricular size and function in patients receiving cardiotoxic chemotherapy. This problem is often encountered after sternotomy and pericardiotomy, after placement of an exteriorized central catheter, or as a result of right ventricular dilatation.

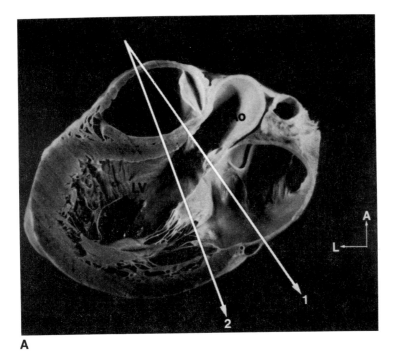

A

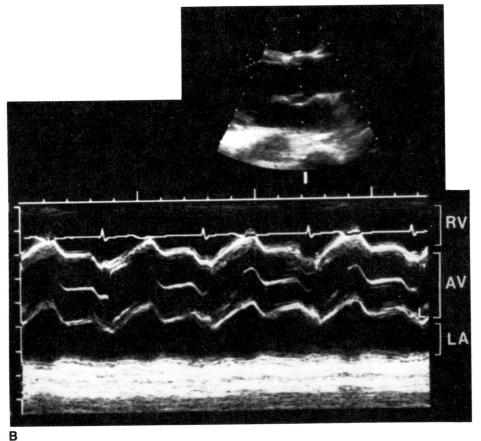

B

FIGURE 4–1. (*A*) Cross section of heart parallel to the long axis of the left ventricle and aorta. Cursor 1 corresponds to the echo beam intersecting the right ventricle, aortic valve, and left atrium; cursor 2 corresponds to the echo beam intersecting the right ventricle, left ventricle, and anterior and posterior leaflets of the mitral valve. (*B*) M-mode echocardiogram corresponding to cursor 1 in (A). The box-like inscription corresponds to systolic motion of aortic leaflets. The wedge-shaped section above illustrates the corresponding two-dimensional echocardiogram image; center dotted line indicates the plane of the M-mode image. *Figure continued on following page*

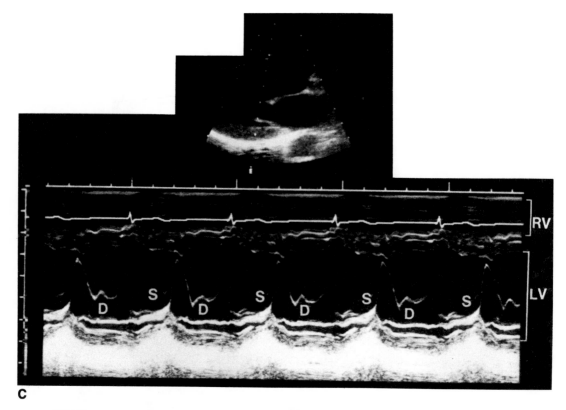

C

FIGURE 4–1. (*continued*) (*C*) M-mode echocardiogram with echo beam directed through the right ventricle, left ventricle, and anterior and posterior leaflets of the mitral valve. The mitral valve is displayed by nonspecific M- and W-shaped inscriptions. The dual peaks of diastole are bordered by the linear systolic closure line. The two-dimensional echocardiogram wedge is at top. A = anterior; Ao = aorta; AV = aortic valve; D = diastole; L = left; LA = left atrium; LV = left ventricle; RV = right ventricle; S = systole.

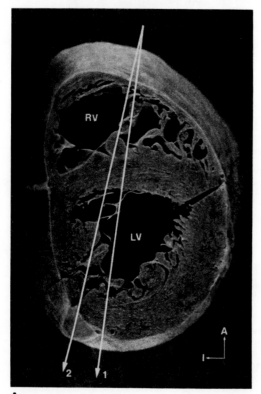

A

FIGURE 4–2. (*A*) Cross section of the right and left ventricle with the echo beam intersecting the left ventricular posterior wall virtually equidistant to both papillary muscles (cursor 1) and closer to the inferolateral papillary muscle (cursor 2). *Figure continued on opposite page*

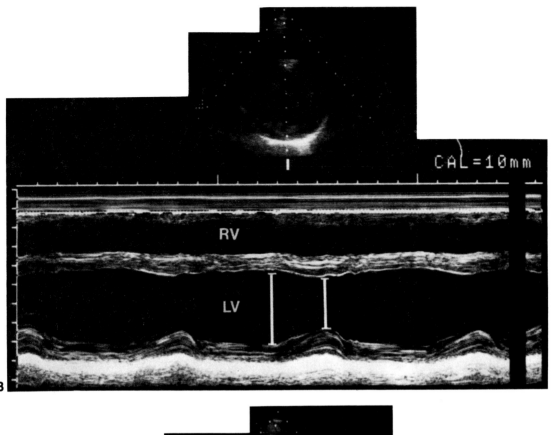

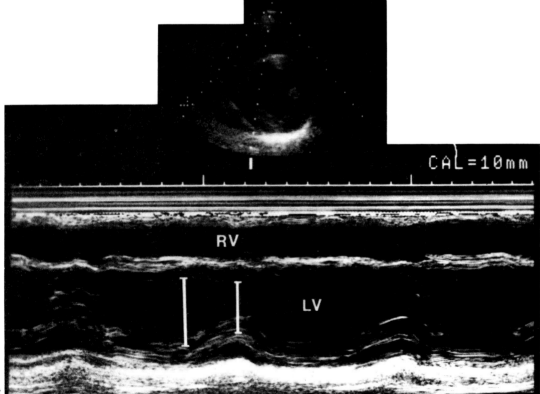

FIGURE 4–2. (*continued*) (*B*) M-mode echocardiogram recording corresponding to the position of cursor 1 in (A). Two-dimensional echocardiogram wedge is at top. (*C*) M-mode echocardiogram recording corresponding to the eccentric position of cursor 2 in (A). This position artificially reduces the end-systolic and end-diastolic dimensions of the left ventricle with an apparent increase in the shortening fraction. The two-dimensional echocardiogram wedge is at top. A = anterior; I = inferior; LV = left ventricle; RV = right ventricle.

TWO-DIMENSIONAL ECHOCARDIOGRAPHY

Two-dimensional echocardiography is the current standard for ultrasound imaging of cardiovascular anatomy. Unlike M-mode, two-dimensional imaging is based on sequential transmission of ultrasound signals by an array of horizontally stacked ceramic crystals. In contrast to the superimposition of contiguous structures on the standard chest roentgenogram and cineangiogram, two-dimensional echocardiography presents a tomographic image similar to that seen with computed tomography and magnetic resonance imaging. The two-dimensional cardiac ultrasound probe functions as an electronic knife that generates serial cross-sectional images displaying the "cut surfaces" in a video format. As with other ultrasound imaging, air, distance to the target, and extremes in acoustic velocities interfere with two-dimensional echocardiography.

Two-dimensional echocardiography shares with conventional photography processing features that influence image quality and detail. Perspective, lighting, film speed, lens aperture, shutter speed, and subject influence the quality of a photograph. With two-dimensional echocardiography, these issues translate into orientation of the echo beam (i.e., projection), focal distance, cardiac probe operating frequency, image rate, and target depth. Perspective in two-dimensional echocardiography is the projection of the echo beam from either a transthoracic, suprasternal notch, subxiphoid, or retrocardiac transesophageal position. The patient's age and body habitus and the clinical question to be answered determine which projections are or can be used. With conventional photography, removal of the lens cap is a fundamental first step when imaging. With all forms of transcutaneous imaging, the lens cap equivalent is the aqueous gel placed on the skin to form an acoustic seal with the cardiac probe.

Patient size and target distance determine the operating frequency (2.25, 3.50, 5.00, or 7.50 MHz) and focal zone of the cardiac probe used for the two-dimensional echocardiography examination. Small subjects require higher-frequency cardiac probes with shorter focal zones. The cardiac probe best suited for an adolescent or adult subject is usually unsuitable for detailed imaging of the neonate, infant, or toddler with congenital or acquired heart disease. When standard imaging from the surface of the thorax or abdomen is compromised by patient size, lung volume, or practicality during cardiothoracic surgery, a retrocardiac transesophageal perspective may be necessary.[14,15] With transesophageal echocardiography, the ceramic crystal elements are mounted on a flexible gastric endoscope.

Anatomic definition with high-frequency two-dimensional cardiac probes permits detailed examination of intracardiac as well as extracardiac structures. The interatrial and interventricular septa, proximal systemic and pulmonary veins, great vessels, and coronary arteries are well visualized using multiple transthoracic and transabdominal projections[16-28] (Fig. 4–3).

Cardiac ultrasonography offers a useful alternative to chest fluoroscopy and roentgenograms for management of general pediatric medicine problems.[29-31] Discrimination between a pleural effusion and lobar atelectasis is quickly accomplished using transthoracic and subxiphoid projections. Two-dimensional echocardiography simplifies pericardiocentesis and thoracentesis by displaying the effusion, adjacent cardiovascular and pulmonary structures, and loculating adhesions. Diaphragmatic paresis with inspiratory rocking of the ipsilateral hemidiaphragm can be identified with subxiphoid projections.

The diagnostic capability of two-dimensional echocardiography is apparent in its use as a definitive preoperative alternative to cardiac catheterization. There is no general agreement regarding this matter, but in some centers quality and specificity of the cardiac ultrasound examination may obviate the need for preoperative cardiac catheterization of interatrial and isolated interventricular septal defects, tetralogy of Fallot, anomalously draining pulmonary veins, *d*-transposition of the great vessels, truncus arteriosus communis, and aortic arch anomalies. Two-dimensional echocardiography identifies aortic and pulmonic valve stenosis, but patients with these abnormalities typically undergo catheterization for therapeutic angioplasty rather than for diagnosis. Neonates may undergo anatomic correction of simple *d*-transposition of the great arteries following its identification with cardiac ultrasonography. In those infants with this anomaly who require balloon atrial septostomy, two-dimensional imaging may avoid delay in treatment by facilitating catheteri-

FIGURE 4–3. (*A*) Two-dimensional echocardiogram in subxiphoid projection demonstrating the left ventricle and ascending aorta with a large, subaortic, membranous interventricular septal defect indicated by arrows. (*B*) Two-dimensional echocardiogram demonstrating the origination of the main pulmonary artery from the left ventricle in *d*-transposition of the great arteries. A membranous-type interventricular septal defect is present below the pulmonary valve (arrows). Ao = aorta; LAA = left atrial appendage; LV = left ventricle; MPA = main pulmonary artery; R = right; RV = right ventricle; S = superior. Arrow marker on the ECG indicates timing of the echocardiographic image.

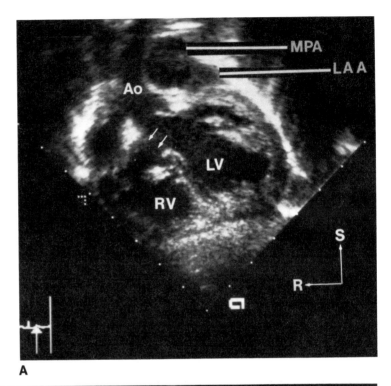

A

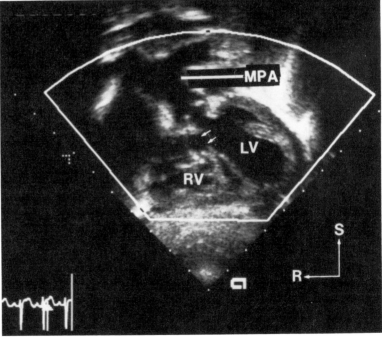

B

zation of these neonates in a special care nursery.[32-34] In a tertiary neonatal intensive care setting, the septostomy catheter, introduced via the umbilical vein or percutaneously via the femoral vein and inferior vena cava, can be advanced into the left atrium under ultrasound guidance.

DOPPLER ECHOCARDIOGRAPHY

Two-dimensional echocardiography displays cardiac anatomy. The contribution of echocardiography to understanding cardiac function has been enhanced with integration of anatomic two-dimensional imaging and Doppler examination of blood flow. Quantitation of transvalvar gradients and cardiac output as well as qualitative grading of atrioventricular and semilunar valve regurgitation has expanded the scope of cardiac ultrasonography.[35-39]

The composite technology that examines both morphology and blood flow uses the same basic principles of ultrasonography. How the reflected ultrasound signal is processed determines the nature of the display. Anatomic two-dimensional imaging processes the signal to measure the distance between the transmitting cardiac probe and the reflecting tissue boundaries. Doppler echocardiography processes the reflected signal to identify changes in the frequency of the originally transmitted signal. The difference between the reference frequency and the frequency of the reflected signal is the Doppler shift frequency.

A common illustration of the Doppler shift phenomenon is the perceived sound of an ambulance siren by a pedestrian observer. Sound of a stationary siren is in part determined by its reference frequency. The apparent or perceived sound of a siren when moving, however, is a function of the reference frequency and the velocity as well as the direction of movement of the ambulance. The siren's reference frequency is constant regardless of the motion of the ambulance or the position of the observer. The perceived frequency of the siren, however, is some increment higher or lower than the reference frequency depending on the speed and direction of the ambulance. The siren of an approaching ambulance has a higher frequency. The difference in frequencies is because each cycle of the signal arrives at the observer's position sooner than

it would if the siren were stationary. As the ambulance passes the observer, the siren is neither approaching or receding, and there is no difference between the perceived and reference frequency. Although the ambulance is moving, momentarily there is no Doppler shift frequency. After the ambulance passes the observer, its direction and velocity again distort the siren signal. The sound perceived by the observer has a lower frequency owing to a lengthening interval between each cycle.

Use of the Doppler shift principle in cardiac ultrasonography parallels the siren illustration. With cardiac Doppler ultrasonography the cardiac probe serves as the transmitter and receiver, and red blood cells are multiple reflectors. Depending on the direction of movement of red blood cells relative to the probe, the reflected ultrasound signal is either greater or less than the transmitted reference frequency. A mathematical relation[1] exists between the Doppler shift frequency (F_D), the reference frequency (F_R), the velocity of sound in the tissue medium (C), and the velocity of a reflecting surface (V_{rbc}):

$$F_D = 2F_R V_{rbc}/C$$

The velocity of the red blood cells is:

$$V_{rbc} = F_D C/2F_R$$

Blood flow velocity is not a commonly used clinical index of cardiac function. Velocity, however, can be used to calculate blood flow (e.g., cardiac output) if the cross-sectional area (A) of the blood vessel (e.g., aorta, main pulmonary artery, umbilical vein) is known:

$$Flow = V_{rbc} \times A$$

Doppler echocardiography also offers noninvasive quantitation of more complex hydrodynamic relations. Simplifying the complex Bernoulli equation describing conservation of energy in a fluid permits estimation of gradients across obstructed or regurgitant valves, interventricular septal defects, or narrowed vessels. This technique measures instantaneous rather than the more common catheterization laboratory peak-to-peak value; the formula for the gradient across an area of accelerated flow is:

$$Gradient \ (mm \ Hg) = 4 \times [V_{rbc} \ (m/s)^2]$$

Continuous-Wave Doppler Echocardiography

Doppler echocardiography is a generic title for all qualitative or quantitative ultrasound techniques displaying flow velocity. Differences in sampling, processing, and display determine which Doppler technique is appropriate to answer a clinical question. Nonimaging, continuous-wave Doppler is the most generally used form of Doppler ultrasonography. This technique is used for electronic auscultation of blood flow in peripheral arteries and veins. The Doppler probe is placed on the skin over a vessel (e.g., brachial, carotid, or popliteal artery) without direct visualization of the channel. The ultrasound signal reflected by moving red blood cells generates an audible Doppler shift signal but does not identify direction or quantitate flow velocity. Nonimaging continuous-wave Doppler has been integrated with two-dimensional echocardiography and modified to quantitate velocity. The uninterrupted interrogation of the reflected signal by continuous-wave Doppler allows quantitation of the higher Doppler shift frequencies encountered with most stenotic valves or restrictive interventricular septal defects. Although continuous-wave Doppler may be performed without two-dimensional guidance, it is customary to target the echo beam and focus on a particular area of interest (see Fig. 4–4, color plate I).

Stenotic gradients (aortic/mitral/pulmonary) are commonly measured by the Doppler technique, which also permits quantitation of regurgitant systolic and diastolic gradients. Noninvasive estimation of right ventricular and pulmonary artery pressure is a typical example of how regurgitant gradients are used clinically.[40–43] Tricuspid valve regurgitation often is associated with elevated right ventricular pressure. The retrograde regurgitant jet offers a noninvasive "window" to right ventricular systolic pressure. In the absence of pulmonic stenosis, the regurgitant systolic gradient across the tricuspid valve is an index of right ventricular and pulmonary artery systolic pressure. Retrograde diastolic gradients may be combined with systolic systemic blood pressure to estimate left ventricular end-diastolic pressure. Retrograde diastolic gradients measured from the aortic insufficiency Doppler waveform combined with systemic systolic blood pressure allow serial noninvasive monitoring of ventricular filling pressures.

Range-Gated Pulsed Doppler Echocardiography

Continuous-wave Doppler may be guided using two-dimensional imaging, but it cannot be focused at a specific site. If the echocardiography beam is aligned with the left ventricular outflow tract, there is no spatial resolution to identify a gradient as subvalvar, valvar, or supravalvar. This limitation of continuous-wave Doppler (i.e., absence of depth perception) is overcome using range-gated pulsed Doppler echocardiography. Range gating permits focusing of the Doppler signal at a specific distance from the ultrasound probe. It is accomplished by sampling the returning reflected ultrasound signal at an operator-determined time interval after transmission. This delay in sampling identifies those Doppler shift frequencies generated at a given distance from the ultrasound probe.

Targeting of the pulsed Doppler sample site is accomplished with standard two-dimensional echocardiography. The range gate slides along a cursor corresponding to the echo beam that is superimposed on the two-dimensional image. The output from a pulsed Doppler recording of transmitral flow velocity is illustrated in Figure 4–5. The pulsed Doppler data, as with continuous-wave Doppler data, are displayed on velocity–time coordinates. Each datum point represents the velocity at an operator-defined distance from the cardiac probe. The M-shaped configuration of diastolic flow velocity corresponds to the early passive and late atrial diastolic components of ventricular filling.[41–44] This flow velocity profile mirrors the M-mode display of the mitral valve generated by the passive, flow-sensitive motion of the leaflets during ventricular diastole.

The ability to gate the Doppler to a specific anatomic site is both an asset and a liability for pulsed Doppler echocardiography. Although range gating coordinates anatomy and flow velocity, the sampling delay it requires limits the peak velocity it can identify. The display of higher velocities associated with semilunar valve stenosis is distorted by this slower sampling rate. Use of continuous-wave or pulsed Doppler echocardiography to evaluate flow velocities

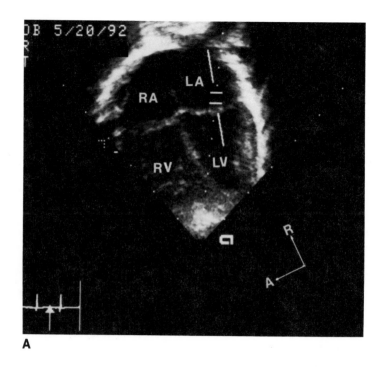

A

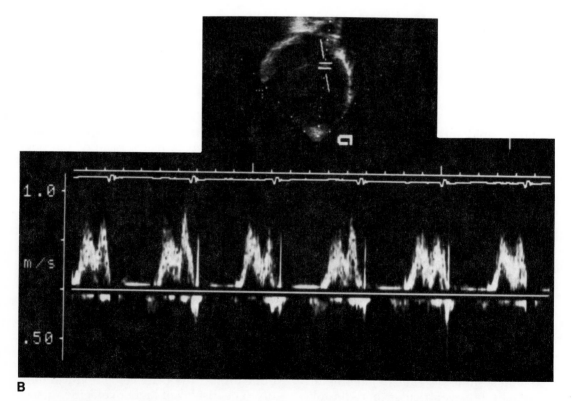

B

FIGURE 4–5. (*A*) Apical four-chamber projection demonstrating the four cardiac chambers with the pulsed Doppler sample volume positioned at the mitral valve. (*B*) Pulsed Doppler echocardiogram of the mitral valve. The biphasic flow velocity configuration of transmitral flow corresponds to early passive and late atrial systolic flow. A = anterior; LA = left atrium; LV = left ventricle; R = right; RA = right atrium; RV = right ventricle. Arrow marker on the ECG indicates timing of the echocardiographic image.

PLATE I

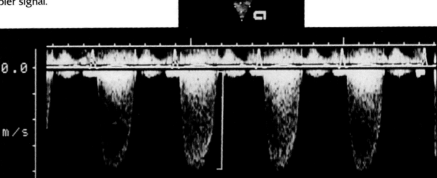

FIGURE 4–4. Apical projection of the left ventricle with continuous-wave Doppler cursor aligned with the left ventricular outflow tract. The continuous wave graph reveals a peak velocity of 4 meters/second, which corresponds to a left ventricular outflow gradient of 64 mm Hg. The two-dimensional wedge above confirms the position of the Doppler signal.

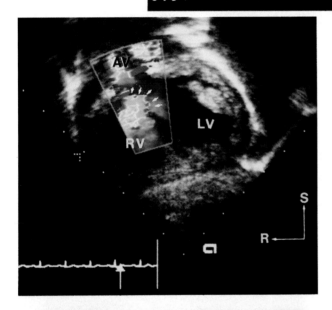

FIGURE 4–6. Subxiphoid two-dimensional echocardiogram of the left ventricle with a superimposed color flow map demonstrating color mosaic corresponding to the left-to-right shunt across the interventricular septal defect (arrowheads); see Figure 4–3A. AV = aortic valve; LV = left ventricle; R = right; RV = right ventricle; S = superior. Arrow marker on the ECG indicates timing of the echocardiographic image.

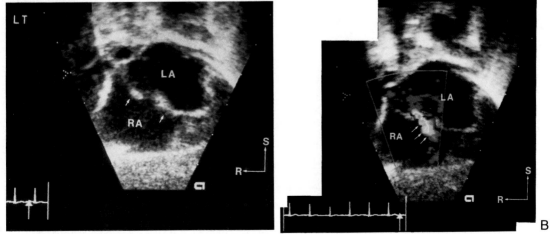

FIGURE 4–7. (A) Subxiphoid two-dimensional echocardiogram demonstrating right and left atria and the interatrial septum (arrows). (B) Same projection as above with superimposed color flow mapping demonstrating a small left-to-right shunt across the foramen ovale (arrows). LA = left atrium; R = right; RA = right atrium; S = superior. Arrow marker on the ECG indicates timing of the echocardiographic image.

PLATE II

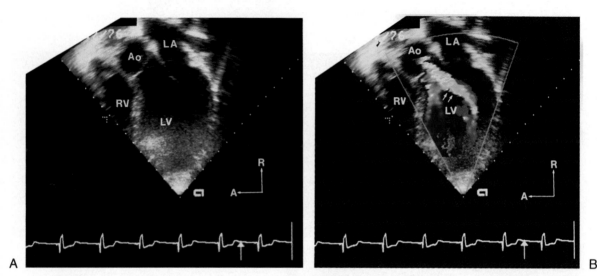

A   B

FIGURE 4–8. (*A*) Two-dimensional apical projection demonstrating the long axis of the left ventricle, left atrium, interventricular septum, and proximal aorta with aortic valve closed. (*B*) Same projection with superimposed color map illustrating aortic regurgitant jet (arrows) deflected off the anterior leaflet of the mitral valve. A = anterior; Ao = aorta; LA = left atrium; LV = left ventricle; R = right; RV = right ventricle. Arrow marker on the ECG indicates timing of the echocardiographic image.

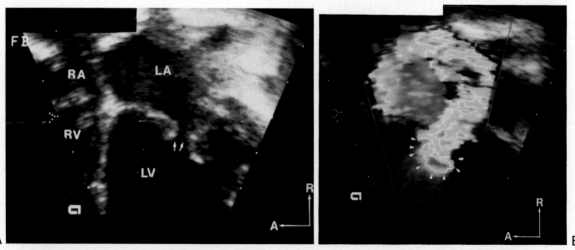

A   B

FIGURE 4–9. (*A*) Magnified four-chamber view of the left atrium, mitral valve, and left ventricular inlet demonstrating systolic separation of the valve leaflets (arrows). (*B*) Superimposed color map revealing large regurgitant jet of severe mitral insufficiency that follows the contour of the posterior left atrial wall. A = anterior; LA = left atrium; LV = left ventricle; R = right; RA = right atrium; RV = right ventricle.

therefore is guided by the specific clinical question to be answered. Evaluation of a stenotic lesion often combines both Doppler applications. The site of obstruction is first pinpointed with gated pulsed Doppler. Continuous-wave Doppler echocardiography is then applied to estimate the peak velocity and gradient.

Color Flow Mapping

Doppler color flow mapping is an extension of pulsed Doppler technology. With conventional range-gated pulsed Doppler echocardiography, velocity and time are displayed in a graph-like manner. With color flow mapping a color rather than a numerical value identifies the direction and magnitude of the velocity. Direction of blood flow, toward or away from the cardiac probe, is assigned a primary color (red or blue). By convention, red corresponds to flow toward the cardiac probe, and blue is flow away from the probe. The magnitude of velocity is identified by a sliding scale of color shades.

Combining the color flow map with two-dimensional echocardiography results in a polychromatic angiogram displaying anatomy and blood flow. Figure 4–6, (see color plate I) illustrates a two-dimensional echocardiogram displaying a large subaortic ventricular septal defect. Superimposition of the color flow map demonstrates the associated left-to-right shunt. Adaptive changes in intracardiac anatomy and blood flow in the neonate, including persistent patency of the foramen ovale with left-to-right shunting, are revealed with combined imaging of anatomy and flow (see Fig. 4–7, color plate I). This application of cardiac ultrasonography to the neonate identifies normal anatomic variants as well as more complex anomalies. Serial two-dimensional and color flow map echocardiograms permit follow-up of medical therapy. Efficacy of treatment to close the ductus arteriosus in a premature infant with indomethacin or preserve its patency using prostaglandin E_1 for control of a ductal-dependent cardiovascular anomaly may be monitored by such serial imaging.

Subtle changes in valve function resulting in mild regurgitation (see Fig. 4–8, color plate II) or more profound distortions of systolic closure resulting in severe regurgitation (see Fig. 4–9, color plate II) are apparent with two-dimensional and color flow map examination. This noninvasive information should guide, but not dictate, clinical management of isolated cardiovascular disease or cardiac pathology secondary to systemic disease. This caveat of ultrasound use is best emphasized by recognizing that color flow mapping can display physiologic regurgitation across anatomically normal atrioventricular or semilunar valves.[44] As a general rule, regurgitant valvar lesions seen on ultrasonography but not audible to the clinician suggest a normal variant of valve function, particularly in the setting of clinically "occult" tricuspid and pulmonic regurgitation. Discrimination between pathologic and physiologic regurgitation of the aortic and mitral valves is more subtle but should be done with consideration of all the clinical data.

OVERVIEW

Combined two-dimensional and Doppler cardiac ultrasonography in pediatric patients continues to evolve in terms of its clinical application. It is a seductive technology that is readily accessible, lends itself to repetition, and has little biohazard in its clinical application.[45–48] When used properly, cardiac ultrasonography expedites diagnosis and permits prompt initiation of appropriate medical and surgical management. Its use has extended the population base of the pediatric cardiologist and perinatologist to the fetus. Fetal cardiology, formerly an exercise confined to the laboratory animal model, has become a practical clinical discipline. Furthermore, advances in ceramic crystal technology and transesophageal imaging allow examination of cardiac anatomy and quantitation of cardiac function during open heart surgery.

Proper utilization of cardiac ultrasonography by the pediatric community requires an understanding of its acquisition and its technical limitations. Echocardiography is a noninvasive technique, but the agitated 2-year-old often does not recognize it as a benevolent alternative to more noxious studies. Echocardiography in the toddler age group often requires sedation to allow a comprehensive examination. Sedation protocols vary among pediatric echocardiography laboratories. The most common approach is the use of chloral hydrate by mouth or rectal suppository. In contrast to the adult, transesophageal echocardiography in pediatric subjects under 12 years of age typically

requires sedation with endotracheal intubation to protect the airway.

Cardiac ultrasonography in the pediatric
population offers invaluable data for the
management of congenital and acquired cardiac disease. Its successful application depends on asking the right question, using
the proper technology, and avoiding its application in a clinical vacuum.

REFERENCES

1. Taylor KJW, Burns PN, Wells PNT (eds): Clinical Applications of Doppler Ultrasound. New York, Raven Press, 1988, pp. 1–25.
2. Schneider AR, Serwer GA: Echocardiography in Pediatric Heart Disease. Chicago, Year Book Medical Publishers, 1990, pp. 1–10.
3. Come PC, Riley MF, Carl LV, Nakao S: Pulsed Doppler echocardiographic evaluation of valvar regurgitation in patients with mitral valve pro-lapse: comparison with normal subjects. J Am Coll Cardiol 8:1355–1364, 1986.
4. Marks AR, Choong CY, Chir MBB, et al: Identifi-cation of high-risk and low-risk subgroups of pa-tients with mitral valve prolapse. N Engl J Med 320:1031–1036, 1989.
5. Ansari A: M-mode echocardiography in supine and standing position in control subjects and pa-tients with auscultatory evidence of mitral valve prolapse but negative supine echocardiography: does sensitivity improve? Clin Cardiol 8:591–596, 1985.
6. Loehr JP, Synhorst DP, Wolfe RR, et al: Aortic root dilatation and mitral valve prolapse in the fragile X syndrome. Am J Med Genet 23:189–194, 1986.
7. Leier CV, Call TD, Fulkerson PK, et al: The spec-trum of cardiac defects in the Ehlers-Danlos syn-drome, types I and II. Ann Intern Med 92:171–178, 1980.
8. Seliem MA, Duffy CE, Gidding SS, et al: Echocar-diographic evaluation of the aortic root and mitral valve in children and adolescents with isolated pectus excavatum: comparison with Marfan pa-tients. Pediatr Cardiol 13:20–23, 1992.
9. Marlow N, Gregg JE, Qureshi SA: Mitral valve disease in Marfan's syndrome. Arch Dis Child 62:960–962, 1987.
10. Wann LS, Grove JR, Hess TR, et al: Prevalence of mitral prolapse by two-dimensional echocardiog-raphy in healthy young women. Br Heart J 49:334–340, 1983.
11. Jeresaty RM: Mitral valve prolapse: definition and implications in athletes. J Am Coll Cardiol 7:231–236, 1986.
12. Maron BJ, Bodison SA, Wesley YE, et al: Results of screening a large group of intercollegiate com-petitive athletes for cardiovascular disease. J Am Coll Cardiol 10:1214–1221, 1987.
13. Franklin RC, Wyse RK, Graham TP, et al: Normal values for noninvasive estimation of left ventricu-lar contractile state and afterload in children. Am J Cardiol 65:505–510, 1990.
14. Shah PM, Stewart S III, Calalang CC, Alexson C: Transesophageal echocardiography and the intra-
15. Ritter SB: Transesophageal real-time echocardi-ography in infants and children with congenital heart disease. J Am Coll Cardiol 18:569–580, 1991.
16. Bierman FZ, Williams RG: Subxiphoid two-di-mensional imaging of the interatrial septum in in-fants and neonates with congenital heart disease. Circulation 60:80–90, 1979.
17. Shub C, Dimopoulos IN, Seward JB, et al: Sensi-tivity of two-dimensional echocardiography in the direct visualization of atrial septal defect utilizing the subcostal approach: experience with 154 pa-tients. J Am Coll Cardiol 2:127–135, 1983.
18. Lieppe W, Scallion R, Behar VS, Kisslo JA: Two-dimensional echocardiographic findings in atrial septal defects. Circulation 56:447–456, 1977.
19. Hatle L: Flow velocity patterns across atrial septal defects recorded with Doppler echocardiography. Acta Paediatr Scand Suppl 329:68–77, 1986.
20. Bierman FZ, Fellows K, Williams RG: Prospec-tive identification of ventricular septal defects in infancy using subxiphoid two-dimensional echo-cardiography. Circulation 62:807–817, 1980.
21. Stevenson JG: Doppler evaluation of atrial septal defect, ventricular septal defect, and complex malformations. Acta Paediatr Scand [Suppl] 329:21–43, 1986.
22. Cheatham JP, Latson LA, Gutgesell HP: Ventric-ular septal defect in infancy: detection with two dimensional echocardiography. Am J Cardiol 47:85–89, 1981.
23. Sutherland GR, Godman MJ, Smallhorn JF, et al: Ventricular septal defects: two dimensional echo-cardiographic and morphological correlations. Br Heart J 47:316–328, 1982.
24. Jaffe CC, Atkinson P, Taylor KJ: Physical param-eters affecting the visibility of small ventricular septal defects using two-dimensional echocardi-ography. Invest Radiol 14:149–155, 1979.
25. Daskalopoulos DA, Edwards WD, Driscoll DJ, et al: Correlation of two-dimensional echocardio-graphic and autopsy findings in complete transpo-sition of the great arteries. J Am Coll Cardiol 2:1151–1157, 1983.
26. Jureidini SB, Appleton RS, Nouri S: Detection of coronary artery abnormalities in tetralogy of Fal-lot by two-dimensional echocardiography. J Am Coll Cardiol 14:960–967, 1989.
27. Pasquini L, Sanders SP, Parness IA, Colan SD: Diagnosis of coronary artery anatomy by two di-mensional echocardiography in patients with transposition of the great arteries. Circulation 57:557–564, 1987.
28. Meyer RA: Echocardiography in Kawasaki dis-ease. J Am Soc Echocardiogr 2:269–275, 1989.
29. Taavitsainen M, Bondestam S, Mankinen P, et al: Ultrasound guidance for pericardiocentesis. Acta Radiol 32:9–11, 1991.
30. Carazo Martinez O, Vargas Serrano B, Rodriguez Romero R: Real-time ultrasound evaluation of tu-berculous pleural effusions. J Clin Ultrasound 17:407–410, 1989.
31. Connell DG, Crothers G, Cooperberg PL: The subpulmonic pleural effusion: sonographic as-pects. J Can Assoc Radiol 33:101–103, 1982.
32. Bullaboy CA, Jennings RB Jr, Johnson DH: Bed-

operative management of pediatric congenital heart disease: initial experience with a pediatric esophageal 2D color flow echocardiographic probe. J Cardiothorac Vasc Anesth 6:8–14, 1992.

side balloon atrial septostomy using echocardiographic monitoring. Am J Cardiol 15:971, 1984.

33. Steeg CN, Bierman FZ, Hayes C, et al: "Bedside" balloon septostomy for infants with transposition of the great arteries: new concepts using two dimensional echocardiographic techniques. J Pediatr 107:944–946, 1985.

34. Baylen BG, Crzeszczak M, Gleason ME, et al: Role of balloon atrial septostomy before early arterial switch repair of transposition of the great arteries. J Am Coll Cardiol 19:1025–1031, 1992.

35. Reeder GS, Currie PJ, Fyfe DA, et al: Extracardiac conduit obstruction. initial experience in the use of Doppler echocardiography for noninvasive estimation of pressure gradient. J Am Coll Cardiol 4:1006–1011, 1984.

36. Fyfe DA, Currie PJ, Seward JB, et al: Continuous-wave Doppler determination of the pressure gradient across pulmonary artery bands: hemodynamic correlation in 20 patients. Mayo Clin Proc 59:744–750, 1984.

37. Murphy DJ Jr, Ludomirsky A, Huhta JC: Continuous-wave Doppler in children with ventricular septal defect: noninvasive estimation of interventricular pressure gradient. Am J Cardiol 57:428–432, 1986.

38. Snider AR, Stevenson JG, French JW, et al: Comparison of high pulse repetition frequency and continuous wave Doppler echocardiography for velocity measurement and gradient prediction in children with valvar and congenital heart disease. J Am Coll Cardiol 7:873–879, 1986.

39. Sullivan ID, Robinson PJ, Wyse RK, et al: Continuous wave Doppler in the evaluation of simple and complex congenital heart disease in infants and children. Int J Cardiol 13:69–80, 1986.

40. Labovitz AJ, Ferrara RP, Kern MJ, et al: Quantitative evaluation of aortic insufficiency by continuous wave Doppler echocardiography. J Am Coll Cardiol 8:1341–1347, 1986.

41. Gidding SS, Snider AR, Rocchini AP, et al: Left ventricular diastolic filling in children with hypertrophic cardiomyopathy: assessment with pulsed Doppler echocardiography. J Am Coll Cardiol 8:310–316, 1986.

42. Appleton CP, Hatle LK, Popp RL: Relation of transmitral flow velocity patterns to left ventricular diastolic function: new insights from a combined hemodynamic and Doppler echocardiographic study. J Am Coll Cardiol 12:426–440, 1988.

43. Takenaka K, Dabestani A, Gardin JM, et al: Pulsed Doppler echocardiographic study of left ventricular filling in dilated cardiomyopathy. Am J Cardiol 58:143–147, 1986.

44. Yoshida K, Yoshikawa J, Shakudo M, et al: Color Doppler evaluation of valvar regurgitation in normal subjects. Circulation 78:840–847, 1988.

45. Skorton DJ, Collins SM, Greenleaf JF, et al: Ultrasound bioeffects and regulatory issues: an introduction for the echocardiographer. J Am Soc Echocardiogr 1:241–251, 1988.

46. American Institute of Ultrasound in Medicine Bioeffects Committee: Bioeffects considerations for the safety of diagnostic ultrasound. J Ultrasound Med 7:S1–S38, 1988.

47. Rabe H, Grohs B, Schmidt RM, et al: Acoustic power measurements of Doppler ultrasound devices used for perinatal and infant examinations. Pediatr Radiol 20:277–281, 1990.

48. Miller DL: Update on safety of diagnostic ultrasonography. J Clin Ultrasound 19:531–540, 1991.

Part II
GENERAL CLINICAL PROBLEMS

5

CYANOTIC NEWBORNS

Benjamin E. Victorica

The pediatric primary care physician is confronted sooner or later by a newborn who has critical congenital heart disease. Once the preliminary diagnosis of heart disease has been established, all efforts should be directed toward determining the hemodynamic status of the patient. In most of these patients clinical deterioration is directly related to progressive closure of the ductus arteriosus. The newborn can be ductal-dependent for one of three hemodynamic reasons: (1) for mixing pulmonary and systemic blood flow; (2) for supplying pulmonary arterial blood flow; (3) for maintaining systemic blood flow. In the first two situations the infant's primary problem is hypoxemia; in the third, the primary problem is low systemic output. These infants are therefore described according to the following clinical presentation: (1) the cyanotic newborn infant; and (2) the newborn infant with low systemic output (cardiogenic shock).

The primary care physician must assess the problem, determine its urgency, and take appropriate steps to stabilize the patient prior to transfer to a tertiary pediatric cardiology center. This chapter addresses the problem of the cyanotic newborn as described above including a third category of cyanotic heart disease characterized by increased pulmonary arterial blood flow, the so-called mixing lesions, a group that is not ductal-dependent. Chapter 6 presents the problem of the infant with low systemic output due to critical heart disease.

CYANOTIC NEWBORN

Cyanosis is an observation not a diagnosis, just as jaundice is an observation not a diagnosis. As there are multiple causes for jaundice, so too are there many causes for cyanosis. The word cyanosis literally means blue blood, accurately describing the color given to blood by unoxygenated (reduced) hemoglobin. Hemoglobin that is fully saturated with oxygen is bright red. If arterial blood contains enough "blue" hemoglobin, the individual appears cyanotic. Detection of cyanosis is in the eye of the beholder, not in a specific laboratory value. The examiner's eye functions as a spectrophotometer, assessing the color of the blood. Accuracy in determining the presence of cyanosis comes from a combination of experience and careful observation.

What is the significance of cyanosis? In and of itself cyanosis is not harmful. The fetus is always "cyanotic," as its systemic arterial oxygen saturation is 60 to 65 per cent. If this situation persisted after birth and nothing else changed, the newborn would still be in no difficulty. It is the implication of cyanosis and its potential for worsening that creates urgency. Persistent cyanosis in the newborn requires investigation. Cyanotic heart disease does not go away by itself. It might be stable, but it might also lead to rapid clinical deterioration. Either way, temporizing management serves no purpose.

To help understand this subject, some basic concepts regarding oxygenation are reviewed, followed by some guidelines for evaluating the patient and a simplified pathophysiologic classification. Specific lesions exemplifying these pathophysiologic types of cyanotic heart disease are presented concluding with management recommendations. No attempt is made to describe all cyanotic heart disease in the newborn. Rather, we propose a method of categorizing the nature and severity of the infant's problem within the framework provided.

Physiologic Concepts

Oxygen is transported in the blood primarily on hemoglobin. The proportion of red blood cell hemoglobin oxygen-carrying sites that actually contain oxygen is called the *per cent oxygen saturation*. Oxygen saturation therefore tells you how much oxygen is in the blood only if you know how much hemoglobin is present. Oxygen attaches to hemoglobin in relation to its availability (*partial pressure*), first from the alveolus, then from what is dissolved in serum. The relation of oxygen partial pressure (PO_2 in millimeters of mercury) and oxygen saturation (per cent) creates the familiar oxygen dissociation curve. Factors such as blood pH, temperature, PCO_2, 2,3-diphosphoglycerate (2,3-DPG), and type of hemoglobin influence this relation, as illustrated in Figure 5–1.[1] For example, at a given PO_2 fetal hemoglobin carries more oxygen (higher saturation) than does adult hemoglobin because fetal hemoglobin has much less affinity for 2,3-DPG than does adult hemoglobin, making fetal hemoglobin behave as if the 2,3-DPG level is low. The oxygen dissociation curve is considered to be shifted to the left. Acidosis (increased hydrogen ion concentration) shifts the curve to the right, resulting in decreased hemoglobin saturation for a given PO_2.

It is important to have a concept of how PO_2 and saturation relate to oxygen content. As already mentioned, the absolute amount of oxygen being transported in blood is a function of hemoglobin level and per cent saturation. One gram of hemoglobin carries approximately 1.39 ml of oxygen[2] if fully saturated (100 per cent). It is a simple calculation to determine that a normal adult with a hemoglobin level of 15 gm/dl, which is fully saturated, has 15 (hemoglobin) × 1.39* × 1.0 (100 per cent saturation) × 10 = 208 ml oxygen/liter blood. This value represents the total oxygen-carrying capacity of hemoglobin in that patient; it cannot go higher. From the oxygen dissociation curve it is apparent that in a normal adult full saturation cannot occur unless arterial PO_2 is more than 80 mm Hg. What happens if PO_2 is lower (e.g., 40 mm Hg)? At that PO_2 saturation is about 70 per cent. In our example the oxygen content is 15 × 1.39 × 0.7 × 10 = 146 ml/liter.

What happens in the newborn? The newborn may have a hemoglobin level of 20 gm/dl. Fetal hemoglobin holds more oxygen for a given PO_2. Thus in our example of arterial PO_2 = 40 mm Hg, the newborn has a saturation of about 75 per cent. Oxygen content for this individual is 20 (hemoglobin) × 1.39 × 0.75 (per cent saturation) × 10 = 208 ml/liter, the exact amount as the case of fully saturated hemoglobin (15 gm/dl).

Other factors also come into play, but from these examples you can see that, by itself, a PO_2 of 40 mm Hg does not mean that oxygen availability is significantly impaired. It should be apparent also that a low hemoglobin level rapidly becomes a problem for the infant operating at PO_2 40 mm Hg and even more so if PO_2 decreases further. For example, in a newborn saturation at PO_2 30 mm Hg is 60 per cent. If hemoglobin is only 12 gm/dl, the oxygen content is 12 × 1.39 × 0.6 × 10 = 100 ml/liter.

A small amount of oxygen is dissolved in serum in proportion to the PO_2. For each 100 mm Hg PO_2, blood carries 3 ml oxygen/liter. This amount is insignificant to the adult breathing room air, who has 208 ml oxygen/liter being carried on hemoglobin.

Clinical Cyanosis

Cyanosis is defined as "blue" arterial blood. How blue must it be to be visible? Experienced observers (and those paying

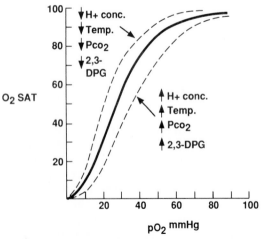

FIGURE 5–1. Oxygen dissociation curve for normal adult human blood (solid line) and curves showing the effect of either an increase (↑) or a decrease (↓) in hydrogen ion concentration, body temperature, PCO_2, and 2,3-DPG level (dotted lines).

---

* Reference 2 provides the data to calculate the value of 1.39 ml oxygen per gram of hemoglobin. It is based on the calculated hemoglobin iron content of 0.347 per cent (w/w).

close attention) see cyanosis at 3 gm of reduced hemoglobin per deciliter of blood. This amount is absolute, not a proportion. Cyanosis does not necessarily indicate lack of oxygen. If the individual has 20 gm of hemoglobin per deciliter, 5 gm can be reduced and 15 gm remain saturated. The patient appears cyanotic but still has as much oxygen available as the person with a hemoglobin level of 15 gm/dl who is 100 per cent saturated.

Cyanosis can occur because of slow blood flow, which permits greater extraction of oxygen. This problem is the cause of acrocyanosis, or blue hands and feet, in the newborn. It should be apparent now that polycythemia makes it easier to be cyanotic, and that if the total hemoglobin level is high per cent saturation need fall only a small amount to create 3 gm of reduced hemoglobin per deciliter. Conversely, anemia requires much lower saturation to cause cyanosis. The individual with a hemoglobin of 10 gm/dl does not appear even slightly cyanotic until saturation falls to 70 per cent.

It should be apparent also that cyanosis can occur if blood is not fully oxygenated as it traverses the lung. Pulmonary causes of cyanosis are common in the newborn. Differentiating respiratory disease from cardiac abnormality as a cause for cyanosis can be difficult. Pulmonary causes include respiratory distress syndrome, persistent fetal circulation, pneumonia, and mechanical abnormalities such as diaphragmatic hernia. Cyanosis can originate from hypoventilation, leading to inadequate oxygenation. Intracranial hemorrhage and sepsis may cause this problem. Abnormal hemoglobin configuration (e.g., methemoglobinemia) can prevent uptake of oxygen, also leading to cyanosis.

Evaluation of the Cyanotic Newborn

Detection of cyanosis may be obvious because of its severity; or it may be subtle, in which case some objective measurement may be necessary to confirm what your eyes are telling you. An arterial blood gas assay is helpful but the diagnosis can also be made more simply, without trauma, and at less cost using a transcutaneous oximeter. The normal newborn has an oxygen saturation of more than 85 per cent and does not appear cyanotic centrally. Saturation of 70 per cent or less should be readily detectable as clinical cyanosis unless the infant has a low hemoglobin level. Between these two percentages the oximeter may tip the diagnosis one way or the other. Once the infant has been identified as cyanotic, evaluation should proceed in an orderly and expeditious manner. First obtain at least a brief history, as it can be informative. Is the infant's mother a diabetic? Has she been febrile? Was delivery difficult or stressful, and what were the 1-minute and 5-minute Apgar scores? Is there a family history of congenital heart disease?

Physical Examination

Examine the infant. Critical components of the physical examination are appearance, respiratory rate and pattern, cardiovascular examination, and neurologic status. Look for key observations.

Appearance. Does the infant appear distressed? Is the infant anxious or irritable? Is the infant, in fact, cyanotic centrally or just in the periphery?

Respiration. Respiratory rate and pattern are of critical importance. Respiratory disease is more likely in an infant who is tachypneic with intercostal or subcostal retractions, nasal flare, or grunting. An infant who is cyanotic because of heart disease generally breathes normally except for mild tachypnea or hyperpnea.

Cardiovascular Examination. Assess arterial pulses in all four extremities and in the neck or head if extremity pulses are all weak. Check the circulatory status by evaluating skin temperature and capillary refill time. Check precordial activity especially for a thrill at the lower left sternal border, which would suggest tricuspid regurgitation. A loud murmur along the left sternal border also would suggest tricuspid regurgitation or possibly right ventricular outflow tract obstruction as in tetralogy of Fallot. Is S_2 split, confirming the presence of two great arteries (and likely two semilunar valves)? Is there a soft, continuous murmur at the left base, suggesting a patent ductus arteriosus as in tetralogy of Fallot with pulmonic atresia? If the cardiac examination is "normal," with single S_1, single S_2, and no murmur, consider transposition of the great arteries. A hyperactive heart with vigorous precordial impulses, tachycardia, abnormal heart sounds, and murmurs suggests lesions with increased pulmonary blood flow. All of these elements are described below in more detail in regard to specific types of cardiac abnormality. Check the abdomen for liver size and symmetry.

Neurologic Examination. Evaluate the infant's neurologic status particularly for evidence of central nervous system abnormality.

At this point reassess the situation. You should have a reasonably good idea what category of abnormality is causing the infant's cyanosis, assuming that your examination has confirmed that central cyanosis is in fact present. It is now appropriate to consider some laboratory testing.

Laboratory Studies

All infants who are cyanotic require some laboratory tests. Obtain a complete blood count, including hemoglobin and hematocrit, blood glucose, transcutaneous oxygen saturation or arterial blood gas (or both), and a chest radiograph. If there is evidence of poor perfusion, arterial PO_2 is less than 30 mm Hg, or oxygen saturation is less than 60 per cent, measure blood lactic acid and follow this indicator, as an elevation of more than 2 mmol/liter reveals metabolic acidosis before the blood pH falls. If you believe the infant has heart disease, obtain an electrocardiogram. Its usefulness is described later in the chapter. A hyperoxia test improves discrimination between cardiac and pulmonary disease and helps separate types of heart abnormality. Place the infant in 100 per cent oxygen by mask or hood and repeat the arterial PO_2 in 5 to 10 minutes. (Measurement of oxygen saturation alone is not sufficient, as an increase to 95 to 100 per cent does not discriminate.) The patient should be monitored carefully during this test, as oxygen can stimulate ductal closure, which can be detrimental. In the infant with neither significant respiratory disease nor cyanotic heart disease, 100 per cent oxygen breathing increases the PO_2 dramatically, reaching or exceeding 300 mm Hg. This level rules out cyanotic congenital heart disease. (*Note:* Arterial PO_2 of more than 300 mm Hg does not mean there is absolutely no right-to-left shunt, as some could exist; it does mean that the patient cannot have an obligatory cyanotic lesion.) With most lung diseases, despite significant alveolar/capillary block, atelectasis, or other causes of incomplete oxygenation within the pulmonary capillary bed, administration of 100 per cent oxygen increases pulmonary venous PO_2 to levels higher than 150 mm Hg. This condition rules out most types of cyanotic heart disease, especially those with obstruction to pulmonary blood flow, although an occasional patient with cyanotic heart disease has a PO_2 of up to 200 mm Hg. Similarly, not all lung disease responds to high inspired oxygen levels by correcting the arterial PO_2. Persistent fetal circulation with large ductal right-to-left shunt is one example. The hyperoxia test also can discriminate within types of cyanotic congenital heart disease. Infants with cyanotic heart disease in whom the systemic arterial PO_2 does not increase significantly have either transposition of the great arteries or obstructive pulmonary blood flow; infants in whom the arterial PO_2 rises moderately (75 to 150 mm Hg) have lesions with increased pulmonary blood flow and mixing of the pulmonary and systemic circulations.

The hyperoxia test can provide additional information if arterial blood is sampled from more than one site. For example, simultaneous right radial artery and umbilical arterial sampling may indicate ductal right-to-left shunt. (With the patient breathing room air transcutaneous oxygen saturations may provide the same information.)

At this point another decision is indicated. You should have enough information to make a diagnosis of cyanotic heart disease (or rule it out) with more than 90 per cent probability. If cyanotic heart disease is diagnosed, arrangements for referral to a pediatric cardiology tertiary center should be initiated. Other management decisions are described later in the chapter.

Throughout the process of evaluating the infant with cyanosis, the health care team should remain alert to possible abrupt clinical deterioration. If the latter occurs, treatment with prostaglandin E_1 should be started without delay as described in the management section of this chapter.

PATHOPHYSIOLOGIC CLASSIFICATION

Cyanotic congenital heart disease can be categorized according to the following scheme: (1) independent pulmonary and systemic circulation; (2) inadequate pulmonary blood flow; (3) admixture of pulmonary and systemic circulations. Lesions characterized either by independent pulmonary and systemic circulation or by inadequate pulmonary blood flow present with severe

TABLE 5–1. CARDIAC CAUSES OF CYANOSIS IN THE NEWBORN

Independent pulmonary and systemic circulations (severe cyanosis)
  Transposition of the great arteries with an intact ventricular septum
Inadequate pulmonary blood flow (severe cyanosis)
  Tricuspid valve atresia
  Pulmonary valve atresia with an intact ventricular septum
  Tetralogy of Fallot
  Ebstein anomaly of the tricuspid valve
Admixture lesions (moderate cyanosis)
  Total anomalous pulmonary venous return

TABLE 5–2. DIAGNOSIS OF THE CYANOTIC NEWBORN

Severe cyanosis (arterial PO_2 breathing 100% O_2 = 20–50 mm Hg)
  Chest radiograph: normal or shunt vascularity with little or no cardiomegaly
    Transposition of the great arteries
  Chest radiograph: decreased pulmonary vascularity
    Tricuspid valve atresia
    Pulmonary valve atresia
    Tetralogy of Fallot
    Ebstein anomaly
Moderate cyanosis (arterial PO_2 on breathing 100% O_2 = 75–200 mm Hg)
  Chest radiograph: increased pulmonary arterial vascularity and cardiomegaly
    Total anomalous pulmonary venous return (unobstructed)

cyanosis unresponsive to additional oxygen in inspired air. Admixture lesions have increased pulmonary blood flow and manifest mild cyanosis.

Transposition of the great arteries with intact ventricular septum exemplifies independent pulmonary and systemic circulations. Examples of lesions with inadequate pulmonary blood flow are tricuspid valve atresia, pulmonic valve atresia with intact ventricular septum, tetralogy of Fallot, and Ebstein anomaly of the tricuspid valve. Admixture lesions are represented by total anomalous pulmonary venous return. Table 5–1 summarizes this approach to classification. Each of the representative lesions mentioned is described in the next section.

SPECIFIC LESIONS

You have now made a diagnosis of cyanotic congenital heart disease and wish to categorize further the type of abnormality. Combining severity of cyanosis, results of the hyperoxia test, and analysis of the chest radiograph provides a diagnostic approach, summarized in Table 5–2. The electrocardiogram adds to the diagnostic framework, particularly in patients with inadequate pulmonary blood flow (Fig. 5–2).

Specific diagnostic information is obtained by performing two-dimensional echocardiography and Doppler echocardiography, provided experienced personnel are responsible for its recording and interpretation. Echocardiography is seldom necessary outside the tertiary pediatric cardiology center. Tertiary level neonatal intensive care units, however, may be faced with diagnostic dilemmas that require echocardiography. Differentiation of persistent fetal circu-

lation from primary heart disease and ruling out heart disease in a newborn infant being considered for extracorporeal membrane oxygenation are two examples. These units must establish methods for resolving the diagnosis and management of these infants.

Newborn With Severe Cyanosis

Normal or Increased Pulmonary Vascularity on Chest Radiograph

Transposition of the Great Arteries with an Intact Ventricular Septum. ANATOMIC AND HEMODYNAMIC FEATURES. Transposition of the great arteries (TGA), produced by a single embryologic defect, results from abnormal septation of the truncus arteriosus. The anterior aorta originates from the right ventricular infundibulum, and the posterior pulmonary artery originates from the left ventricle (Fig. 5–3). The pulmonary and systemic circulations are in parallel. This anomaly is not a problem before birth, where the circulation is always in parallel, but it cannot be survived after birth when a series circuit is required unless bidirectional mixing is possible at one or more sites. Mixing can occur between the aorta and the pulmonary artery via the ductus arteriosus and between the left atrium and the right atrium across a stretched open foramen ovale or true atrial septal defect.

CLINICAL FEATURES. Infants with TGA usually appear otherwise normal, as they have a low incidence of other associated congenital anomalies. They are cyanotic and mildly tachypneic but in no respiratory distress. With inadequate mixing they develop

Cyanotic Newborn with Decreased Pulmonary Vascularity
Electrocardiogram

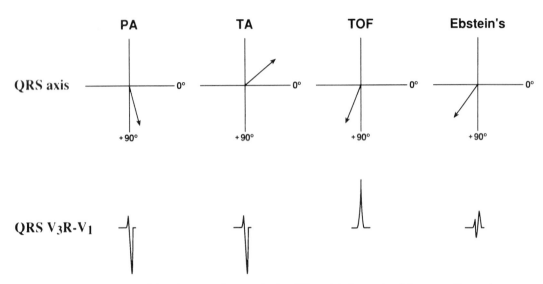

FIGURE 5–2. Use of the electrocardiogram in the differential diagnosis of the cyanotic newborn with decreased pulmonary vascularity on chest roentgenogram. Pulmonary valve atresia with intact ventricular septum and tricuspid valve atresia both have hypoplastic right ventricles. This abnormality manifests in the electrocardiogram by a left QRS axis and small r waves in V_3R and V_1. The difference is that pulmonary valve atresia has a mean QRS in the left inferior quadrant, whereas tricuspid valve atresia has a mean QRS in the left superior quadrant. Tetralogy of Fallot typically has a right QRS axis and right ventricular hypertrophy, usually depicted by 100% R waves in V_3R and V_1. Ebstein anomaly has mild right QRS axis deviation and low-voltage rsR′ complexes in V_3R and V_1. It is the only anomaly in the group that combines right QRS axis with marked right atrial enlargement, which is shown by tall, peaked P waves sometimes taller than the QRS complexes.

severe hypoxemia, and progressive metabolic acidosis may ensue. Cardiac auscultation demonstrates single S_1 and S_2, no clicks or diastolic sounds, and no murmur.

CHEST RADIOGRAPH. Immediately after birth the chest radiograph likely is normal. Essential to the diagnosis is the observation that pulmonary vascularity appears normal or is perhaps even increased in the presence of severe cyanosis (Fig. 5–4). Heart size is normal or slightly increased, but the cardiac contour demonstrates an abnormal "egg" shape created by a narrow mediastinum that is due to abnormal position of the pulmonic trunk.

ELECTROCARDIOGRAM. The electrocardiogram usually is normal.

HYPEROXIA TEST. The resting PO_2 breathing room air is 30 to 40 mm Hg with adequate mixing, less if mixing is poor. With 100 per cent oxygen breathing, the peak PO_2 seldom is more than 50 mm Hg with adequate mixing. With inadequate mixing the PO_2 might not rise above 30 mm Hg.

Decreased Pulmonary Vascularity on Chest Radiograph

Tricuspid Valve Atresia. ANATOMIC AND HEMODYNAMIC FEATURES. With tricuspid valve atresia (TA) the tricuspid valve is absent or nearly so; the right ventricle therefore has no inflow portion and consists only of the right ventricular outflow tract (infundibulum). The pulmonic valve and pulmonic trunk may be small but can be reasonably normal in size. The great arteries are normally related. All of the right atrial flow must cross the atrial septum, usually through a large atrial septal defect. A ventricular septal defect, usually small, provides the only source of pulmonary blood flow after closure of the ductus arteriosus (Fig. 5–5).

CLINICAL FEATURES. Infants with TA often are deeply cyanotic. Auscultation demonstrates a harsh systolic murmur characteristic of a ventricular septal defect. The pulmonic component of S_2 is soft or absent owing to diminished pulmonary arterial

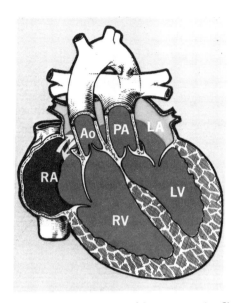

FIGURE 5–3. Transposition of the great arteries. Shading in the heart and vessel lumens indicates relative oxygen saturations. The lightest shading, in the pulmonary veins and superior left atrium, indicates fully oxygenated blood; the darkest shading, in the right atrium, indicates low oxygen saturation of systemic venous blood and intermediate shading indicates mixing of high and low. Bidirectional mixing at the atrial level is indicated by the two arrows. Ao = aorta; LA = left atrium; LV = left ventricle; PA = pulmonary artery; RA = right atrium; RV = right ventricle.

pressure and low-velocity pulmonary blood flow.

CHEST RADIOGRAPH. The heart size is frequently normal, and the pulmonic trunk is absent. Pulmonary arterial vascularity is markedly diminished (Fig. 5–6). The right atrial shadow appears cut off.

ELECTROCARDIOGRAM. (See Fig. 3–11.) There is right atrial enlargement. Characteristically, the mean frontal QRS axis is directed to the left and superiorly between 0 and -90 degrees. The precordial leads show decreased right ventricular forces with small r waves in V_3R and V_1, reflecting the hypoplastic right ventricle. Leads V_6 and V_7 demonstrate dominant R waves.

HYPEROXIA TEST. Arterial PO_2 is low (30 to 50 mm Hg) and does not increase significantly with oxygen breathing.

Pulmonary Valve Atresia With Intact Ventricular Septum. ANATOMIC AND HEMODYNAMIC FEATURES. With pulmonic valve atresia (PA) the pulmonic valve probably becomes atretic early during cardiac development. In some individuals it results in a hypoplastic tricuspid valve and a tiny right ventricular cavity; there may be myocardial

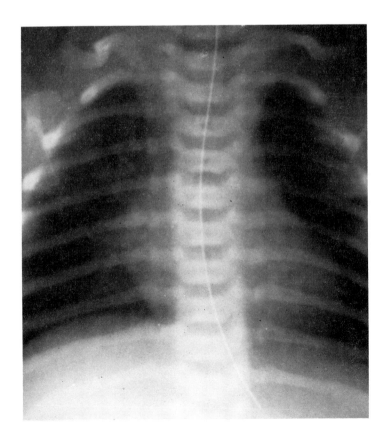

FIGURE 5–4. Chest radiograph of a newborn with transposition of the great arteries. There is minimal cardiomegaly, and pulmonary arterial vascularity is normal to slightly increased. A nasogastric tube is present.

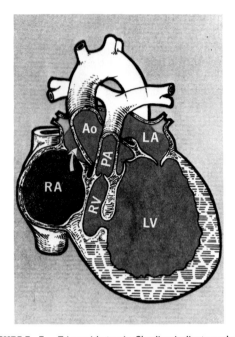

FIGURE 5–5. Tricuspid atresia. Shading indicates relative oxygen saturation as described in Figure 5–3. Systemic venous blood must cross the atrial septum (arrow). The left ventricle is dilated. A small ventricular septal defect gives access to the right ventricular infundibulum and pulmonary artery. Abbreviations are as in Figure 5–3.

sinusoids connecting the right ventricular cavity with the coronary arteries; right ventricular pressure is suprasystemic and sometimes provides retrograde flow into the coronary arteries via these sinusoids. Alternatively, some of these individuals develop a grossly incompetent tricuspid valve, in which case the right ventricular cavity may enlarge and be of any volume up to and including higher than normal. Right ventricular systolic pressure is not as high if tricuspid regurgitation is marked. Both of these types have an obligatory atrial level right-to-left shunt through a stretched foramen ovale or an atrial septal defect. The pulmonic trunk usually is of normal size, as are the branch pulmonary arteries. Pulmonary blood flow is supplied only by the ductus arteriosus.

CLINICAL FEATURES. Infants with PA are severely cyanotic and are prone to sudden clinical deterioration because of ductal dependency. Auscultation may reveal no murmurs in patients with a competent tricuspid valve, as flow through the ductus arteriosus may not be turbulent. There can be a systolic thrill and a grade IV to VI early holosystolic murmur at the lower left sternal edge indicating tricuspid valve regurgitation. S_2 is single.

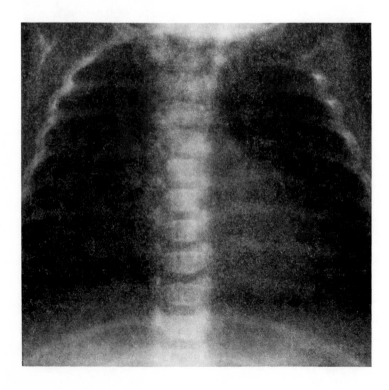

FIGURE 5–6. Chest radiograph of a newborn with tricuspid valve atresia. Heart size is normal, and the pulmonary vascularity is markedly decreased.

CHEST RADIOGRAPH. (See Fig. 2–32.) There is usually cardiomegaly with evidence of right atrial enlargement in proportion to the degree of tricuspid regurgitation. The lung fields are significantly hypovascular.

ELECTROCARDIOGRAM. There is marked right atrial enlargement. The mean frontal QRS axis is usually normal. The precordial leads show absent right ventricular forces and dominant left ventricular forces. Electrocardiographic findings of tricuspid atresia and PA with intact ventricular septum are similar with the exception of the frontal QRS axis (Fig. 5–2).

HYPEROXIA TEST. Added oxygen does little or nothing to the arterial PO_2. Maximal arterial PO_2 is dependent on total pulmonary blood flow but seldom is higher than 50 mm Hg.

Tetralogy of Fallot. ANATOMIC AND HEMODYNAMIC FEATURES. Tetralogy of Fallot results from anterior displacement of the conus septum, the structure that divides the ventricular outflow tracts. Displacement ranges from mild to complete, with the effect of producing degrees of stenosis of the right ventricular infundibulum and pulmonic valve ranging from mild to complete atresia. In regard to right ventricular outflow tract obstruction, therefore, tetralogy of Fallot has a spectrum of severity. Presentation with significant cyanosis at birth implies severe stenosis or atresia. Anterior displacement of the conus septum results in the presence of a large, nonrestrictive, basilar ventricular septal defect (Fig. 5–7). Tetralogy of Fallot cannot have a small or restrictive ventricular septal defect. Total pulmonary blood flow is controlled by the infundibular and valvar stenosis. In patients with pulmonic atresia pulmonary blood flow is supplied by the ductus arteriosus.

CLINICAL FEATURES. The infant with significant stenosis or atresia is cyanotic from birth. Often the baby is small for gestational age, and there is a high incidence of associated anomalies (e.g., VACTERL syndrome). The presence of a high-frequency ejection systolic murmur in the third left intercostal space at the sternal border implies patency of the right ventricular outflow tract. With atresia, there is no right ventricular outflow tract murmur, although a soft, continuous murmur of the patent ductus arteriosus or bronchial collateral vessels may be audible.

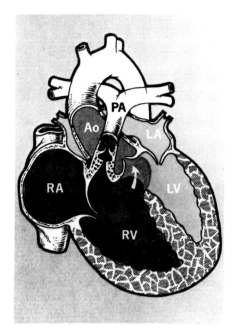

FIGURE 5–7. Tetralogy of Fallot. Shading indicates relative oxygen saturations as in Figure 5–3. There is a large ventricular septal defect that allows shunting from the right ventricle into the aorta (arrow). Right ventricular infundibular stenosis is illustrated underneath the pulmonic valve. Abbreviations are as in Figure 5–3.

An aortic ejection sound due to augmented ejection volume into a large anterior aorta is common. S_2 is single due to the absence of P_2 as a result of low pulmonic trunk diastolic pressure and low pulmonic trunk flow velocity.

CHEST RADIOGRAPH. (See Fig. 2–20.) The heart size is normal, but it has an upturned apex and a concave right ventricular outflow tract–pulmonic trunk area. A right aortic arch (illustrated in Figure 2–12) is present in 25 per cent of cases. Skeletal anomalies are frequently present. The pulmonary arterial vascularity is diminished.

ELECTROCARDIOGRAM. (See Fig. 3–9.) There is often right atrial enlargement. The mean frontal QRS axis is to the right but within the normal range. The precordial pattern, even in newborns, shows right ventricular hypertrophy of the pressure overload type either with pure R waves, rR′, or a qR pattern in the right precordial leads (Fig. 5–2).

HYPEROXIA TEST. Added oxygen does little or nothing to the arterial PO_2. Maximal arterial PO_2 is dependent on total pulmonary blood flow but is seldom higher than 50 mm Hg.

Ebstein Anomaly of the Tricuspid Valve. ANATOMIC AND HEMODYNAMIC FEATURES. The tricuspid valve cusps are derived from the right ventricular myocardium by a process of undermining that separates the inner layer from the rest of the wall. With Ebstein anomaly this process is incomplete and does not reach the valve annulus, leaving part of the leaflet still "attached" to the wall. The redundant free portion of the valve leaflets originates from the right ventricular wall some distance from the tricuspid annulus. The portion of the right ventricle between the annulus and the downward-displaced valve functionally becomes part of the right atrium and is called the "atrialized right ventricle." When severe, the remaining right ventricle is functionally impaired. An atrial septal defect is present in 50 per cent of cases. The risk of Ebstein anomaly is increased in infants born to mothers who take lithium during pregnancy.

CLINICAL FEATURES. These infants may resemble those with pulmonic valve atresia with an intact ventricular septum. Occasionally, they present with supraventricular tachycardia. Shortly after birth the ductus arteriosus is patent, shunting left to right and producing near systemic pulmonary artery systolic pressure. If there is significant tricuspid regurgitation, as is often the case with Ebstein anomaly, the functionally impaired right ventricle might not be able to generate high enough systolic pressure to open the pulmonic valve. This situation makes the tricuspid valve regurgitation worse, and there is a total atrial level right-to-left shunt. The clinical situation therefore mimics pulmonic atresia with intact ventricular septum. As pulmonic resistance drops and the ductus closes, pulmonic trunk pressure falls, and there is a progressive increase of forward pulmonary blood flow, less tricuspid regurgitation, and less right-to-left shunt with spontaneous improvement of the degree of cyanosis. The systolic murmur of tricuspid valve regurgitation is not as loud as it is in the patient with pulmonic atresia and intact ventricular septum; and sometimes it is surprisingly soft because with Ebstein anomaly the right ventricular systolic pressure generally is low. S_2 is variable depending on the pulmonic trunk pressure and the source of pulmonary blood flow. It may be single but can be widely split if there is significant right ventricular conduction delay. Often prominent S_3 and S_4 are present along the lower left sternal border, reflecting right

ventricular filling events. A mid-diastolic right ventricular filling murmur may be present.

CHEST RADIOGRAPH. (See Fig. 2–14.) Cardiomegaly varies from mild to massive depending on the degree of tricuspid regurgitation. The latter also controls the degree of right atrial dilation. Pulmonary arterial vascularity is decreased.

ELECTROCARDIOGRAM. There is marked right atrial enlargement with a P wave that occasionally is taller than the QRS complex; the PR interval is prolonged. There is right axis deviation of the QRS and a right ventricular conduction delay pattern with rsR' complexes in leads V_3R and V_1 and low-voltage R' (Fig. 5–8). Occasionally the electrocardiogram shows Wolff-Parkinson-White syndrome (see Fig. 11–6), with a precordial pattern simulating left ventricular conduction delay, a short PR interval, and initial slowing of the QRS complexes (delta wave). The precordial QRS forces are posterior with dominant S waves in V_3R and V_1.

HYPEROXIA TEST. Added oxygen does little or nothing to the arterial PO_2. Maximal arterial PO_2 is dependent on total pulmonary blood flow but seldom is higher than 50 mm Hg.

Newborn With Moderate Cyanosis

Moderate cyanosis of cardiac origin most likely is due to an admixture lesion. These defects are characterized by mixing of pulmonary and systemic circulations at some level. They have increased pulmonary arterial blood flow resulting in mild systemic desaturation. Representative examples of admixture lesions include various forms of single ventricle (e.g., double-inlet left ventricle) and truncus arteriosus. The scope of this chapter does not allow detailed discussion of each of them. Total anomalous pulmonary venous return (TAPVR) also is a mixing lesion. Its importance derives from the fact that it is a common defect in this group and that it is the only one amenable to complete anatomic surgical correction.

Total Anomalous Pulmonary Venous Return

Anatomic and Hemodynamic Features. The definitive left atrium is formed as the pulmonary veins gain connection to the common pulmonary vein, which arises

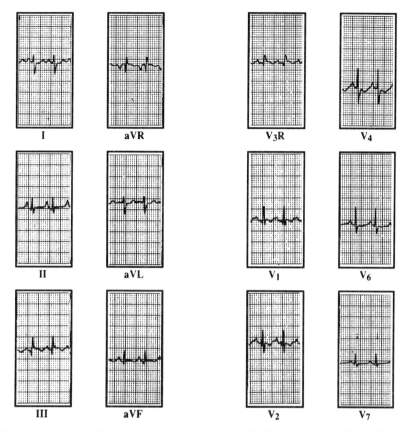

FIGURE 5–8. Electrocardiogram of a 1-day-old infant with Ebstein anomaly of the tricuspid valve. There is right atrial enlargement (tall, peaked P waves in lead II) and right ventricular conduction delay (slow terminal R wave in V_3R). Septal forces are normal showing small q waves in V_6 and V_7.

from the embryonic left atrium. Failure of development of the common pulmonary vein results in TAPVR because the pulmonary veins then must develop some other connection in order to reach the heart. Pulmonary venous return may connect to the left anterior cardinal system and drain via the left superior vena cava either superiorly toward the left innominate vein and right superior vena cava (supracardiac) or inferiorly into the coronary sinus (cardiac); return may be via a long vein that descends behind the heart, through the diaphragm, and eventually into the portal venous system (infracardiac). The pulmonary and systemic circulations mix in the right atrium; blood reaches the left heart only by way of an atrial level right-to-left shunt.

Clinical Features. With cardiac or supracardiac TAPVR the newborn is usually asymptomatic and shows no obvious cyanosis. Systemic oxygen saturation may be as high as 90 per cent. Pulmonary arterial blood flow increases progressively, ulti-

mately causing congestive heart failure, usually by 4 to 6 weeks of age. There is marked volume overload of the right heart, producing auscultatory findings that are similar to those of an atrial septal defect. There is a pulmonary flow murmur and a mid-diastolic right ventricular filling murmur. S_2 is split but not widely, and P_2 is accentuated because of elevated pulmonary arterial pressure. Respiratory variation of S_2 splitting is inapparent.

Newborns with the less common infradiaphragmatic form develop obstruction to pulmonary venous return and become symptomatic within the first few days of life with clinical features that resemble those of severe hyaline membrane disease. Differentiation of these two conditions often is a challenge to the neonatologist and pediatric cardiologist.

Chest Radiograph. Patients with supradiaphragmatic TAPVR show cardiomegaly and widening of the superior mediastinum, producing a characteristic "figure of eight" or "snowman" appearance of the cardiac silhouette (see Fig. 2–19). The pulmonary vascularity is increased of the shunt type. With the obstructive type there is evidence of pulmonary venous obstruction (see Fig. 2–30).

Electrocardiogram. There is right atrial enlargement and usually severe right ventricular hypertrophy, sometimes producing a qR pattern in V_3R and V_1.

Hyperoxia Test. With the supracardiac or cardiac type of TAPVR, the PO_2 may increase to 150 to 200 mm Hg. With obstructed total pulmonary venous return, as in the infradiaphragmatic type, the PO_2 ordinarily does not rise above 75 to 100 mm Hg. Higher levels due to patency of the ductus venosus have been documented, however; and they allow streaming of the oxygenated blood entering the portal system across the ductus venosus and atrial septum into the left atrium. Rarely, the PO_2 in such an individual may reach 200 mm Hg.

MANAGEMENT OF THE CYANOTIC NEWBORN

Prostaglandin E₁

Prostaglandin E_1 (PGE_1) has revolutionized the care of newborns with critical congenital heart disease.[3,4] It is possible to open and maintain patency of the ductus arteriosus with constant intravenous infusion of PGE_1. This regimen is the first line of treatment in any newborn with suspected cyanotic congenital heart disease. The open ductus arteriosus supplies pulmonary blood flow in patients with right heart obstructive lesions. With transposition of the great arteries, mixing improves significantly when the ductus is opened. In situations where cardiologic evaluation is not immediately available, PGE_1 infusion on an empiric basis may be indicated. The usual beginning dosage is 0.1 µg/kg/min, reduced to 0.05 µg/kg/min after a response is obtained. It is important to obtain a clinical result, documented by improved PO_2 prior to reducing the infusion rate. It is advisable to have a transcutaneous oximeter for constant monitoring of systemic saturation. The infusion line should be secure; and it is best to have two functioning intravenous lines.

Side effects of PGE_1 occur.[5] The most important is central apnea, which occurs in approximately 10 per cent of patients. Apnea is more frequent in smaller infants and at the beginning of the infusion; if it occurs,

endotracheal intubation and mechanical ventilation should be performed. It is wise to intubate infants receiving PGE_1 prior to transport to a tertiary center in order to obviate the risk of apnea. Temperature elevation is common in patients receiving PGE_1. It usually is not necessary to reduce the infusion rate. Fever should not be attributed to PGE_1, however, without a negative septic workup.

Oxygen

Increasing the inspired concentration of oxygen to 40 per cent may reduce hypoxemia; it also reduces pulmonary resistance, enhancing pulmonary blood flow.

Intubation and Mechanical Ventilation

As mentioned, cyanotic patients receiving PGE_1 may require intubation and mechanical ventilation. Supraphysiologic positive end-expiratory pressure (PEEP) increases resistance to pulmonary blood flow. Because most cyanotic infants require increased pulmonary blood flow to maintain adequate systemic saturation, PEEP is contraindicated. The only exception is the presence of pulmonary venous obstruction, as in infracardiac TAPVR.

Blood Transfusion

Cyanotic newborns are helped by a high hemoglobin level (15 gm/dl or higher), which can maintain an adequate oxygen-carrying capacity. Correction of a relative anemia results in improvement in the systemic oxygen content.

Several cyanotic lesions, particularly tetralogy of Fallot and truncus arteriosus, are associated with the DiGeorge syndrome. This disorder is characterized by defective T cell immunity and an absence of thymus and parathyroids. In a newborn with any risk of DiGeorge syndrome, in order to prevent graft-versus-host disease, irradiated blood products must be used until a definite diagnosis can be made by assessing T cell function. Serum calcium should be monitored; hypocalcemia should be corrected.

REFERENCES

1. Singer RB: Respiration and circulation. *In* Altman PL, Dittmer DS (eds): Proceedings of the Federation of the American Society of Experimental Biology, Bethesda, 1971, p. 139.
2. Eilers RJ: Notification of final adoption of an inter-

national method and standard solution for hemoglobinometry: specification for preparation of standard solution. Am J Clin Pathol *47*:212–214, 1967.

3. Freed MD, Heyman MA, Lewis AB, et al: Prostaglandin E_1 in infants with ductus arteriosus dependent congenital heart disease. Circulation *64*: 899–905, 1981.

4. Hallidie-Smith KA: Prostaglandin E_1 in suspected ductus dependent cardiac malformation. Arch Dis Child *59*:1020–1026, 1984.

5. Lewis AB, Freed MD, Heyman MA, et al: Side effects of therapy with prostaglandin E_1 in infants with critical congenital heart disease. Circulation *64*:893–898, 1981.

6

NEWBORNS WITH LOW SYSTEMIC OUTPUT

Benjamin E. Victorica

The problem addressed in this chapter is the sudden appearance of totally inadequate systemic arterial blood flow in the newborn. This situation usually is urgent, and rapid management is necessary. Other, less critical causes of congestive heart failure in the newborn are reviewed in Chapter 7. Here the emphasis is on recognition and stabilization of the specific hemodynamic abnormality.

The neonate who presents with low systemic output and congestive heart failure most likely has a left heart obstructive lesion. Onset of cardiovascular collapse immediately after birth strongly suggests that systemic blood flow (often including coronary artery flow) is dependent on patency of the ductus arteriosus (Table 6–1).

ANATOMIC AND HEMODYNAMIC CONSIDERATIONS

The hypoplastic left heart syndrome typically is characterized by the presence of aortic valve atresia, with marked hypoplasia of the mitral valve, left ventricle, and ascending aorta. All pulmonary venous blood crosses the atrial septum to the dilated right atrium where it mixes with systemic venous return. If the atrial septum is intact (prenatal closure of the foramen ovale), the infant also has severe pulmonary venous obstruction. Survival in this setting is rare regardless of therapy. From the markedly dilated right ventricle, blood enters both pulmonary arteries and crosses the ductus arteriosus to supply systemic arterial flow, both distally and proximally, with retrograde flow into the tiny ascending aorta to supply the coronary artery circulation.

Aortic atresia is the most common form of hypoplastic left heart syndrome. Some infants have critical aortic stenosis with minimal forward flow that is inadequate to provide systemic output. A few have severe aortic stenosis with marginally adequate forward flow. This condition therefore is a syndrome in which total left ventricular capacity is determined by the volume flow that has been able to cross the aortic valve during fetal development. In some newborns with critical aortic stenosis the left ventricle is still of small capacity, incapable of providing effective cardiac output even if the aortic obstruction could be relieved. In other infants, however, left ventricular capacity may be reasonable. In this group the left ventricle may even be dilated as well as hypertrophied, although ventricular contractility may be poor with inadequate forward cardiac output through the obstructed aortic valve. Flow patterns in the heart in this situation are identical with aortic atresia; pulmonary venous return crosses the atrial septum, and systemic flow is supplied almost entirely by the right ventricle via the ductus arteriosus. These infants can be helped dramatically by opening the aortic valve even a small amount.

Severe, discrete coarctation of the aorta may present with hemodynamic features similar to those of hypoplastic left heart syndrome—except that if the ductus arteriosus is patent, flow from the pulmonic trunk supplies only the descending aorta. The left ventricle pumps fully saturated blood into the proximal aorta; thus even though left ventricular function may be poor, the right arm and sometimes even the left arm can have higher systolic blood pressure and higher oxygen saturation than the lower ex-

TABLE 6–1. CARDIAC LESIONS WITH DUCTAL-DEPENDENT SYSTEMIC BLOOD FLOW

Hypoplastic left heart
Critical aortic valve stenosis
Severe coarctation of the aorta
Interrupted aortic arch, type B

tremities. The presence of intracardiac left-to-right shunts via an atrial septal defect, a ventricular septal defect, or both significantly influences the oxygen saturation findings.

A specific form of aortic obstruction that is important to understand is true interruption of the aortic arch in which the interruption occurs between the left common carotid artery and the left subclavian artery. This abnormality therefore represents atresia of the left fourth aortic arch, not a true coarctation of the aorta. It is always accompanied by a large ventricular septal defect and often is associated with DiGeorge syndrome. Interruption of the aortic arch of this type has been labeled interrupted aortic arch type B in a classification that considers type A interruption to be that occurring at the usual site of aortic coarctation, that is, distal to origin of the left subclavian artery. Type A, however, is a severe, total (if you will) coarctation of the aorta. It is not necessarily accompanied by a ventricular septal defect and is not associated with DiGeorge syndrome. Lumping these two types of aortic obstruction together has been a source of confusion. Patients with true interrupted aortic arch are totally dependent on right-to-left ductal flow to supply the lower body and left arm. The right subclavian artery may arise aberrantly, distal to the interruption, in which case it too is supplied by the ductus; the left ventricle and ascending aorta provide flow only to the coronary arteries, neck, and head. Because of the large ventricular septal defect and the presence of heart failure, oxygen saturation data may not reflect higher saturations in areas supplied by the left ventricle.

CLINICAL FEATURES

The clinical presentation is similar for all these lesions. The infant seems normal immediately after birth and perhaps for some hours thereafter. As soon as the ductus arteriosus begins closing, however, clinical deterioration is rapid. Initially, the symptoms

and signs are subtle. Lethargy, tachypnea, tachycardia, sweating, and poor suck appear and progressively worsen. Decreased peripheral perfusion is manifested by weak pulses, delayed capillary filling, and ashen skin color perhaps with mild cyanosis. Dyspnea with intercostal and subcostal retractions, nasal flaring, and wheezing indicate severe pulmonary congestion. As the right heart fails, hepatomegaly develops.

Cardiac examination demonstrates a forceful right ventricular impulse. Arterial pulses and blood pressure likely are poor in all locations, but differences can be helpful. With aortic atresia all pulses are equally poor, and extremity blood pressures are equal. With severe coarctation with a closed or closing ductus arteriosus, pulses in the arms, especially the right arm, may be detectably greater than those in the legs, and systolic blood pressure may be higher as well. These abnormalities depend on cardiac output, however. If cardiac output is poor, there may be no detectable difference. After treatment that improves cardiac output, the difference may become apparent; thus reexamination of the infant at regular intervals is essential. With severe coarctation, symptoms and physical findings may be obscured by a widely patent ductus arteriosus. For true interruption of the aortic arch, pulses and blood pressure may be normal only in the right arm. If the right subclavian artery is aberrant, pulses may be present only in the head and neck; these pulses must therefore be examined whenever all the pulses in the extremities are poor.

An aortic ejection sound may be heard in the presence of critical aortic valve stenosis, as may an aortic ejection systolic murmur. With aortic atresia usually no significant murmur is present. S_2 is single with increased intensity of P_2. An occasional patient with severe aortic stenosis may have a narrowly split S_2.

Diastolic sounds, particularly an S_4 or an S_3-S_4 summation sound, are likely. Murmurs from an intracardiac shunt are manifest only if cardiac output is sufficient to generate them.

The chest radiograph shows that cardiomegaly is always present. Pulmonary vascularity is increased owing to a combination of left-to-right shunt and pulmonary venous obstruction.

On the electrocardiogram severe right axis deviation of the QRS, right atrial enlargement, and right ventricular hypertrophy are

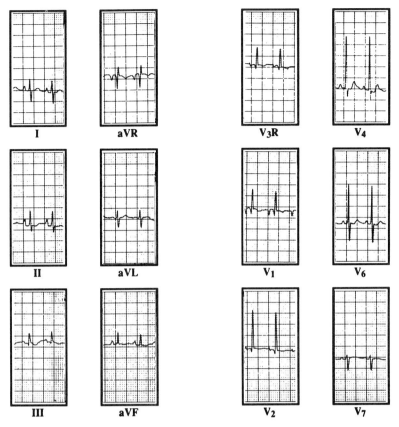

FIGURE 6–1. Electrocardiogram of a 2-day-old infant with a hypoplastic left heart. There is right atrial enlargement (tall P waves in lead II) and severe right ventricular hypertrophy (qR pattern in V_3R–V_1). There are ST-T changes reflecting myocardial abnormality.

almost constant findings (Fig. 6–1). Left ventricular hypertrophy may be seen in the presence of critical aortic valve stenosis with a functioning left ventricle.

LABORATORY FINDINGS

1. *Lactic acid:* Low systemic blood flow with poor peripheral tissue perfusion causes progressive metabolic acidosis that is most rapidly detected by measuring blood lactic acid. In fact, lactic acid may start to increase before arterial pH begins to decrease. Close monitoring of lactic acid levels (arterial or venous) is of great value in the management of these infants.[1] The test requires a minimal amount of blood (0.25 to 0.50 ml), and the results are immediately available (2300 STAT L-lactate Analyzer, Yellow Spring Instruments, Yellow Springs, OH). A blood level of less than 2.0 mmol/liter is normal.

2. *Arterial blood gases:* This vital measurement provides information regarding metabolic acidosis (pH), pulmonary function (PCO_2), and arterial oxygen (PO_2).

3. *Blood glucose:* This measure should be monitored closely, as these patients often develop severe hypoglycemia.

4. *Hematocrit/hemoglobin:* Relative anemia, primary or iatrogenic, can contribute to cardiac failure. Hematocrit should be maintained above 45 to 50 per cent.

5. *Ionized calcium:* It is useful to evaluate the ionized calcium level particularly if DiGeorge syndrome is considered to be a possible complicating factor.

6. *Serum electrolytes:* Many therapeutic manipulations affect electrolyte homeostasis, and the disease process itself may affect renal perfusion. Electrolytes, blood urea nitrogen, and creatinine should be evaluated as often as the patient's condition indicates.

MANAGEMENT

Prostaglandin E₁

Prostaglandin E_1 should be given to newborns with low systemic output caused by left heart obstructive lesion.[2] Reopening and maintaining patency of the ductus arteriosus improves systemic perfusion by allowing unobstructed ductal flow from pulmonic trunk to the aorta, recreating fetal circulation. The starting dose is 0.1 µg/kg/min IV. Systemic perfusion is monitored by physical findings indicating improved peripheral arterial blood flow and by following lactic acid levels. Side effects (apnea, fever) are discussed in Chapter 5.

Intubation and Mechanical Ventilation

Endotracheal intubation and mechanical ventilation is effective treatment for low systemic output with increased pulmonary blood flow and pulmonary congestion, as with left heart obstructive lesions. Supraphysiologic end-expiratory pressure (PEEP) of 8 to 10 and up to 15 cm H_2O increases resistance to pulmonary arterial blood flow and inhibits and possibly reverses alveolar capillary leak.[3] Reduction of pulmonary edema allows better gas exchange and reduces the work of ventilation.

Oxygen

Oxygen is a potent pulmonary vasodilator, a disadvantage when used in patients with ductal-dependent systemic blood flow. Dilation of the pulmonary arterial bed would increase pulmonary arterial blood flow, thereby reducing flow across the ductus into the systemic circulation. For this reason oxygen is contraindicated in these patients.

Diuretics

Diuretics play an important role in the treatment of congestive heart failure. A commonly used diuretic in infants is furosemide, a loop diuretic (1 to 2 mg/kg IV). Dopamine stimulates vasodilator receptors in the kidney, facilitating diuresis. Continuous intravenous infusion in doses ranging between 2 and 5 µg/kg/min increases renal blood flow in patients who have severe cardiac failure and decreased urine output. Preparation of the infusion solution is done by formula: 6 × body wt (kg) equals the milligrams of drug to be added to 100 ml of an intravenous solution. Infusion of this solution at the rate of 1 ml/hour delivers 1 µg/kg/min.[4]

Digoxin

Digoxin (Lanoxin) is commonly used for the treatment of chronic congestive heart failure. It is of limited use in the acute treatment of cardiac failure. Digoxin should not be used in patients with poor systemic perfusion and reduced renal function, as the possibility of digitalis intoxication is significantly increased. This point is particularly true in patients in whom elevated lactic acid levels identify compromised systemic perfusion.

Inotropes

Rapid-acting inotropic agents are of great help in the emergency treatment of heart failure.[5] Dobutamine is a synthetic catecholamine whose mechanism of action is direct stimulation of myocardial beta-1 receptors. It has a more prominent inotropic than chronotropic effect. This drug should be used particularly when there is evidence of significant left ventricular dysfunction.[6,7] The therapeutic dose is a continuous intravenous infusion at 5 to 10 µg/kg/min. Preparation of infusion solution is the same as for dopamine.

Blood Transfusion

Anemia can make cardiac failure worse by placing an extra load on the heart. Hemodynamic improvement can be seen after transfusing packed red blood cells to increase the hematocrit above 45 per cent. Irradiated blood products should be used when there is the possibility of DiGeorge syndrome, as with true interrupted aortic arch.

CONCLUSION

Initial management and stabilization of infants with ductal-dependent pulmonary or systemic blood flow is a challenge to the primary care physician. It is critical, however, to successful definitive care of the cardiac abnormality. Table 6–2 summarizes the basic approach to management of these problems.

TABLE 6–2. MANAGEMENT OF THE NEWBORN WITH CRITICAL CONGENITAL HEART DISEASE

Treatment	Ductal-Dependent Pulmonary Blood Flow	Ductal-Dependent Systemic Blood Flow
PGE_1	Yes; follow PO_2	Yes; follow lactic acid
Intubation	If needed and for transport	Yes
PEEP	No	Yes; 8–10 cm H_2O
Oxygen	Yes	No
Diuretics	If needed	Yes
Digoxin	No	No
Inotropic agents	If needed	If needed
Blood (irradiated)	Hct > 45%	Hct > 45%

REFERENCES

1. Frommer JF: Lactic acidosis. Med Clin North Am 67:815–829, 1983.
2. Jonas RA, Lang P, Mayer JE, et al: The importance of prostaglandin E_1 in resuscitation of the neonate with critical aortic stenosis [letter]. J Thorac Cardiovasc Surg 89:314–315, 1985.
3. Alexander JA, Rodgers BM: Diagnosis and management of pulmonary insufficiency. Surg Clin North Am 60:983–1001, 1980.
4. Committee on Drugs, American Academy of Pediatrics: Emergency drug dose for infants and children. Pediatrics 81:462–465, 1988.
5. Maskin CS, LeJemtel TH, Kugler J, Sonnenblick EH: Inotropic therapy in the management of congestive heart failure. Cardiac Reviews and Reports, June 1992, p. 8–23.
6. Stopfkuchen H, Schranz D, Huth R, Jungst B: Effects of dobutamine on left ventricular performance in newborns as determined by systolic time intervals. Eur J Pediatr 146:135–139, 1987.
7. Martinez AM, Padbury JF, Thio S: Dobutamine pharmacokinetics and cardiovascular responses in critically ill neonates. Pediatrics 89:47–51, 1992.

7

CONGESTIVE HEART FAILURE

Ira H. Gessner

Heart failure is a clinical syndrome characterized by inadequate cardiac performance under existing workload conditions. In other words, the heart is unable to pump enough blood to meet the body's metabolic needs. The condition can be thought of in simple terms as either a primary abnormality of cardiac muscle so the heart cannot manage even a reasonable workload (e.g., primary dilated cardiomyopathy) or an excessive workload that cannot be managed even by intrinsically normal myocardium (e.g., a large ventricular septal defect); it may even be a combination of the two situations. The heart and body attempt to adapt to this set of circumstances by several means, including cardiac dilation and hypertrophy. Systemic and pulmonary venous congestion follow, producing the primary clinical symptoms and signs that in conglomeration are labeled congestive heart failure.

This chapter reviews general physiologic concepts of heart failure, clinical presentation, principles of management, and etiology by age of onset. Some specific cardiac abnormalities that produce congestive heart failure are reviewed as clinical entities. Finally, specific classes of drugs are reviewed, and tables of dosages are provided for commonly used agents. Problems facing the primary care pediatric physician are recognition of the presence of heart failure, initial evaluation and management, and monitoring the status of patients with chronic heart failure.

PHYSIOLOGY OF HEART FAILURE

It is important to have a general comprehension of the physiologic basis of heart failure. This knowledge can aid understanding of the several clinical settings in which heart failure is seen in infants and children and may make therapeutic measures more meaningful. Detailed presentation of this complex subject would be excessive for this book. The interested reader can review appropriate chapters in several textbooks.[1-3]

The primary problem that occurs in heart failure is inadequate systemic output for metabolic demands of the body. The heart may actually be pumping an excessive total quantity of blood, but the amount reaching the body is not sufficient for metabolic demands. This situation occurs in an infant with a large left-to-right shunt (e.g., a large ventricular septal defect). In this case heart muscle is not primarily at fault. Inability of the myocardium to function, on the other hand, or primary pump failure, results in low total cardiac output.

Cardiac output is controlled by several factors: (1) ventricular filling volume, or preload; (2) force acting on ventricular muscle during systole, or afterload; (3) ventricular contractile state; and (4) heart rate. Two heart failure states have already been suggested, and they describe most clinical heart failure in pediatric patients. So-called high-output failure results from conditions that produce excessive volume loading (e.g., a large ventricular septal defect or severe atrioventricular valve regurgitation). Affected chambers are dilated, and ventricular end-diastolic pressure (filling pressure) is elevated. Measures of myocardial contractility may be reasonably normal, and the ejection fraction may be increased.[4] Conditions that affect systemic perfusion predominantly, such as primary pump failure and left heart obstruction, also demonstrate elevated ventricular filling pressure, but ventricular contractility is decreased and systemic perfusion is poor.

The presence of either excessive hemodynamic demands, a primary myocardial abnormality, or both results in several adaptive responses. Most important are (1) the Frank-Starling mechanism, which states that an increase in preload (end-diastolic ventricular volume) results in a greater ejection (stroke) volume; (2) myocardial hypertrophy, sometimes with ventricular dilation; and (3) adrenergic events brought about by increased release of catecholamines. Each of these areas is discussed briefly followed by some additional adaptive mechanisms.

An increase in end-diastolic ventricular volume results in increased stroke volume even though the ejection fraction may decrease. For example, a ventricle with a 30 per cent increase in end-diastolic volume (e.g., from 100 ml to 130 ml) can decrease its ejection fraction from 60 per cent to 50 per cent and still increase its stroke volume from 60 ml to 65 ml. Maintaining ventricular systolic pressure, however, requires an increase in wall stress and in myocardial oxygen demand. It is worth noting that the newborn heart has less diastolic reserve than does the adult heart, and it has decreased compliance, both factors limiting this adaptive response.

Myocardial hypertrophy develops as an adaptive mechanism to maintain systolic wall stress within normal limits.[5,6] Studies in adult patients with compensated left heart failure due to either pressure overload or volume overload have demonstrated that left ventricular systolic stress, end-diastolic pressure, and mass are increased approximately equally in both groups.[7] Ventricular geometry (wall thickness and chamber radius) changes so as to maintain systolic stress within normal limits. Myocardial hypertrophy is an important compensatory mechanism to maintain systolic emptying of the overloaded ventricle, but as a result there may be interference with the ventricle's ability to fill; the result may be diastolic dysfunction. Systolic and diastolic failure are important concepts and are reviewed further.

Heart failure, whether due to ventricular overload or myocardial dysfunction, activates the sympathetic nervous system. Catecholamines released from synaptic terminals stimulate both heart rate and contractility and regulate vascular tone, thereby increasing cardiac output and maintaining satisfactory blood pressure. A decrease in renal perfusion stimulates renin production, which in turn stimulates production of angiotensin II and aldosterone, leading to systemic vasoconstriction and renal salt and water retention. This change causes increased intravascular volume, which by the Frank-Starling mechanism initially improves cardiac contractility and cardiac output. Undesirable effects of these neurohumoral responses include pulmonary and systemic congestion, increased wall stress, and increased myocardial energy requirements.

Other adaptive consequences of heart failure can be mentioned. Heart failure causes an increase in 2,3-diphosphoglycerate resulting in a shift to the right of the oxygen-hemoglobin dissociation curve[8] (see Fig. 5–1). By this mechanism oxygen unloading in the tissues is facilitated, widening the arteriovenous oxygen difference. Atrial natriuretic peptide (ANP) is released from the atrial wall in response to atrial stretch. ANP promotes urinary loss of sodium and water. ANP, a vasodilator, reduces tachycardia by altering baroreceptor function.[9] With chronic heart failure ANP also is synthesized in the ventricles.[10]

Heart failure can be considered, as Parmley has done, to be the end result of a series of hemodynamic alterations and intrinsic compensatory mechanisms.[11] These compensatory mechanisms initially are beneficial, but they frequently exceed the boundaries of improvement, resulting in deleterious effects. These harmful outcomes are what we see clinically as the symptoms and signs of congestive heart failure. Table 7–1 lists the hemodynamic alterations that are common in heart failure. Patients with heart failure due primarily to myocardial disease rather than to excessive workload

TABLE 7–1. HEMODYNAMIC CHANGES IN HEART FAILURE

Increased heart rate

Increased ventricular end-diastolic volume

Increased ventricular end-diastolic pressure

Increased atrial pressure

Increased systemic vascular resistance

Decreased systemic blood flow

TABLE 7–2. COMPENSATORY ADAPTATION DURING HEART FAILURE

Increased heart rate

Frank-Starling mechanism

Sympathetic nervous system activation
  Increased sympathetic tone
  Renin-angiotensin system activation

Increased 2,3-diphosphoglycerate

Increased atrial natriuretic peptides

Myocardial hypertrophy

---

also would demonstrate decreased blood pressure and decreased ejection fraction.

Compensatory mechanisms are summarized in Table 7–2. An increase in heart rate, use of the Frank-Starling mechanism, and beneficial effects of catecholamines on myocardial contractility eventually give way to increased ventricular end-diastolic volume and pressure and to increased systemic vascular resistance as the system is overwhelmed. Myocardial hypertrophy begins quickly and initially is helpful, although eventually chronic hypertrophy leads to decreased contractility.

If the end result of these interactions is overshoot of the compensatory mechanisms, heart failure occurs and if not interrupted therapeutically tends to be self-perpetuating. Compensation for decreased ventricular function and systemic blood flow by an increase in systemic vascular resistance adds to the load on the heart. The renin-angiotensin system causes salt and water retention and systemic vasoconstriction, resulting in excessive intravascular volume thereby inducing tissue fluid accumulation. Medical therapy of congestive heart failure is directed, therefore, at enhancing the beneficial compensatory effects and counteracting the harmful effects.

SYSTOLIC AND DIASTOLIC DYSFUNCTION

Systolic dysfunction, characterized by a dilated left ventricle with reduced ejection fraction, is the most common heart failure syndrome. Diastolic dysfunction is characterized by restricted ventricular filling with preserved ejection fraction. It is recognized now that diastolic dysfunction also is a common heart failure syndrome, although it is due less often to congenital heart defects than to acquired heart disease. A typical example of diastolic dysfunction is hypertrophic cardiomyopathy in which there is marked ventricular hypertrophy, decreased left ventricular lumen, and increased ejection fraction. Hypertrophy, however, is a common response of the failing heart from any cause, therefore a component of diastolic dysfunction occurs in almost all patients with systolic dysfunction. Ventricular compliance (the relation between wall stress and chamber volume) decreases with ventricular hypertrophy.[12] As chamber volume increases, the ventricular diastolic pressure increases, causing higher left atrial and pulmonary venous pressures, promoting further pulmonary congestion.

The newborn ventricle has decreased diastolic function compared to the adult ventricle.[13] This characteristic may make the newborn more susceptible to heart failure.

Diastolic filling of the ventricle also is limited by tachycardia and by elevated end-systolic volume that can come about by pump failure. It is apparent that interaction of systolic and diastolic ventricular function is present in virtually all patients with heart failure.

CLINICAL FEATURES

History

In the newborn the history is seldom useful for the diagnosis of heart failure, as the presentation usually is acute and severe, as discussed in Chapter 6. Knowledge that delivery was stressful or that the mother is diabetic may be important, however. The infant with heart failure has a history that reflects predominantly feeding difficulties. Parents report that the infant seems hungry and sucks vigorously but has difficulty because of rapid breathing and seems to tire readily. The infant rests frequently, prolonging the feeding and then falls asleep only to awaken after a shorter than normal interval and repeat the process. The result is inadequate caloric intake and therefore poor weight gain. This situation creates anxiety and frustration for the parent, compounding the feeding difficulty. Excessive sweating during feeding and sleep is common.

Wheezing and a nonproductive cough are noted often in infants with heart failure, particularly in infants with an enlarged left atrium and increased left atrial pressure, that is, conditions associated with left ventricular failure. Left ventricular failure leads to increased left atrial and pulmonary venous pressure, which causes interstitial pulmonary edema and small airway compression resulting in wheezing respiration. The child with congestive heart failure gives a history of decreased exercise tolerance, fatigue, decreased appetite, and respiratory difficulties such as rapid rate and discomfort on lying down.

Acute onset of heart failure in the child, as may occur with acute rheumatic heart disease, viral myocarditis, or bacterial endocarditis, has historical features pertinent to the etiology as discussed in Chapters 10, 12, and 15. Rather abrupt onset of respiratory symptoms, such as orthopnea, coughing, fatigue, and evidence of fluid accumulation, may be reported.

Infants and children with chronic heart failure that is compensated under medical treatment may develop symptoms of worsening heart failure when stressed by an acute infectious illness. This is true particularly for respiratory infections, to which these patients are especially susceptible.

Physical Examination

The hallmarks of congestive heart failure on physical examination are tachypnea, tachycardia, cardiomegaly, and hepatomegaly. These findings are so common that absence of any one bears explanation whenever a diagnosis of congestive heart failure is made otherwise.

The infant with congestive heart failure breathes rapidly; and if there is significant pulmonary venous congestion, the infant may demonstrate nasal flare, intercostal retractions, and an expiratory grunt. The latter is an attempt by the infant to create positive end-expiratory pressure as the physician might want to do with a mechanical ventilator. Rales are heard rarely. Cyanosis is seldom apparent, although the infant may appear pale with cool, mottled extremities if peripheral perfusion is poor. Arterial pulses are decreased in amplitude if systemic blood flow is decreased. They may seem increased in amplitude because of increased left ventricular stroke volume in a patient with a large ventricular septal defect in whom failure is not severe. Peripheral edema does not occur, although puffiness of the eyelids can be observed. Heart rate is increased and

tends to be fixed in regard to respiration. Cardiac auscultation reflects the particular heart disease or defect. Diastolic sounds, either S_3 and S_4 or an S_3-S_4 summation sound, are present. Absence of all diastolic sound would be unusual in an infant with heart failure.

Enlargement of the liver occurs in all infants with heart failure whether the cause is excessive volume load or inadequate myocardial function. It is important to distinguish between a normal size liver that is displaced down into the abdomen by hyperinflated lungs and a liver that is engorged by venous congestion. The normal liver has a soft, sharp edge, and the liver mass can be pushed up easily by gentle pressure from below. The enlarged liver has a firm, rounded edge and cannot be pushed up more than 1 to 2 cm.

Evidence of heart failure in the child is similar to that just discussed. The child may have dilated veins in the neck and is apt to have rales. Liver tenderness may be apparent, and peripheral edema can occur.

Laboratory Examination

Chest radiography demonstrates cardiomegaly with rare exceptions. In all patients with heart failure the examination is abnormal. If the heart is not enlarged overall, its shape may be abnormal. Pulmonary vascularity (arterial, venous, or both) is abnormal; and pulmonary parenchymal abnormalities such as patchy atelectasis or infiltrates are common. There may be fluid in the fissures and hyperinflation of the lungs; pleural fluid is seen rarely in the child. The pattern of pulmonary edema can be seen with severe left heart failure.

An electrocardiogram is useful for evaluating an infant or child with suspected congestive heart failure. If heart failure is present, the electrocardiogram is not normal. In addition to revealing chamber enlargement, the electrocardiogram may suggest myocardial disease or pericardial disease.

Echocardiography is vital for evaluation of a pediatric patient with congestive heart failure; but as mentioned elsewhere (see Chapters 4 and 8), echocardiography is not part of the evaluation responsibility of the primary pediatric physician. There is one exception to this admonition: the infant in whom acute purulent pericarditis with impending tamponade is suspected (discussed later in the chapter).

Additional laboratory tests can be helpful for the initial evaluation of an infant or child with congestive heart failure, particularly if the patient is unstable. Blood gas assay, pH, and lactic acid determination are important, as discussed in Chapter 6. Serum electrolytes help manage the patient in chronic failure, particularly the patient receiving diuretic therapy. Blood glucose should be measured in all infants with heart failure, as undiscovered hypoglycemia can be devastating. Serum calcium also should be assayed in the newborn or young infant. Hypocalcemia may be a clue to DiGeorge syndrome or to diabetes in the mother. Treatment of congestive heart failure may be impeded if calcium is low. Hemoglobin, hematocrit, and white blood cell count also can provide useful information. Anemia worsens heart failure; and heart failure due to any etiology can cause leukocytosis. Urinalysis may demonstrate albuminuria and microscopic hematuria. Total urine output is reduced in heart failure, and urine specific gravity is high.

MANAGEMENT PRINCIPLES AND ETIOLOGY OF CONGESTIVE HEART FAILURE IN INFANTS AND CHILDREN

Congestive heart failure has many causes in the pediatric age range, but all causes have one of two final common pathways: myocardial damage or excessive workload demands. Specific diseases or defects vary with patient age and therefore are presented here accordingly. Principles of management pertinent to initial therapy by the primary care pediatric physician are reviewed in tandem with etiology for congestive heart failure occurring in the fetus, the first week of life, the infant, and the child or adolescent. These patients should be referred to a tertiary care pediatric cardiology center. Survival, especially of the infant, may depend on successful emergency treatment and prompt referral.

Heart Failure in the Fetus

Heart failure can and does occur in the fetus.[14] It no doubt occurs also in the embryo in which case death and spontaneous abortion probably are the result. Methods for recognizing and treating heart failure in the fetus now exist, and the primary care pediatrician should be aware of it. Table 7–3 lists

TABLE 7–3. CONGESTIVE HEART FAILURE IN THE FETUS

Volume Load
Erythroblastosis fetalis

Arteriovenous malformation

Myocardial Abnormality
Supraventricular tachycardia

examples of causes of congestive heart failure in the fetus. Remember that the fetal circulation is a parallel circuit. Both sides of the heart deliver their blood volume to the aorta, the right side via the ductus arteriosus. It is possible, therefore, for either side to be missing or severely obstructed. As a result, these abnormalities ordinarily do not affect hemodynamic stability in the fetus.

Supraventricular tachycardia leads to myocardial failure in the fetus if it persists just as it does in the infant (see Chapter 11). The obstetrician may recognize the problem by counting the fetal heart rate (usually >300 beats/minute) or by recognizing polyhydramnios. Fetal echocardiography reveals the diagnosis. Administration of digitalis to the mother has been used successfully to convert the fetus to normal sinus rhythm.[15]

For management of a fetus with heart failure the role of the pediatric physician is to act as consultant to the obstetrician. If possible, the mother should be referred for delivery to a high-risk pregnancy facility at which pediatric cardiology consultation is immediately available.

Heart Failure During the First Week of Life

Conditions causing heart failure during the first week of life can be divided into those that depend on patency of the ductus arteriosus for survival and those that result in heart failure regardless of ductal status (Table 7–4).

Etiology and emergency treatment of conditions that are dependent on ductal patency for systemic blood flow have been discussed in Chapter 6. Restoration of ductal patency by administration of intravenous prostaglandin E_1 is the only therapy of significant value. Severe or complete right heart obstruction manifests by critical hypoxemia when the ductus closes, in which case the infant succumbs to hypoxemia before heart failure occurs.

TABLE 7–4.   CONGESTIVE HEART FAILURE DURING THE FIRST WEEK OF LIFE

Ductal-dependent Abnormalities
  Hypoplastic left heart (aortic atresia)
  Critical aortic valve stenosis
  Severe coarctation of the aorta
  Interrupted aortic arch, type B

Non-ductal-dependent Abnormalities
  TAPVR with obstruction
  Arteriovenous malformation
  Myocardial dysfunction syndrome
  Supraventricular tachycardia
  Sepsis

TAPVR = total anomalous pulmonary venous return.

Table 7–4 also lists several conditions that do not require ductal patency for survival. Principles of primary management are directed by specific diagnosis.

Total anomalous pulmonary venous return to the portal vein manifests as severe pulmonary venous obstruction because the common pulmonary vein must descend through the diaphragm, and in doing so it is narrowed. In addition, once the ductus venosus closes, pulmonary venous blood must travel with portal venous blood through the liver. The result is severe respiratory distress, hypoxemia, and heart failure. This condition, however, is one of the few in which heart failure is associated with normal heart size on chest radiograph (see Fig. 2–30). Distinguishing this condition from primary lung disease requires expert echocardiography. These patients, though not dependent on the ductus arteriosus for survival, may benefit from maintaining ductal patency, as it allows some right-to-left shunt from pulmonic trunk to aorta thereby improving systemic blood flow. Mechanical ventilation with room air and some positive end-expiratory pressure are advisable.

A *cerebral arteriovenous malformation* in the newborn can cause severe heart failure. Therapeutic measures are available but depend for their success on rapid diagnosis and referral. The infant presents with heart failure manifested by dilation of all four cardiac chambers, nonspecific flow murmurs with prominent diastolic sounds, and massive hepatomegaly. The chest radiograph shows generalized cardiomegaly with venous and arterial vascular prominence, and the electrocardiogram demonstrates generalized chamber enlargement. The key to diagnosis lies in the physical examination. Arterial pulses are uniformly poor in all four extremities in the presence of congestive heart failure but are increased in amplitude in the neck. Auscultation over the head reveals a continuous murmur. The message is clear. Physical examination of a newborn in congestive heart failure must include palpation of pulses in the neck as well as auscultation of the head. There is no primary therapy of value for this condition other than mechanical ventilation.

Abnormalities that occur in proximity to birth can stress the fetal or neonatal heart, resulting in the *myocardial dysfunction syndrome*. First described by Rowe and Hoffman in 1972,[16] this syndrome affects the entire heart and frequently is characterized by tricuspid valve regurgitation, as first described by the Divisions of Cardiology and Neonatology at the University of Florida.[17] Heart failure can occur with electrocardiographic evidence of global ischemia (again more apparent in the right ventricle) and elevation of myocardial-bound creatine phosphokinase.[18] The syndrome seems to be related to significant hypoglycemic or hypoxemic stress (or both). Primary therapy includes correction of any hypoglycemia and hypocalcemia that may be present. Minimal supplemental inspired oxygen is useful. Mechanical ventilation is seldom required. The principle of avoiding excessive treatment is important because this condition is self-limited and almost all patients recover without sequelae.

Supraventricular tachycardia is discussed in Chapter 11. An infant who is hemodynamically unstable should be electrically cardioverted.

Sepsis is not a cardiac diagnosis but is so important in the differential diagnosis of a critically ill newborn that it must be mentioned as a reminder to maintain vigilance about this possibility.

Heart Failure in the Infant

Heart failure beginning after the first week or two of life can be due to severe left heart obstruction. Particularly important is coarctation of the aorta. Abnormalities that increase pulmonary blood flow (left-to-right shunts and mixing lesions) become the most common cause of heart failure in the infant soon thereafter. Myocardial abnormalities

TABLE 7–5. CONGESTIVE HEART FAILURE IN THE INFANT

Obstruction to Systemic Blood Flow
Coarctation of the aorta
Severe aortic valve stenosis

Left-to-right Shunts
Ventricular septal defect
Endocardial cushion defect
Patent ductus arteriosus

Mixing Lesions
TAPVR without obstruction
Single functioning ventricle without PS
TGA with a large VSD
Truncus arteriosus

Myocardial/pericardial Abnormalities
Supraventricular tachycardia
Myocarditis
Cardiomyopathy
Anomalous left coronary artery
Acute purulent pericarditis

PS = pulmonic stenosis; TAPVR = total anomalous pulmonary venous return; TGA = transposition of the great arteries; VSD = ventricular septal defect.

account for a small number of these patients (Table 7–5).

Severe *coarctation of the aorta* manifests by congestive heart failure that can begin toward the end of the first week of life but often is not recognized until later when it becomes more severe. The infant goes home on the second day of life seemingly well but begins to exhibit rapid respiration, fretfulness, and poor feeding. Recognition that this infant, who is not "doing well" and who shows vague symptoms, may be in congestive heart failure is the absolute key to early recognition of severe coarctation of the aorta. Physical examination by the primary pediatric physician is critical to making this diagnosis. Physical examination must include careful assessment of arterial pulses in all four extremities, assessment of liver size, and thoughtful cardiac auscultation. Diastolic sounds and tachycardia may be present, but a significant heart murmur is not heard. Remember that heart failure severe enough to reduce systemic blood flow substantially may obscure a difference in pulse amplitude and blood pressure between the arms and legs. The lower the cardiac output, the less is this difference. If systolic blood pressure in the right arm is only 60 mm Hg, a systolic blood pressure of 50 mm Hg in the legs may represent a significant difference. Once supportive treatment is begun and systemic blood flow improves, these pressures may rise to 100 mm Hg and 60 mm Hg, respectively. Keep in mind that

physical findings are not absolutes. They must be interpreted in the context of the patient's total picture. Initial management of the infant with heart failure due to coarctation is directed at stabilization prior to transfer to a pediatric cardiology center. If onset of symptoms has been abrupt and the infant is in the first few weeks of life, recent closure of the ductus arteriosus may have occurred, in which case administration of prostaglandin E_1 can be valuable. Hypoglycemia should be corrected and an intravenous diuretic is indicated. Do not give digitalis. The critically ill infant should be managed with mechanical ventilation and intravenous agents as discussed in Chapter 6. Referral should be expedited.

Left-to-right shunt lesions causing heart failure are exemplified by a large ventricular septal defect, an endocardial cushion defect (particularly complete atrioventricular canal), and a large patent ductus arteriosus. Onset of symptoms and signs of heart failure in these patients is gradual, beginning a few weeks after birth as pulmonary vascular resistance decreases and total pulmonary blood flow increases. Points in the history have been described. Physical findings can be subtle. Cardiac auscultation in the infant with either a large, unrestricted ventricular septal defect or a complete atrioventricular canal without atrioventricular valve regurgitation may reveal only flow murmurs, diastolic sounds, and accentuation of the pulmonic component of S_2. Tachycardia, tachypnea, increased precordial activity, and hepatomegaly usually are present.

Mixing lesions are those that manifest heart failure due to excessive pulmonary blood flow in addition to mild cyanosis caused by intracardiac admixture of systemic and pulmonary venous return. Examples of mixing lesions are total anomalous pulmonary venous return (without pulmonary venous obstruction), various types of single ventricle (without significant pulmonary valve or artery obstruction), transposition of the great arteries with a large ventricular septal defect, and truncus arteriosus. If the parents note mild cyanosis, it usually is by recognizing perioral duskiness, perhaps more severe with prolonged crying. Physical findings reflect the specific defects. Abnormal cardiac auscultation and hepatomegaly are uniformly present.

Respiratory infections are common in these infants, although variation in degree of heart failure may be responsible for some symptoms thought to be infectious. Chest radiographs in infants with increased pulmonary blood flow are illustrated in Figures 2–2, 2–27, and 2–28. The electrocardiogram typically demonstrates atrial and ventricular enlargement with significantly increased QRS voltages. Specific diagnostic points, such as a superior frontal axis in an endocardial cushion defect (see Fig. 3–8) may be noted.

Initial treatment of heart failure due to excessive pulmonary blood flow is similar regardless of the specific diagnosis. Acute management includes use of a diuretic agent, avoidance of hypoglycemia, and correction of anemia, if severe. Humidified oxygen administration overcomes ventilation-perfusion abnormalities produced by pulmonary interstitial and alveolar fluid accumulation. The infant with severe congestive heart failure due to a large net left-to-right shunt may be helped significantly by mechanical ventilation with increased positive end-expiratory pressure: It decreases the work of breathing and forces lung fluid into the circulation.

Treatment of the infant with chronic congestive heart failure due to excessive pulmonary blood flow is a joint undertaking by the pediatric cardiology center and the primary care pediatric physician. Definitive diagnosis and management plans should have been established by the center and communicated to the primary physician and the patient's family. Mild to moderate heart failure may be managed with digoxin and diuretics. Vasodilator drugs can be of benefit, particularly in those patients who also have significant atrioventricular valve regurgitation, as may occur with some endocardial cushion defects. Diet of the infant with chronic congestive heart failure is important. Salt restriction is difficult, as low-sodium formulas have not been successful in terms of patient acceptance and adequate growth. The primary care pediatric physician is in a position of responsibility for day-to-day monitoring of patient status. Intercurrent infectious illnesses must be recognized and treated accordingly. Adequate growth should be taking place; if it is not, measures are taken to ensure that it does. The latter may take the form of formula strengthening by increasing calories per ounce and by carbohydrate and fat additives. If inadequate growth persists, the cardiology center should be stimulated to take more aggressive action to modify the underlying problem if possible. The primary care physician also is in a position to supervise patient compliance. This physician knows the family best and should know if parental involvement and care are adequate or if social or financial problems are interfering with proper treatment of the patient.

Management of the infant with *myocardial abnormalities* has been discussed elsewhere. Supraventricular tachycardia is discussed in Chapter 11 and earlier in this chapter. Myocarditis, cardiomyopathy, and anomalous left coronary artery are reviewed in Chapter 12. Kawasaki disease, a rare cause of congestive heart failure, is discussed in Chapter 13. Bacterial endocarditis is almost unheard of in the infant who has not undergone cardiac surgery or chronic intravascular instrumentation.

A cause of acute heart failure in the older infant that demands the best combined efforts of the primary care physician and the specialist is *acute purulent pericarditis*. A previously well infant presents with rather sudden onset of severe respiratory distress, inability to feed, and fever. Symptoms of an upper respiratory infection may have been noted for a day or two. Physical examination demonstrates signs of heart failure with some liver enlargement. Heart tones are poor. There is marked tachycardia out of proportion to the degree of fever or heart failure, and it is this disproportionate tachycardia that may be the best clue to the diagnosis. Chest radiography demonstrates a large cardiac silhouette and evidence of pneumonitis. The electrocardiogram may show diminished voltages in all leads and ST elevation. Appearance of an acute, severe febrile illness with suggestions of heart failure in an infant known to be normal previously should alert the physician to the possibility of this diagnosis. Rapid confirmation of the diagnosis and treatment are essential, as pericardial tamponade and death are distinct threats. If the infant seems hemodynamically unstable (i.e., with signs of low cardiac output; see Chapter 6), there may not be time for referral to a tertiary care center. Echocardiography from any source should be performed without delay. A significant pericardial effusion should be readily identifiable, in which case emergency drainage is indicated. Simple needle aspiration may not be successful in the presence of thick pus. Removal of as little as 20 to 30 ml of fluid (pus, in this case) can be lifesaving. The fluid should be cultured, antibiotics started (preferably intravenously), and the patient transferred as an emergency case to a tertiary care center where open drainage of the pericardium can be accomplished. Do not do anything that may either decrease the heart rate (e.g., administration of digoxin) or increase intravascular volume (e.g., administration of intravenous fluid bolus for "hypotension"), as either may acutely precipitate fatal tamponade. Few events in the field of pediatric cardiology are as dramatic as this one.

Heart Failure in the Child and Adolescent

Heart failure presenting for the first time in the older child or adolescent implies acquired heart disease as the most likely etiology. Complications of congenital heart disease, naturally occurring in the patient or as the result of surgery, also are important causes (Table 7–6). *Rheumatic fever* is discussed in Chapter 10, *myocarditis* and *cardiomyopathy* in Chapter 12, and *bacterial endocarditis* in Chapter 15. *Lyme disease* is a rare cause of myocarditis.

Neuromuscular diseases such as Friedreich's ataxia and muscular dystrophy can affect the heart, causing congestive heart failure. By the time the heart is significantly involved, the primary disease process has long since been manifest. Cancer therapy with *cardiotoxic drugs* such as doxorubicin and daunorubicin now constitutes a significant cause of cardiomyopathy in the child for which cardiac transplantation is the only effective treatment (see Chapter 18). Heart failure may appear years after completion of cancer therapy; it is uncertain whether there is any time limit beyond which myocardial deterioration cannot occur. Cardiac manifestations of *acquired immunodeficiency syndrome* are seen infrequently in the pediatric age range. Myocarditis has been reported infrequently, and endocarditis is rare except in intravenous drug users.

Substance abuse, such as alcohol and cocaine, can cause myocardial degeneration, although it is a rare cause especially in the young. Alcohol-induced cardiomyopathy ordinarily takes years to develop. Cocaine is much more likely to produce sudden death or myocardial infarction than chronic cardiomyopathy in the young individual.

The primary care physician should be alert to changes in patients who have undergone *surgery for complex congenital heart disease* (see Chapters 18 and 19). Patients who had Fontan-type correction for some type of single ventricle may never be assumed to be stable. Complications, including congestive heart failure due to myocardial deterioration, are possible indefinitely. Patients whose surgery included a homograft, such as correction of complex tetralogy of Fallot and truncus arteriosus, as well as those with prosthetic valves also must be considered at risk for the rest of their lives.

The principles of management of these patients by the primary care pediatric physician are not substantially different from those described for the infant. Recognition and early referral of either previously well patients or those with worsening of established disease are the most important points. Acute, severe heart failure with hemodynamic instability is rare in this age group. It requires aggressive primary management options, including diuretics, mechanical ventilation with added oxygen, intravenous inotropic agents, and intravenous vasodilators.

Management of chronic heart failure in this age group usually includes digitalis, diuretics, and vasodilators. β-Blockade is beneficial in some patients.

TABLE 7–6. CAUSES OF CONGESTIVE HEART FAILURE IN THE CHILD OR ADOLESCENT

Acquired CHF
Myocarditis

Rheumatic heart disease

Idiopathic dilated cardiomyopathy

Neuromuscular disease

Cardiotoxic drug therapy

AIDS

Substance abuse

Complications of Existing Heart Disease
Anemia

Bacterial endocarditis

Effects of surgery

Myocardial deterioration

SPECIFIC DRUG THERAPY

Treatment of congestive heart failure has two objectives. Of most importance is elimination of the cause, if possible. Second is pharmacologic therapy designed to ameliorate the consequences of the hemodynamic alterations and compensatory mechanisms discussed earlier in the chapter. Elimination of the cause of congestive heart failure is implicit in the specific etiology; the best treatment for congestive heart failure due to a large ventricular septal defect is surgical closure of the ventricular septal defect. Drug treatment is reviewed here according to specific types: digitalis, parenteral inotropic agents, vasodilators, diuretics, and β-blocking agents.

Digitalis

Digoxin continues to be given to infants and children with congestive heart failure. Its most significant benefits seem to result from its inotropic effect, that is, its ability to increase the force and velocity of ventricular contraction. Digoxin also ameliorates sympathetic tone, decreasing systemic vascular resistance by causing vasodilation, and it slows the heart rate. Both of these actions are energy-sparing to the failing heart.[19] Digitalis may not be beneficial and may be harmful when given to infants with acute left heart obstruction and low systemic blood flow such as may occur with coarctation of the aorta. These infants seem overly sensitive to digitalis; acute toxic effects, including fatal rhythm disturbance, can occur. It seems true that digitalis probably does not literally save lives, but the opposite can occur. Digoxin dosage varies with patient size as indicated in Table 7–7. Half of the total digitalizing dose is given by mouth or intravenously (do not use digoxin intramuscularly), followed by one fourth of the total dose 8 to 12 hours later and the final one fourth 8 to 12 hours after that. A short electrocardiographic tracing is recommended prior to the final one fourth dose to evaluate cardiac rhythm and intervals. The

maintenance dose is one fourth the total digitalizing dose and is given in divided doses every 12 hours starting 8 to 12 hours after the last one fourth of the initial digitalizing dose. Monitoring the serum digoxin level is not necessary unless there is specific reason to believe that a complicating factor or event is present. The therapeutic digoxin level in infants is 1 to 3 ng/ml when the blood sample is drawn approximately 12 hours after the last oral dose.

Most parents learn readily to use the dropper supplied with commercial digoxin. A 1-cc syringe may be preferable for the small dose required by newborns, especially those born prematurely. Parents should be told not to repeat a dose should the infant vomit soon after administration. It is better to err on the side of too little than to risk giving too much. Cessation of digoxin therapy appears to be haphazard. Pediatric cardiologists as a group seem to be reluctant to discontinue the drug, with the result that many infants taking digoxin eventually outgrow their dose. At some point someone finally determines that the maintenance dose is less than therapeutic, the patient is doing well, and the drug is discontinued. It seems likely that most patients over 1 year of age taking digoxin for treatment of volume overload problems would do just as well without it.

In the adult population there is now evidence that inotropic drugs may be detrimental for the treatment of chronic heart failure.[20] It is possible that inotropic agents, by increasing energy expenditure, can increase myocardial cell damage. The literature on adults suggests that pure inotropic agents shorten survival in patients with chronic congestive heart failure.[21] Whether these observations have applicability for pediatric patients remains to be determined.

Parenteral Inotropic Agents

Severe congestive heart failure in the infant or child may require more aggressive acute inotropic therapy (Table 7–8). Several agents are available for parenteral administration by constant infusion. Dobutamine is a sympathomimetic agent that has a predominantly inotropic effect, increasing contractility with little effect on heart rate. It causes an increase in cardiac output and a decrease in systemic vascular resistance.[22]

Dopamine is a catecholamine precursor of epinephrine. In low doses (<5 μg/kg/min) it

TABLE 7–7. DIGOXIN DOSAGE

Age	Total Digitalizing Dose (μg/kg PO or IV)
Newborn	
Premature	20
Full term	30
Infant	40
Child	20–30
Maximum	1 mg

TABLE 7–8. PARENTERAL INOTROPIC AGENTS: DOSAGE

Agent	Dose (µg/kg/min)
Dobutamine	5–10
Dopamine (renal effects)	2–5
Amrinone	5–10 (after 0.75 mg/kg loading dose)

TABLE 7–9. VASODILATORS: DOSAGE

Agent	Route	Dose
Captopril	PO	Infants and children: 0.1–2.0 mg/kg/dose q6–12h (6 mg/kg/day max.)
		Adolescents: 6.25–25 mg/dose q8–12h (50–75 mg/day max.)
Enalapril	PO	Adolescents: 2.5 mg qid to 15 mg bid

acts primarily to increase renal blood flow, promoting loss of sodium and water.[23] In doses of 10 to 20 µg/kg/min, dopamine has primarily inotropic effects, but it can cause rhythm disturbances. For this reason it is not advisable to use dopamine as an inotropic agent.

A new class of inotropic agents has proved beneficial for management of severe heart failure, particularly heart failure due to myocardial abnormality.[24] These drugs, of which amrinone is the best known, are chemically different than either digitalis glycosides or sympathomimetic agents. Amrinone acts by inhibiting phosphodiesterase activity, resulting in buildup of cyclic adenosine monophosphate (cyclic AMP). This action appears to be responsible for both positive inotropic and vasodilator effects of this drug. In the myocardium, cyclic AMP results in increased intracellular calcium, thereby enhancing contractility. As mentioned above when discussing digitalis, however, agents that increase cellular levels of cyclic AMP increase energy expenditure by the cell and in the long run may be detrimental. Amrinone also has noteworthy side effects including thrombocytopenia and liver toxicity, warranting close monitoring. Despite these admonitions, amrinone has proved to be an exceptionally valuable agent for acute treatment of severe congestive heart failure.

Vasodilators

Direct-acting vasodilating agents have been of considerable use for acute and chronic management of congestive heart failure. Vasodilator therapy includes arteriolar dilation, which decreases afterload and thereby increases cardiac output, and venous dilation, which decreases preload and thereby decreases pulmonary congestion.

An important class of vasodilators is the angiotensin-converting enzyme (ACE) inhibitors exemplified by captopril and enalapril[25] (Table 7–9). These agents inhibit formation of angiotensin II, which is the end result of the renin-angiotensin adaptive mechanism; angiotensin II is a potent vasoconstrictor. This inhibition also decreases aldosterone secretion, thereby promoting renal secretion of sodium and water. Captopril decreases systemic vascular resistance and increases venous capacitance, thereby increasing cardiac output. Enalapril has been reported to be more effective in its renal actions.[26] ACE inhibitors seem to have beneficial effects in the adult that exceed their vasodilation activity. How the benefit occurs and whether it is useful for treating the young patient is undetermined. Medical supervision with the patient at bed rest is required at the initiation of these agents because occasionally severe hypotension occurs.

Other vasodilator agents such as nitroglycerin, hydralazine, and calcium channel blocking agents are not discussed. The interested reader is referred to textbooks of pediatric cardiology for further description.[1-3]

Diuretics

Diuretics are designed to promote excretion of salt and water, whose retention is a consequence of the adaptive mechanisms set in motion by the onset of congestive heart failure (Table 7–10). Diuresis is promoted by improving renal blood flow, as just described under vasodilators. Increased flow delivers salt and water to the renal tubules; and diuretic agents act directly to promote their loss.

Furosemide is the most commonly used diuretic in the pediatric group. It is a loop diuretic that acts on the ascending loop of Henle to block sodium and free water reabsorption. Furosemide has the undesirable effect of promoting potassium loss, however,

TABLE 7–10. DIURETICS: DOSAGE

Agent	Route	Dose
Furosemide	IV	1 mg/kg/dose q8–12h
	PO	2–5 mg/kg/day divided bid or tid
Chlorothiazide	PO	<6 months age: 20–30 mg/kg/day divided q8–12h
		>6 months age: 10–20 mg/kg/day divided q12h (max. 2 gm/day)
Spironolactone	PO	1.5–3.5 mg/kg/day divided q12h

and supplemental potassium usually is given with it.

Thiazide diuretics also impede sodium reabsorption and promote free water loss. Potassium loss also occurs with these agents.

Spironolactone is a specific aldosterone antagonist. It impairs reabsorption of sodium and secretion of potassium; therefore potassium loss is not a consequence of its use. Spironolactone is effective only if aldosterone levels are increased. It does not promote free water loss. Spironolactone is used most commonly in association with other diuretics that do cause potassium loss.

Diuretic therapy successfully removes salt and water, but effective diuresis in patients with severe congestive heart failure can produce significant volume depletion resulting in low cardiac output that could lead to renal and hepatic failure. It is important to monitor patient status carefully and often. Serum electrolytes, blood urea nitrogen, and creatinine should be evaluated regularly. Hyponatremia is a risk if the patient ingests excessive water. Potassium loss enhances hydrogen ion loss, which may lead to metabolic alkalosis. Hyponatremia and metabolic alkalosis can be managed conservatively by withholding the diuretic and allowing some additional salt intake for a few days. Rapid elevation of sodium by intravenous administration of hypertonic salt solution should not be undertaken. Here again it is important to know the patient and not to simply react to a laboratory value.

β-Blockade Therapy

β-Blockade has been used for treatment of heart failure associated with diastolic dys-

function as might occur in hypertrophic obstructive cardiomyopathy. There is evidence that β-blockade is beneficial in adult patients with chronic systolic congestive heart failure such as dilated cardiomyopathy.[27] Indeed, Katz suggested that β-blockers may become the most important agents for treating mild congestive heart failure in the adult and in those with severe left ventricular dysfunction who can tolerate this form of therapy.[20] Katz pointed out that β-blockade slows energy expenditure in myocardial cells and may reduce maladaptive myocardial cell growth by blunting cyclic AMP stimulation. Once again, usefulness of this therapy in pediatric patients remains to be determined.

REFERENCES

1. Garson A, Bricker JT, McNamara DG (eds): The Science and Practice of Pediatric Cardiology. Philadelphia, Lea & Febiger, 1990.
2. Adams FH, Emmanouilides GL, Riemenschneider TA (eds): Moss' Heart Disease in Infants, Children, and Adolescents. 4th Ed. Baltimore, Williams & Wilkins, 1989.
3. Braunwald E (ed): Heart Disease: A Textbook of Cardiovascular Medicine. 4th Ed. Philadelphia, WB Saunders, 1992.
4. Sahn DJ, Vaucher Y, Williams DC, et al: Echocardiographic detection of large left-to-right shunts and cardiomyopathies in infants and children. Am J Cardiol 38:73–79, 1976.
5. Gunther S, Grossman W: Determinants of ventricular function in pressure overload hypertrophy in man. Circulation 59:679–688, 1979.
6. Donner R, Carabello BA, Black I, Spann JF: Left ventricular wall stress in compensated aortic stenosis in children. Am J Cardiol 51:946–951, 1983.
7. Grossman W, Jones D, McLaurin LP: Wall stress and patterns of hypertrophy in the human left ventricle. J Clin Invest 56:56–64, 1975.
8. Versmold HT, Linderkamp O, Dohlemann C, et al: Oxygen transport in congenital heart disease: influence of fetal hemoglobin, red cell pH and 2,3-diphosphoglycerate. Pediatr Res 10:566–570, 1976.
9. Kikuchi K, Nishioka K, Ueda J, et al: Relationship between plasma atrial natriuretic polypeptide concentration and hemodynamic measurements in children with congenital heart diseases. J Pediatr 111:335–342, 1987.
10. Takemura G, Fujiwara H, Korike K, et al: Ventricular expression of atrial natriuretic polypeptide and its relations with hemodynamics and histology in dilated human hearts. Circulation 80:1137–1147, 1989.
11. Parmley WW: Pathophysiology of Congestive Heart Failure. Clin Cardiol (Suppl I):I5–I12, 1992.
12. Grossman W, Barry WH: Diastolic pressure-volume relations in the diseased heart. Fed Proc 39:148–155, 1980.

13. McPherson RA, Kramen MF, Covell JM, et al: A comparison of the active stiffness of fetal and adult cardiac muscle. Pediatr Res *10*:660–664, 1976.

14. Kleinman CS, Donnerstein R, DeVore G, et al: Fetal echocardiography for evaluation of in utero congestive heart failure. N Engl J Med *306*: 568–575, 1982.

15. Harrigan JT, Kangos JJ, Sikka A, et al: Successful treatment of fetal congestive heart failure secondary to tachycardia. N Engl J Med *304*:1527–1529, 1981.

16. Rowe RD, Hoffman T: Transient myocardial ischemia of the newborn infant: a form of severe cardiorespiratory distress in full-term infants. J Pediatr *81*:243–250, 1972.

17. Bucciarelli RL, Nelson RM, Egan EA, et al: Transient tricuspid insufficiency of the newborn: a form of myocardial dysfunction in stressed newborns. Pediatrics 59:330–337, 1977.

18. Nelson RM, Bucciarelli RL, Eitzman DV, et al: Serum creatine phosphokinase MB fraction in newborns with transient tricuspid insufficiency. N Engl J Med 298:146–149, 1978.

19. Ferguson DW, Berg WJ, Sanders JS, et al: Sympathoinhibitory responses to digitalis glycosides in heart failure patients: direct evidence from sympathetic neural recordings. Circulation *80*: 65–77, 1989.

20. Katz AM: Heart failure in 2001: a prophecy. Am J Cardiol *70*:126c–131c, 1992.

21. Packer M, Carver JR, Rodheffer RJ, et al: Effect of oral milrinone on mortality in severe chronic heart failure. N Engl J Med *325*:1468–1475, 1991.

22. Driscoll DJ, Gillette PC, Duff DF, et al: Hemodynamic effects of dobutamine in children. Am J Cardiol *43*:581–585, 1979.

23. Goldberg LI, Rajfer SI: Dopamine receptors application to clinical cardiology. Circulation *72*: 245–248, 1985.

24. Colucci WS, Wright RF, Braunwald E: New positive inotropic agents in the treatment of congestive heart failure. N Engl J Med *314*:349–358, 1986.

25. Artman M, Graham TP: Guidelines for vasodilator therapy of congestive heart failure in infants and children. Am Heart J *113*:994–1005, 1987.

26. Hirsch AT, Talsness CE, Smith AD, et al: Differential effects of captopril and enalapril on tissue renin-angiotensin systems in experimental heart failure. Circulation 86:1566–1574, 1992.

27. Gilbert EM, Anderson JL, Deitchman D, et al: Long-term β-blocker vasodilator therapy improves cardiac function in idiopathic dilated cardiomyopathy: a double-blind, randomized study of bucindolol versus placebo. Am J Med 88: 223–229, 1990.

8

EVALUATION OF THE INFANT AND CHILD WITH A HEART MURMUR

Ira H. Gessner

The most common reason for referring an infant or child to a pediatric cardiologist is the presence of a heart murmur. The most common final diagnosis for these patients is an innocent (normal) heart murmur. It is important therefore to review this topic in detail because it is here that a significant impact can be made on the quality of health care including costs. It would be unreasonable to suggest that the primary care physician should be able to diagnose all heart murmurs as either innocent or pathologic. It is possible, on the other hand, to improve on current medical practice, which is one of the foremost objectives of this book.

How frequently does a murmur, any murmur, occur in the pediatric age group? Studies have suggested that virtually all children demonstrate a heart murmur at some time during childhood.[1] Acting on this knowledge, you should begin a routine physical examination in a child with the expectation that a heart murmur will be heard. Just as you examine the ears expecting that you will need to evaluate the structure of the eardrums, you should listen to the precordium with the expectation that you will hear and need to evaluate a heart murmur. Probabilities are that it is a systolic murmur and that it is a vibratory Still's murmur, a pulmonic flow murmur, or both. Just as you know the landmarks on an eardrum so you can recognize any deviation from normal, you should know the characteristics of these innocent murmurs so you can recognize a different, perhaps pathologic, murmur. It is the challenge to the primary care physician to make

this yes–no decision, innocent or not, that is at the core of primary pediatric cardiovascular diagnosis.

The problem addressed in this chapter is the evaluation of an asymptomatic infant or child with a heart murmur, emphasizing murmur recognition, interpretation, and management, including the decision regarding referral to a pediatric cardiologist. Referral of normal infants and children for specialist evaluation is common, and many factors influence the decision to do so. An innocent murmur can be accentuated by circumstances that increase cardiac output. Fever is probably the most common such cause, and anemia and patient anxiety are others. Chest pain and palpitations are common complaints in children and adolescents, as discussed in Chapters 9 and 11. These symptoms focus attention on the heart, with the result that a murmur that might not otherwise have been considered potentially significant is now noted, resulting in anxiety for the doctor as well as for the parent. Request for clearance to play sports is another significant source of these referrals, as the examining primary physician may be unwilling to sign an authorization after having heard a heart murmur. This situation is particularly true after casual examinations by physicians unfamiliar with the patient, as might occur in the now ubiquitous walk-in clinics; the examining physician reports to the parents that a murmur is present but does not want to evaluate it further. Some physicians may be insecure about making a diagnosis of an innocent murmur. Such insecurity, resulting in referral, may derive from lack of training or lack of readily available support from colleagues.

It is appropriate here to discuss the usefulness of laboratory tests for evaluating an asymptomatic heart murmur. It is just such tests that hold the potential for greatly increasing the cost of evaluation. There have been several studies of this question, two of which suffice to make the point that laboratory tests add almost nothing to the initial diagnosis by an experienced listener that a murmur is either innocent or pathologic. Newburger et al., in a study from Boston Children's Hospital published in 1983, found that performing routine electrocardiography, chest radiography, and M-mode echocardiography in 142 children diagnosed as normal by physical examination identified only five patients with probable heart disease, three of whom were thought to have mitral valve prolapse, a diagnosis that could be challenged as inadequate by echocardiography alone.[2] The other two patients had a stable asymptomatic cardiomyopathy. In the second study Smythe and colleagues, at Children's Hospital of Eastern Ontario, in 1990 described 1061 patients age 1 month to 17 years (median 3.2 years).[3] They compared the clinical diagnosis of a heart murmur by a pediatric cardiologist after physical examination alone with the diagnosis after electrocardiography and two-dimensional echocardiography that included Doppler and color Doppler flow analysis. After electrocardiography alone, no diagnosis was changed. After two-dimensional echocardiography the clinical diagnosis of "normal" in 109 patients was changed to "pathologic" in only two: one with a small ventricular septal defect and one with a small atrial septal defect. The latter diagnosis likely cannot be made by physical examination. In 46 patients thought to be abnormal by physical examination, the diagnosis was changed to innocent murmur in three patients after addition of laboratory studies. These two studies provide strong support for the contention that skilled evaluation of a heart murmur is sufficient to allow a yes–no, normal–abnormal decision in almost 100 per cent of patients. The physical examination in these studies was done by a pediatric cardiologist. It is hoped that an experienced, motivated children's physician can do almost as well.

The remainder of this chapter addresses the observation that a murmur is present.

You have heard the murmur and you have made some fundamental decisions regarding its characteristics, particularly its timing and location on the chest. It is assumed that you have an initial impression as to etiology of the murmur. The discussion that follows therefore is organized according to timing and diagnosis.

SYSTOLIC MURMURS

Figure 8–1 expands on the four etiologies of systolic murmur described in Chapter 1. Each is discussed further in this chapter. All innocent systolic murmurs are caused by blood flow in response to ventricular contraction and therefore must be mid-systolic in timing, as they cannot occupy isovolumetric contraction (see Chapter 1).

Innocent Systolic Murmurs

Vibratory (Still's) Murmur

The vibratory murmur initially reported by Still in 1909[4] has been described by a plethora of adjectives, including twangy-string, violin string, and harmonic. Vibratory is a useful term because the murmur tends to have uniform frequency characteristics and to be much less noisy than most other heart murmurs, as clearly demonstrated by phonocardiography (Fig. 8–2). The murmur can be of almost any pitch. It usually is of medium to low frequency, and it is always harmonic. Its point of maximal intensity is located most often in the 4th to 5th intercostal space a few centimeters to the left of the sternal border, that is, over the midprecordium. Occasionally it is maximal at the apex. This murmur, heard best with the stethoscope bell, begins well after S_1, is rarely louder than grade 2, and often has a distinctive double peak (Fig. 8–2) that gives it a groaning character. The murmur tends to disappear with sitting or standing and with exercise.

The *cause* of the vibratory murmur remains at issue. Evidence exists that the murmur may originate either from turbulence in the left ventricular outflow tract[5] or as a result of fibrous bands that cross the left ventricular lumen.[6] It also has been suggested that vibrations of chordae tendineae of the tricuspid valve are responsible, the sound being generated by Aeolian tones.[7]

The *differential diagnosis* of the vibratory

SYSTOLIC MURMUR

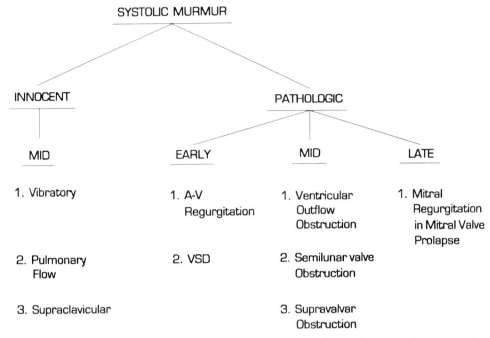

FIGURE 8–1. Differential diagnosis of systolic murmurs by time of onset during systole. A-V = atrio-ventricular valve; VSD = ventricular septal defect.

murmur is concerned most often with distinguishing it from the murmur of either a small ventricular septal defect or mitral regurgitation, both of which begin early during systole, occupying isovolumetric contraction. This pattern is never seen with the vibratory murmur. The murmur of a small ventricular septal defect is harsh and noisy and tends to radiate to the right sternal edge. The mur-

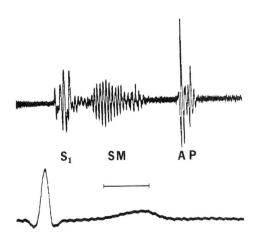

S_1 SM A P

FIGURE 8–2. Phonocardiogram from a child with a vibratory (Still's) innocent murmur. Note the multiple components of S_1, the uniform frequency of the systolic murmur, and the split S_2. Systole is approximately 0.24 seconds in duration. S_1 = first heart sound; SM = systolic murmur; A = aortic component of S_2; P = pulmonic component of S_2; horizontal line = 0.1 second.

mur of mitral regurgitation is of higher frequency, does not have a groaning character, is maximal at the apex, and radiates toward the left axilla or left base. Murmurs of either right or left ventricular outflow tract obstruction might be considered in the differential diagnosis of a vibratory murmur. With both of these conditions the murmur is rougher and noisier and does not have the harmonic quality of a vibratory murmur. In all of the pathologic conditions mentioned, additional findings, such as a palpable thrill or lift, an ejection sound, or abnormal splitting of S_2, would differentiate between an innocent murmur and a pathologic murmur.

Management of an innocent vibratory murmur has been alluded to earlier. No laboratory tests are necessary. What do you tell the parents? In simple terms you tell them that the child has an innocent heart murmur, there is no evidence of heart disease or defect, and no further evaluation is needed. You may explain to parents that the word murmur simply means noise, and that normal movement of blood through the heart and great vessels creates sound, as does water flowing through a garden hose, a phenomenon familiar to almost everyone. Mention that the murmur likely will become less obvious with advancing age as the resting heart rate slows and the chest wall becomes thicker. It is important to make this explanation with confidence. Do not be wishy-washy. It may be helpful to use a brochure on innocent heart murmurs such as that published by the American Heart Association; or you may want to write your own. Do not send the patient to a traveling echocardiography service or to a cardiologist who does not care for children on a regular basis. Doing so would only create problems and cause expense. If you cannot make a decision on the basis of physical examination alone, ask for a specialist consultation. You may elect to obtain an electrocardiogram provided either that you are able to interpret it or you have pediatric electrocardiographic interpretation readily available, and provided that a normal electrocardiogram will convince you that your diagnosis of innocent murmur is correct.

Pulmonic Flow Murmur

The pulmonic flow murmur is described as a mid-systolic, midfrequency ejection murmur best heard in the second or third left intercostal space at the sternal border with radiation to both right and left lung fields. It begins well after S_1 and usually is no louder than grade 2, never more than grade 3. It ends before either component of S_2. The murmur is common in children and is frequently observed in premature infants for reasons related to its etiology. The murmur is accentuated by conditions that increase cardiac output, particularly fever or anemia. The murmur decreases when the child sits and decreases during inspiration.

This murmur is *caused* by turbulent flow in the pulmonic trunk and at the origins of the right and left pulmonary arteries. Turbulence at the latter locations is often prominent in premature infants, explaining the increased incidence and prominence of this murmur in those patients.

The *differential diagnosis* of the murmur is best accomplished by evaluating the company it keeps. In other words, no pathologic findings are associated with the innocent pulmonic flow murmur. The location of the murmur directs the diagnosis to either an innocent murmur or some abnormality associated with right ventricular ejection, for example, pulmonic stenosis or an atrial septal defect. Pulmonic valve stenosis, described further later in the chapter, may produce a murmur loud enough to cause a systolic thrill in the second left intercostal space; but if so, the observer seldom confuses it with an innocent murmur. Even with mild stenosis and a softer murmur, there is a pulmonic ejection sound, the murmur is both low frequency and noisy, and S_2 splits more widely than normal (while maintaining normal respiratory variation). None of these features occurs with an innocent pulmonic flow murmur. The innocent pulmonic flow murmur may not be distinguishable from mild anatomic obstruction of the pulmonary arteries, so-called coarctation of the pulmonary artery. This point is discussed further later in the chapter.

An atrial level left-to-right shunt (e.g., *atrial septal defect*) detectable by auscultation causes a right ventricular parasternal lift due to a dilated right ventricle. It causes a systolic murmur at the second left intercostal space that is, in fact, the same murmur as the innocent pulmonic flow murmur, usually somewhat louder but still no more than grade 2 to 3. It is louder for the same reason that the innocent murmur increases with fever or exercise (i.e., greater flow). S_2 is widely split, does not vary with respiration, and the intensity of both components is normal (see Fig. 1–8). There is a mid-diastolic right ventricular filling murmur at the lower left sternal border, but you must listen specifically for it; it does not immediately come to your attention. Of the three auscultatory features of an atrial level left-to-right shunt—systolic murmur, widely split fixed S_2, and diastolic murmur—least specific is the systolic murmur. The systolic murmur, however, is what you notice first because it is the most obvious. When you hear this murmur, your evaluation should specifically focus your attention both on S_2 and on early diastole at the lower left sternal border. If your findings suggest that an atrial level left-to-right shunt is present, a chest radiograph and electrocardiogram should readily clarify the issue. You cannot hear the auscultatory effects of an atrial septal defect that is too small to cause changes on both the chest radiograph and electrocardiogram. The chest radiograph (Fig. 8–3) demonstrates increased pulmonary arterial vascularity with prominence of the pulmonic trunk and right heart enlargement. The electrocardiogram (see Fig. 3–22) demonstrates right ventricular enlargement. It is not necessary to differentiate between types of atrial level shunts. Once you make the initial diagnosis, specialist referral is indicated.

Management of the innocent pulmonic flow murmur is simple explanation of nor-

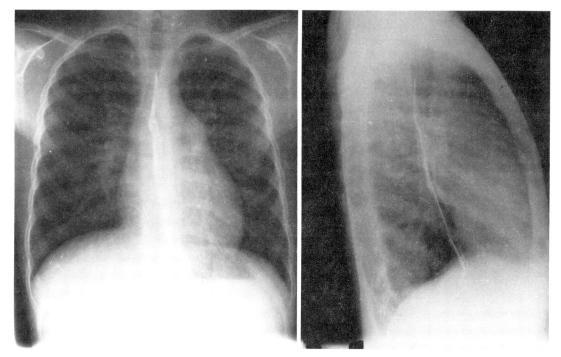

FIGURE 8–3. Posteroanterior and lateral chest roentgenograms with barium in the esophagus of a child with an atrial septal defect. Note the rounded, upturned cardiac apex, indicating right ventricular enlargement, prominent pulmonic trunk and pulmonary arterial vascularity, and an absence of left atrial enlargement.

mality to the parents and avoidance of additional tests. Most patients with an innocent pulmonic flow murmur are readily identified as such.

Supraclavicular Systolic Murmur

The supraclavicular systolic murmur is described as an early systolic ejection murmur that is of short duration and best heard underneath the right clavicle with radiation to the neck, particularly on the right.[8] The murmur is grade 2, occasionally grade 3. Murmur intensity can be decreased substantially by asking the child to sit and hyperextend the shoulder by bringing the arms back.

The murmur is *caused* by turbulence in the major brachiocephalic arteries as they arise from the aorta. It seldom creates a problem of differential diagnosis in the child.

Pathologic Systolic Murmurs

Early Systolic Murmur

If the physical examination has convinced you that the patient has an early systolic murmur (see Fig. 1–9), consider two possible explanations: atrioventricular valve re-

gurgitation or a ventricular septal defect. These conditions are the only ones of significance that produce a murmur occupying isometric contraction. Distinction between these two abnormalities ordinarily is not difficult.

Ventricular Septal Defect. Characteristic findings in a child with a moderate ventricular septal defect include a systolic thrill at the lower left sternal border, a grade 4 to 5 noisy, harsh holosystolic murmur in the same location, and no significant changes in S_2. A mid-diastolic apical left ventricular filling murmur suggests that flow through the defect is large enough that pulmonary blood flow is at least twice systemic blood flow with the child at rest. Occasionally, it is possible to hear an early systolic ejection sound at the lower left sternal border with the child sitting, caused by filling of a so-called aneurysm of the ventricular septum; the latter is formed by tissue on the right ventricular side of the defect, which creates a windsock through which the left-to-right shunt flows. As this windsock billows into the right ventricle during early systole, it causes a snapping sound identical with an ejection sound. It is considered a good sign, as formation of the aneurysm is thought to be a mechanism of spontaneous closure of a membranous ventricular septal defect. It is important to listen carefully for an early diastolic murmur of aortic regurgitation, especially in the infant and toddler. Some ventricular septal defects are associated with an abnormal aortic valve or can cause the development of aortic valve abnormality, resulting in aortic regurgitation. The latter usually is considered to be an indication for more aggressive evaluation and management to prevent progressive aortic valve abnormality. Remember that the loudest murmur of a ventricular septal defect comes from the small to moderately sized defect. As the defect becomes even smaller, the murmur becomes progressively less intense and shorter until it disappears entirely. It does, however, always start with S_1.

The typical murmur of a ventricular septal defect is caused by turbulent flow through a restrictive defect, that is, one in which there is significant systolic pressure difference between the two ventricles. It means that the defect is no more than moderate in size. Large ventricular septal defects are associated with murmurs generated by the large volume flow and are more likely to be identified in infants, in whom they may be a cause of congestive heart failure. This phenomenon is described in Chapter 7.

The child with a small to moderate ventricular septal defect often has a normal chest radiograph, although a mild increase in pulmonary arterial vascularity may be present. The electrocardiogram likely is normal as well. A larger ventricular septal defect can cause biventricular hypertrophy, as illustrated in Figure 3–27. Significant abnormality on the electrocardiogram, such as dominant right ventricular hypertrophy or severe left ventricular hypertrophy, should lead you to reconsider interpretation of the murmur as representing a small to moderate ventricular septal defect. In this case further evaluation is indicated.

In the infant and young child with a rapid heart rate, assuring yourself that the murmur is early systolic can be difficult. It is possible to confuse the murmur of a ventricular septal defect with right ventricular infundibular stenosis or the murmur of subvalvar aortic stenosis. Careful physical examination may distinguish these conditions, and the electrocardiogram also is helpful. If the patient with "a small ventricular septal defect" has an electrocardiogram showing systemic pressure right ventricular hypertrophy (see

Fig. 3–15), consider the possibility of tetralogy of Fallot and that you have misinterpreted the ejection murmur of right ventricular infundibular stenosis. If the electrocardiogram shows excessive left ventricular hypertrophy (see Fig. 3–25), and particularly if you feel a significant apical heave, consider subvalvar aortic stenosis.

The murmur of mild mitral regurgitation may be difficult to distinguish from the murmur of a small muscular ventricular septal defect, as the latter tends to be located more toward the midprecordium than the lower left sternal border. Characteristics and causes of mitral regurgitation are described further here as well as in other chapters.

Tricuspid Regurgitation. Tricuspid regurgitation is rare as an isolated lesion beyond the first month of life and need not be considered to any great extent in the diagnosis of an early systolic murmur.

Mitral Regurgitation. The murmur of mitral regurgitation is described as beginning with S_1, and it is best heard at the apex. It is of higher frequency and softer than the murmur of a ventricular septal defect or that of ventricular outflow stenosis, but it is not as harmonic as the innocent vibratory murmur. The murmur of rheumatic mitral regurgitation radiates toward the left axilla and back, whereas the murmur of congenital mitral regurgitation (especially that due to an endocardial cushion defect) radiates toward the pulmonic area and left sternal border. The murmur of mild mitral regurgitation begins with S_1 (except for that due to mitral valve prolapse) and may end at mid-systole. The murmur of moderate to severe chronic mitral regurgitation is holosystolic. Moderate to severe mitral regurgitation can cause a mid-diastolic left ventricular filling murmur (see Fig. 1–10) owing to augmented left ventricular filling. Chronic mitral regurgitation usually does not affect the intensity of the pulmonic component of S_2 unless congestive heart failure also is present.

Causes of mitral regurgitation include rheumatic fever (see Chapter 10), myocarditis and cardiomyopathy (see Chapter 12), and anomalous origin of the left coronary artery from the pulmonic trunk (see Chapter 12). Mitral valve prolapse is reviewed in Chapter 9.

The presence of a murmur of mitral regurgitation together with other auscultatory findings suggesting an atrial level left-to-right shunt (e.g., atrial septal defect) indicates the possibility of the *ostium primum*

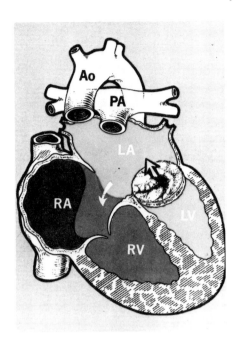

FIGURE 8–4. Ostium primum complex. Note the cleft anterior mitral valve leaflet, with the outlined arrow indicating mitral regurgitation. The white arrow indicates left-to-right shunt through an ostium primum atrial septal defect. Shading indicates relative oxygen saturation: Dark shading indicates systemic venous blood; light shading indicates fully saturated arterial blood; and intermediate shading indicates the effect of the shunt. Ao = aorta; PA = pulmonary artery; RA = right atrium; RV = right ventricle.

complex form of an endocardial cushion defect. With this condition there is an ostium primum type of atrial septal defect and a cleft anterior leaflet of the mitral valve (Fig. 8–4). The electrocardiogram reveals a superior QRS axis as illustrated in Figure 3–8, with right ventricular hypertrophy of the type illustrated in Figure 3–22. The chest radiograph demonstrates increased pulmonary arterial vascularity and right heart dilation. Left atrial enlargement is not present unless the atrial septal defect is small and the mitral regurgitation at least moderate.

Mid-Systolic Murmur

An ejection murmur has been identified and is considered pathologic. The next decision is to determine whether it is caused by left or right ventricular ejection. Innocent ejection murmurs and those associated with an atrial septal defect are described earlier in the chapter.

Right Ventricular Outflow Tract Obstruction. Right ventricular outflow tract obstruction can be infundibular, valvar, or su-

pravalvar. Physical examination again provides substantial information. Significant stenosis causes right ventricular hypertrophy, which in turn produces a lift along the left sternal border. A systolic thrill may be felt in the second and third left intercostal space with pulmonic valve stenosis but is less common with other types of obstruction. The thrill of pulmonic valve stenosis also may be felt in the suprasternal notch; but, if so, it is almost always much more prominent on the chest wall. A pulmonic ejection sound is heard with pulmonic valve stenosis but not with other forms of obstruction. Remember that the pulmonic ejection sound is best heard during expiration. It decreases significantly with inspiration and may disappear entirely. The high-frequency systolic murmur of infundibular stenosis is located in the third left intercostal space at the sternal border. It begins well after S_1 but then peaks rapidly. It continues throughout systole and can override the aortic component of S_2 if the right ventricular ejection time is significantly prolonged. The murmur of pulmonic valve stenosis is best heard in the second left intercostal space. It is rougher, of lower frequency, and peaks later during systole, usually no earlier than mid-systole. It radiates well over the lungs, more so on the left. With severe stenosis murmur peaking can be late during systole as it takes longer for right ventricular pressure to reach its maximum. The murmur of pulmonary artery coarctation is maximal over the pulmonary arteries and radiates to both lungs and into the axillae when the obstruction is bilateral. With severe stenosis of a pulmonary artery, the murmur can extend into diastole and then is correctly designated continuous. Severe pulmonary artery stenosis can be associated with such disorders as postrubella and Alagille syndrome.[9] It may be difficult to distinguish the murmur of mild pulmonary artery stenosis from an innocent pulmonic flow murmur. In the absence of right ventricular hypertrophy this distinction is of no consequence.

The S_2 is of considerable diagnostic help. With right ventricular infundibular obstruction the pulmonic component of S_2 is absent if the obstruction is at least moderately severe. With pulmonic valve stenosis the pulmonic component of S_2 is delayed and decreased in intensity (see Fig. 1–8) but is audible until the stenosis becomes severe. The greater the degree of stenosis the more delayed and softer is this sound.[10] With pulmonary artery stenosis the pulmonic component of S_2 may be delayed by prolonged right ventricular ejection time, but intensity is normal to slightly increased because diastolic pressure in the pulmonic trunk proximal to the obstruction is normal to slightly increased. Diastole is silent except for the occasional patient with pulmonic valve stenosis who has mild pulmonic valve regurgitation.

TETRALOGY OF FALLOT. It is important to identify the infant with tetralogy of Fallot (see Fig. 5–7) not only because eventual surgical correction is required but because of the threat of *hypercyanotic spells* in some of the patients. Tetralogy of Fallot has a spectrum of severity based on the severity of right ventricular infundibular obstruction as discussed in Chapter 5. It is the patient with less severe infundibular stenosis who is more likely to have hypercyanotic spells. This is true because the dynamic nature of the infundibular obstruction has a greater range of variability in these patients and because they have no more than mild cyanosis and mild hematocrit elevation; therefore they have minimal tolerance for a drop in arterial oxygen saturation.

A hypercyanotic spell is thought to be due either to an acute increase in right ventricular outflow tract obstruction caused by contraction of the musculature surrounding the outflow tract or to a sudden decrease in systemic arteriolar resistance. Either condition increases right-to-left shunting, decreasing systemic arterial saturation and thereby causing systemic hypoxemia and stimulating hyperpnea. The infant may become quiet and can exhibit a decreased level of consciousness. Irritability also can occur. An older infant or toddler may learn either to assume the knee-chest position or to squat. Most spells stop spontaneously, but it takes only one severe spell to cause hypoxemic brain damage or death. It is therefore essential that the parent or guardian be questioned carefully at each medical encounter regarding symptoms that could be due to a hypoxemic spell. Onset of spells indicates the need for immediate referral or re-referral to a tertiary care center.

Hypercyanotic spells can be precipitated by dehydration because decreased circulating blood volume may decrease right ventricular filling volume. Systemic vasodilation also can precipitate a spell because decreasing systemic arteriolar resistance promotes right-to-left shunting through the ventricular septal defect. This phenomenon is responsible for the increased frequency of spells during the morning shortly after the patient awakens. Bathing in hot water also can cause systemic vasodilation.

Acute treatment of a hypercyanotic spell is directed at decreasing right ventricular outflow tract obstruction and increasing systemic arteriolar resistance. Home treatment is limited. Knee-chest position or squatting increases peripheral resistance. Comforting the infant, thereby decreasing anxiety, is helpful. Persistence of a spell for more than a few minutes requires immediate medical attention. Parents of an infant with tetralogy of Fallot should be advised regarding both the threat of spells and measures that may reduce their likelihood. Hot water baths should be avoided especially in the morning. The infant should be given something to drink shortly after arising and certainly before bathing.

The best *management* for hypercyanotic spells is to prevent them by surgically correcting the defect. Some surgical groups repair tetralogy of Fallot in infants at any age.[11] Others prefer to delay total repair until 6 to 12 months of age or later if the infant remains asymptomatic. Symptomatic infants can be managed by placing a systemic artery to pulmonary artery shunt, for example, the Blalock-Taussig shunt (see Chapter 19). Acute infundibular obstruction due to contraction of the surrounding musculature can be treated medically with β-blockade (e.g., propranolol). Long-term treatment with propranolol of a patient with tetralogy of Fallot who is having spells, even minor spells, is not recommended. It can be done, but there is hazard in having a patient critically dependent on daily oral medication.

PULMONIC VALVE STENOSIS. Chest radiography of pulmonic valve stenosis (see Fig. 2–16) usually demonstrates nothing more than dilation of the pulmonic trunk and left pulmonary artery. More severe stenosis may change heart shape to reflect more significant right ventricular hypertrophy. The overall heart size seldom is increased unless some associated abnormality is present. Pulmonary arterial vascularity is normal. The electrocardiogram usually reflects some degree of right ventricular hypertrophy. Mild pulmonic stenosis may produce nothing more than a positive T wave in right precordial leads (see Fig. 3–14); more severe stenosis produces more severe change (see Fig. 3–16).

Management of pulmonic valve stenosis is based on its severity. Mild pulmonic valve stenosis (pressure difference <25 mm Hg) remains mild indefinitely,[12] and it is likely that the patient can live a normal life with no need for therapeutic intervention. More significant valvar stenosis usually can be managed by balloon pulmonic valvuloplasty.[13] Results of this procedure are excellent; and once the obstruction is decreased to the mild category, it remains at that level. Some patients with pulmonic valve stenosis have a dysplastic valve that may not respond to balloon valvuloplasty, in which case surgical valvotomy may be necessary, a common occurrence in patients with Noonan syndrome.[14]

OTHER RIGHT VENTRICULAR OUTFLOW TRACT OBSTRUCTIONS. *Right ventricular infundibular stenosis* may be isolated or may be associated with a small ventricular septal defect. This combination is not tetralogy of Fallot. Relief of the obstruction requires surgery. *Pulmonary artery stenoses* often are multiple, and therapeutic intervention frequently is unsuccessful. Discrete obstruction of a pulmonary artery sometimes can be relieved by balloon dilation. Expandable stents also are used in some patients to prevent recurrence of the obstruction at that site.[15]

Left Ventricular Outflow Tract Obstruction. Left ventricular outflow tract obstruction may be due to obstruction within the body of the left ventricle (obstructive hypertrophic cardiomyopathy), in the left ventricular outflow tract (discrete or tubular subvalvar aortic stenosis), at the aortic valve, or in the proximal aorta (supravalvar). Physical examination provides essential information. If the obstruction is severe enough to produce left ventricular hypertrophy, the apex impulse may be increased in amplitude (left ventricular lift), displaced to the left, or both. Palpate for a systolic thrill. A systolic thrill in the suprasternal notch is almost diagnostic of aortic valve disease. This thrill may be present with either supravalvar or subvalvar aortic stenosis but is not felt with obstructive cardiomyopathy. A systolic thrill at the right base caused by aortic valve stenosis suggests that the systolic pressure difference between the left ventricle and aorta is at least 35 to 40 mm Hg in a resting patient

of normal body build. Supravalvar aortic stenosis is often associated with Williams syndrome, in which case the patient demonstrates distinct facial features that suggest this diagnosis.

Listen carefully for an aortic ejection sound, as its presence indicates aortic valve abnormality. It is the only physical finding that clearly differentiates between valvar and subvalvar aortic stenosis. Neither hypertrophic obstructive cardiomyopathy nor supravalvar aortic stenosis causes an aortic ejection sound. Each type of left ventricular outflow tract obstruction can produce a low-frequency, rough ejection systolic murmur that is audible along the left ventricle–aorta listening area that runs from the apex across the third left intercostal space at the sternal border to the second right intercostal space at the sternal border (see Fig. 1–5). Location of the point of maximal intensity of the murmur depends on the specific type of obstruction. The murmurs of hypertrophic obstructive cardiomyopathy and subvalvar aortic stenosis are usually maximal over the midprecordium. That of aortic valve stenosis can likely be best heard in the second right intercostal space at the sternal edge, which is true also for the murmur of supravalvar aortic stenosis. The intensity of the murmur varies with the severity of the obstruction. Subvalvar and valvar aortic stenoses generate more noise for a given degree of obstruction than do either obstructive cardiomyopathy or supravalvar aortic stenosis.

The S_2 narrows with left ventricular outflow tract obstruction as left ventricular ejection time is increased (see Fig. 1–8). S_2 narrows also with aortic valve stenosis even if the obstruction is trivial, provided there is poststenotic dilation of the aorta. S_2 narrowing occurs here because dilation of the aorta increases capacitance of the arterial bed, thereby prolonging aortic hangout interval and delaying aortic valve closure.[16] With severe stenosis of any type the aortic component of S_2 may be delayed enough to make S_2 single at all times. Paradoxical splitting of S_2 in the pediatric patient occurs only with severe obstructive cardiomyopathy (see Fig. 1–8).

Two types of diastolic murmur may be heard in patients with left ventricular outflow tract obstruction. An early diastolic murmur of aortic regurgitation is heard often with subvalvar aortic stenosis and occasionally with aortic valve stenosis, particularly in patients with a bicuspid aortic valve without significant stenosis. Aortic regurgitation is rare with obstructive cardiomyopathy or supravalvar stenosis. A mid-diastolic apical left ventricular filling murmur may be caused by decreased left ventricular compliance. This murmur is more common with obstructive cardiomyopathy than with the other types of left ventricular outflow tract obstruction. S_3 and S_4 also are more common with obstructive cardiomyopathy.

Chest radiographs (see Figs. 2–13 and 12–1) demonstrate a change in heart shape, suggesting left ventricular hypertrophy. Some degree of pulmonary venous obstructive pattern may be seen with more severe forms of obstruction. Overall heart size may be increased with obstructive cardiomyopathy and in patients with significant aortic regurgitation but not in those with other forms of pure obstruction. The electrocardiogram (see Fig. 3–25) may demonstrate left ventricular hypertrophy with all forms of left ventricular outflow tract obstruction, although it is surprising how much stenosis can be present without significant electrocardiographic changes. Obstructive cardiomyopathy causes more dramatic electrocardiographic changes, as discussed in Chapter 12.

Management of all forms of left ventricular outflow tract obstruction should include referral for specialist evaluation and decisions regarding further diagnostic procedures and treatment. Sudden death is a risk for patients with obstructive cardiomyopathy, as described in Chapter 12. Sudden death is rare in pediatric patients with aortic valve stenosis, but it does occur. Anginal-type chest pain and syncope or presyncope with exercise are ominous events in a patient with aortic stenosis and indicate the need for urgent referral (or re-referral of an established patient) for definitive therapy. Aortic valve stenosis in the child and adolescent frequently can be relieved by balloon valvuloplasty.[17,18] Subvalvar and supravalvar obstructions require surgery. Obstructive cardiomyopathy management is discussed in Chapter 12.

COARCTATION OF THE AORTA.   It would be useful to digress for a moment and review the clinical findings of coarctation of the aorta in an asymptomatic child. This condition in the critically ill newborn is reviewed in Chapter 6 and in the infant with heart failure in Chapter 7. The child with coarctation of the aorta usually manifests mild resting systemic systolic hypertension that seldom is higher than 125 mm Hg. The diagnosis should be straightforward. In a patient with mild hypertension, compare the brachial artery pulses with those in the feet, specifically the posterior tibial and dorsalis pedis pulses, and measure systolic blood pressure in both arms and at least one leg. Use the largest cuff that can be placed on the arm and calf, a mercury manometer, and a Doppler flow detector to indicate systolic pressure. Systolic pressure in the feet should be approximately 10 mm Hg higher than that at the brachial artery because of the artifact of distal pulse amplification. If significant coarctation is present, systolic pressure in the feet likely is no more than 70 to 80 mm Hg when that in the arm is 125 mm Hg.

Many patients with coarctation of the aorta have a bicuspid aortic valve; therefore one should expect to hear an aortic ejection sound. There may be an aortic ejection murmur, but most such patients do not have significant aortic valve stenosis. Often there is a midfrequency systolic ejection murmur heard in the second left intercostal space, the left axilla, at the apex, and posteriorly just to the left of the spine over the upper back. This murmur is generated by turbulence at the coarctation site. Chest radiography in a child with coarctation of the aorta is shown in Figure 2–15. The electrocardiogram may show left ventricular hypertrophy similar to that shown in Figure 3–25, but it may also be normal. In many patients with coarctation of the aorta there is a pattern of right ventricular conduction delay for reasons that are not determined.

Detection of this lesion by the primary care physician is the cornerstone of *management* of the child with coarctation of the aorta because the patient's abnormality is not otherwise recognized. Coarctation of the aorta should be corrected early during childhood. There is some evidence that repair is advisable as soon as it is discovered after age 1 year.[19]

Late Systolic Murmur

The only late systolic murmur (see Fig. 1–9) of significance is that due to mitral valve prolapse, which is discussed in detail in Chapter 9. In a patient who is supine, the murmur of mitral valve prolapse typically begins during mid-systole after a mid-systolic click or clicks. The murmur is crescendo and is maximal at the apex, seldom louder than grade 2. The murmur begins earlier during systole when the patient sits up. In a few patients with mitral valve prolapse the murmur has a distinctive high-frequency quality with beat-to-beat intensity variation that has the onomatopoeic designation "whoop."

The mitral regurgitation of mitral valve prolapse is of importance because it requires prophylaxis against bacterial endocarditis and because it is associated with connective tissue abnormalities such as Marfan syndrome.

DIASTOLIC MURMURS

It is unusual to note an isolated diastolic murmur in a patient not previously known to have a cardiovascular abnormality. Few patients initially are referred to a pediatric cardiologist for this problem.

All diastolic murmurs should be considered abnormal (Fig. 8–5). There is one innocent diastolic murmur located at the lower left sternal border, but this murmur is seldom identified even by cardiologists and, if heard, can be difficult to evaluate without substantial experience.[20]

The primary care physician may be the first individual to confront a diastolic murmur and therefore would have the important responsibilities of recognizing its presence, evaluating its significance, and planning initial management. If you hear a diastolic murmur, the most important observation is to accurately time the murmur as either early, mid, or late diastolic. This information sets the stage for categorizing both hemodynamic and etiologic considerations for the murmur (Fig. 8–5).

Early Diastolic Murmur

An early diastolic murmur (see Fig. 1–10) is defined as one that starts with its respective component of S_2; that is, it occupies isovolumetric relaxation. Only semilunar valve regurgitation can produce this murmur; therefore an early diastolic murmur indicates either pulmonic or aortic regurgitation.

The murmur of *pulmonic regurgitation* is most commonly a short, low-frequency murmur that begins with the pulmonic component of S_2 (sometimes replacing it) and is best heard in the third left intercostal space radiating down along the left sternal border over the right ventricle sound distribution area (see Fig. 1–5). It may be accentuated by inspiration. Congenital pulmonic regurgitation is uncommon, although mild regurgitation may occur with pulmonic valve stenosis. Absent pulmonic valve syndrome in the newborn creates a loud murmur of pulmonic regurgitation. The murmur of pulmonic regurgitation is common following either surgery for tetralogy of Fallot or bal-

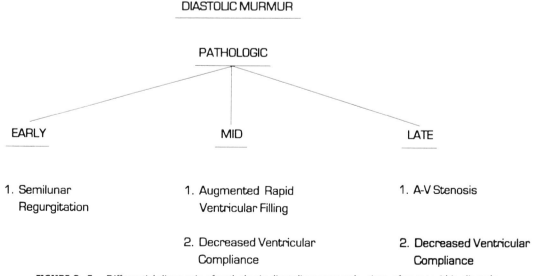

FIGURE 8–5. Differential diagnosis of pathologic diastolic murmurs by time of onset within diastole. A-V = atrioventricular valve.

loon pulmonic valvuloplasty for pulmonic valve stenosis.

The murmur of pulmonic regurgitation in the presence of pulmonary hypertension is of high frequency because high diastolic pressure in the pulmonic trunk causes high-velocity pulmonic regurgitation. There is a direct relation between diastolic pressure in the pulmonic trunk and murmur frequency. Pulmonary artery pressure may be elevated owing to high pulmonary vascular resistance or to left heart disease that causes increased pulmonary venous pressure (e.g., mitral stenosis or severe mitral regurgitation). This type of pulmonic regurgitation murmur, originally described by Graham Steell, bears his name.[21]

Findings on chest radiograph and electrocardiogram associated with pulmonic regurgitation reflect the primary cause rather than the regurgitation directly. Severe pulmonic regurgitation can cause dilation of both right ventricle and pulmonic trunk.

The murmur of *aortic regurgitation* begins with the aortic component of S_2; it is of high frequency and decrescendo in shape. The murmur is best heard in the third left intercostal space at the sternal border and radiates over the left ventricular distribution area (see Fig. 1–5) to the apex. Its duration and loudness generally are directly related to the severity of the regurgitation. Detecting a minimal murmur of aortic regurgitation is difficult, even for the experienced observer. One must make a conscientious effort to listen carefully along the left sternal border. The stethoscope diaphragm is pressed firmly against the chest wall, and a cooperative child is asked to suspend breathing at end-expiration. Occasionally, the murmur is detected best by having the patient sit up and lean forward against the examiner's hand as the stethoscope head is applied.

Several etiologic considerations should be mentioned. Aortic regurgitation may be produced by a bicuspid aortic valve, in which case other clinical findings (discussed earlier in this chapter) reflect the abnormality. There may be a suprasternal notch thrill, and an aortic ejection sound should be present. There may be no more than a grade 1 aortic ejection murmur.

Aortic regurgitation is often present in patients with subvalvar aortic stenosis but seldom when the obstruction is mild. Clinical findings due to obstruction therefore dominate.

Aortic regurgitation may be associated with a membranous ventricular septal defect. The systolic murmur caused by the ventricular septal defect usually is much louder, and one must deliberately listen as just described for the diastolic murmur. Aortic regurgitation due to rheumatic heart disease usually is associated with mitral regurgitation, although it can be isolated; this subject is discussed in Chapter 10. Acute, severe aortic regurgitation can be produced by bacterial endocarditis. In this case the diastolic murmur is short because of rapidly increasing left ventricular end-diastolic pressure in an undilated ventricle. The murmur also is more midfrequency.

Aortic regurgitation usually causes widened pulse pressure because of the decreased diastolic pressure, resulting in so-called bounding arterial pulses. Auscultatory blood pressure in the arms often indicates systolic hypertension, but most of this apparent elevation is an artifact due to exaggerated pulse amplification.

Chest radiographic changes directly related to aortic regurgitation are present only when regurgitation is at least moderate, in which case a left ventricular dilation and pulmonary venous obstructive vascular pattern is noted. Electrocardiographic findings suggesting left ventricular dilation (deep q, tall R, and tall T waves in left precordial leads) may be seen with chronic aortic regurgitation.

Mid-Diastolic Murmurs

Most mid-diastolic murmurs (see Fig. 1–10) are generated by a mismatch between volume flow across the mitral or tricuspid valve and compliance of the respective ventricles during the rapid (passive) phase of ventricular filling (see Chapter 1). The murmur rarely occurs in isolation and therefore is unlikely to be identified as a primary problem. It is, however, an important means of evaluating both structure and ventricular function. Various names have been given to this murmur, including functional or relative mitral/tricuspid stenosis and mitral/tricuspid flow rumble. These names seem inappropriate, as they direct attention to the valve as the source of the murmur, whereas in most instances I believe the sound comes from vibrations of the ventricular wall during rapid ventricular filling. The designation ventricular filling murmur therefore seems more useful. A mid-diastolic murmur can be caused by atrioventricular valve stenosis, but in this case the murmur is not confined to mid-diastole as is the ventricular filling murmur. Tricuspid valve stenosis is an exceptionally rare lesion and is not discussed here. Mitral valve stenosis is unusual in infants and children and is reviewed briefly.

Right Ventricular Filling Murmurs

The right ventricular filling murmur is heard in the presence of a large left-to-right atrial level shunt (e.g., an atrial septal defect) or with significant tricuspid regurgitation, both of which cause excessive early diastolic filling of the right ventricle. The murmur is of midfrequency and maximal at the lower left sternal border. It is never loud, rarely more than grade 2, and it is increased during inspiration. This murmur is essential for the auscultatory diagnosis of an atrial level left-to-right shunt; this diagnosis cannot be made with certainty in its absence.

Tricuspid valve regurgitation is seldom of sufficient severity to cause a right ventricular diastolic filling murmur. Some patients with Ebstein anomaly demonstrate it.

Unlike decreased left ventricular compliance, which often causes a left ventricular diastolic filling murmur, decreased right ventricular compliance seldom is recognized as a cause of a right ventricular diastolic filling murmur. Marked right ventricular hypertrophy, caused by severe pulmonic valve stenosis or pulmonary vascular disease, may generate such a murmur. Another, even more obscure, cause is impaired right ventricular filling due to constrictive pericarditis. This condition, however, is more likely to produce a loud mid-diastolic sound (pericardial knock) than a murmur.

Left Ventricular Filling Murmur

The left ventricular filling murmur is heard in the presence of conditions that either increase volume flow across the mitral valve (e.g., ventricular septal defect, patent ductus arteriosus, and mitral regurgitation) or decreased left ventricular compliance (e.g., left ventricular cardiomyopathy, aortic stenosis, or coarctation of the aorta).

The murmur is located at the apex. It is of low frequency, grade 2 at most, and usually short. Distinguishing between a short mid-diastolic murmur and a prominent S_3 is

sometimes difficult. Distinction depends on both the duration of the sound (S_3 is discrete) and associated findings, because a left ventricular diastolic filling murmur occurs most commonly with other abnormal physical findings pointing to its cause.

Significant *mitral stenosis* produces a diastolic murmur that begins during mid-diastole. The murmur continues, however, with atrial contraction producing late diastolic accentuation. The murmur is maximal at the apex. Congenital mitral stenosis is an uncommon lesion and is rare as an isolated abnormality. Rheumatic mitral stenosis now also is rare in the United States.

The murmur of mitral stenosis is distinctive. It is a long, low-frequency rumbling murmur that increases in intensity just prior to S_1. The murmur can be loud enough to cause a diastolic thrill, a rare observation from any cause. The child's heart rate is fast enough that most observers, including cardiologists, might assume that such a loud murmur is systolic. Taking care when identifying S_1 and S_2 should prevent this error. Significant mitral stenosis increases pulmonary artery pressure and thus affects S_2, making the pulmonic component louder and earlier, thereby reducing the duration of S_2 splitting. An opening snap is heard only with rheumatic mitral stenosis and therefore is rare in children.

Late Diastolic Murmur

The late diastolic murmur (see Fig. 1–10) is generated by atrial contraction. It can be caused by anatomic stenosis of an atrioventricular valve, restricted ventricular filling (decreased compliance), or semilunar valve regurgitation. The murmur begins after the P wave of the electrocardiogram and therefore implies sinus rhythm. A long PR interval, a rapid heart rate, or both cause this murmur to appear earlier during diastole, but it continues until S_1.

Right Heart Late Diastolic Murmur

Tricuspid stenosis is a rare lesion, and most physicians never see such a patient. The murmur is located at the lower left sternal border. It is a low-frequency crescendo-shaped murmur that peaks at S_1. A prominent jugular venous a wave may be detectable.

A late diastolic murmur in association with high pressure pulmonic valve regurgitation has been described.[22] This murmur is analogous with the Austin Flint murmur, described below and in Chapter 1, and probably is similarly produced. It is of mid-frequency and is heard best during expiration. It is an uncommon observation in an uncommon circumstance, and most cardiologists probably have not heard it.

Left Heart Late Diastolic Murmur

Mitral stenosis has been mentioned briefly above. The murmur is generated by turbulence at the narrowed mitral valve and is analogous with the murmur of semilunar valve stenosis. Remember that congenital mitral stenosis can be associated with an atrial septal defect, in which case the physical findings may reflect primarily the effects of the left-to-right atrial shunt. There may be little murmur at the mitral valve, as its flow may be decreased significantly. Rheumatic mitral stenosis is rare in children, as mentioned; when associated with an atrial septal defect, the combination is termed Lutembacher syndrome.[23,24]

In some patients with severely decreased left ventricular compliance, there may be little filling of the left ventricle during the rapid (i.e., passive) phase of ventricular filling. In this situation atrial contraction drives a larger volume of blood into the stiff left ventricle, producing a late diastolic murmur identical with that described above for the mid-diastolic left ventricular filling murmur. It is particularly apparent when the PR interval is long and diastole is short (i.e., faster heart rate).

A late diastolic, low-frequency crescendo murmur at the apex is heard in some individuals with significant aortic regurgitation. This murmur was described in 1862 by Austin Flint and is commonly referred to by his name.[25] Flint proposed that the murmur is generated by atrial contraction forcing blood through the mitral valve, which is partially closed by the stream of aortic regurgitation; that is, the murmur is caused by vibrations of the anterior mitral valve leaflet. One study suggested that the murmur is generated by vibration of the ventricular wall, and that its presence correlates with the severity of the aortic regurgitation or perhaps with the severity of the decreased left ventricular compliance.[26] If the latter explanation is correct, it would be important to recognize the development or change in intensity of the Austin Flint murmur.

CONTINUOUS MURMURS

Characteristics of continuous murmurs are described in Chapter 1 (see Fig. 1–10). A continuous murmur is one that begins during systole and continues through S_2, ending during diastole. Causes of continuous murmur are indicated in Figure 8–6. Every primary care physician should be familiar with the innocent venous hum and should easily recognize the characteristic murmur of a patent ductus arteriosus.

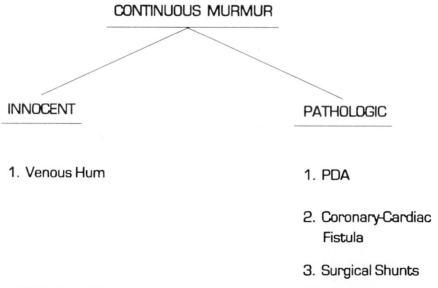

FIGURE 8–6. Differential diagnosis of continuous murmurs. PDA = patent ductus arteriosus.

Innocent Continuous Murmur

The *venous hum* is caused by turbulence in the major veins as they drain into the superior vena cava. Characteristically, a venous hum is located at the right sternoclavicular junction and is heard most often with the patient sitting. The murmur is soft and of midfrequency; it has one intensity peak during systole and a louder peak during diastole when the tricuspid valve opens. The murmur can be obliterated by compressing the right jugular vein, rotating the head, or placing the child supine. A venous hum is heard on the left occasionally, and uncommonly when the patient is supine. Compressing the neck veins obliterates at least the diastolic component, providing distinction between a venous hum and the murmur of a patent ductus arteriosus. No further investigation of this murmur is necessary.

Patent Ductus Arteriosus

The murmur of an uncomplicated patent ductus arteriosus (PDA) in a child is a rough, noisy, continuous murmur that peaks at S_2; the diastolic component is of higher frequency and decrescendo in shape. Intensity is usually grade 2 to 3, occasionally louder, in which case a systolic thrill may be felt in the second left intercostal space (where the murmur is maximal) and in the suprasternal notch. S_2 splitting is normal if it can be heard through the peak of the murmur. A mid-diastolic left ventricular filling murmur may be present at the apex if the left-to-right shunt is large. Peripheral arterial pulse amplitude is increased because pulse pressure is increased by the diastolic aortic runoff into the pulmonary arterial bed.

The chest radiograph often is normal but may show increased pulmonary arterial vascularity, left atrial enlargement, and mild cardiomegaly if the shunt is moderately large. More significant radiographic changes (see Fig. 2–28) are seldom observed beyond infancy. The electrocardiogram likely is normal, even with a moderate shunt. Left ventricular hypertrophy may be present (see Fig. 3–24), and some patients have left atrial enlargement. Biventricular hypertrophy is seldom seen beyond infancy, and dominant right ventricular hypertrophy indicates additional abnormalities or complications.

Management of an asymptomatic PDA in a child is closure to eliminate the risk of bacterial endocarditis and possible aneurysm formation during adulthood. Surgical closure remains the most common method; device closure by transcatheter technique is currently being introduced and may become the treatment of choice for most patients.[27]

Other Continuous Murmurs

Other atrioventricular malformations produce continuous murmurs that might be detected on routine cardiovascular examination. A *fistula* between a coronary artery and a cardiac chamber causes a continuous murmur that is heard best over the chamber into which the fistula drains. Almost all of these patients are asymptomatic. The murmur has two peaks—one during systole and one during diastole—of approximate equal intensity and rarely louder than grade 3. The murmur is of midfrequency and not nearly as noisy as the typical murmur of a PDA. Drainage into the right or left atrium may generate a mid-diastolic filling murmur over the respective ventricle. The chest radiograph and electrocardiogram are usually normal. Treatment consists in closure of the defect, now possible by transcatheter device occlusion techniques.[28] Where this procedure is not possible, surgical closure can be accomplished by closed heart technique.

Cerebral *arteriovenous malformation*, a problem of the newborn, is discussed in Chapter 7. A pulmonary arteriovenous malformation may be heard as a soft continuous murmur over a peripheral lung field, particularly on the back. Often these lesions are noted first because of a density on the chest radiograph. Closure by transcatheter device occlusion is possible.[29]

Surgical systemic artery to pulmonary artery shunts, using either the subclavian artery (Blalock-Taussig shunt) or synthetic material (e.g., Gore-Tex), produce continuous murmurs. The examiner should be aware of these shunts by having obtained the history prior to auscultation or at least should be suspicious on the basis of a surgical scar.

REFERENCES

1. Perloff JK: The clinical recognition of congenital heart disease. 2nd Ed. Philadelphia, WB Saunders, 1978.
2. Newburger JW, Rosenthal A, Williams RG, et al:

Noninvasive tests in the initial evaluation of heart murmurs in children. N Engl J Med 308:61–64, 1983.

3. Smythe JF, Teixeira OHP, Vlad P, et al: Initial evaluation of heart murmur: are laboratory tests necessary? Pediatrics 86:497–500, 1990.

4. Still GF: Common Disorders and Diseases of Childhood. London, H Frowde, Hodder and Stroughton, 1909.

5. Klewer SE, Donnerstein RL, Goldberg SJ: Still's-like innocent murmur can be produced by increasing aortic velocity to a threshold value. Am J Cardiol 68:810–812, 1991.

6. Darazs B, Hesdorffer CS, Butterworth AM, Ziady F: The possible etiology of the vibratory systolic murmur. Clin Cardiol 10:341–346, 1987.

7. McKusick VA, Murray GE, Peeler RG, Webb GN: Musical murmurs. Bull Johns Hopkins Hosp 97: 136–176, 1955.

8. Perloff JK: Heart sounds and murmurs: physiological mechanisms. In Braunwald E (ed): Heart Disease. A Textbook of Cardiovascular Medicine. 4th Ed. Philadelphia, WB Saunders, 1992.

9. Alagille D, Estrada A, Hadchouel M, et al: Syndromic paucity of interlobular bile ducts (Alagille syndrome or arteriohepatic dysplasia): review of 80 cases. J Pediatr 110:195–200, 1987.

10. Gamboa R, Hugenholtz PG, Nadas AS: Accuracy of the phonocardiogram on assessing severity of aortic and pulmonic stenosis. Circulation 30: 35–46, 1964.

11. Groh MA, Meliones JN, Bove EL, et al: Repair of tetralogy of Fallot in infancy: effect of pulmonary artery size on outcome. Circulation 84(Suppl III): III-206–III-212, 1991.

12. Hayes CJ, Gersony WM, Driscoll DJ, et al: Second natural history study of congenital heart defects: results of treatment of patients with pulmonary valvar stenosis. Circulation (Suppl): 1993 (in press).

13. Kan JS, White RI, Mitchell SE, et al: Percutaneous balloon valvuloplasty: a new method for treating congenital pulmonary valve stenosis. N Engl J Med 307:540–542, 1982.

14. Noonan JA: Hypertelorism with Turner's phenotype: a new syndrome with associated congenital heart disease. Am J Dis Child 116:373–380, 1968.

15. O'Laughlin MP, Mullins CE: Balloon dilation and stenting of hypoplastic pulmonary arteries: a new area of cooperation between interventional pediatric cardiologists and cardiac surgeons. Tex Heart J 19:185–189, 1992.

16. Kumar S, Luisada AA: Mechanism of changes in the second heart sound in aortic stenosis. Am J Cardiol 28:162–172, 1971.

17. O'Connor BK, Beekman RH, Rocchini AP, Rosenthal A: Intermediate-term effectiveness of balloon valvuloplasty for congenital aortic stenosis: a prospective follow-up study. Circulation 84: 732–738, 1991.

18. Roth SJ, Keane JF: Balloon aortic valvuloplasty. Prog Pediatr Cardiol 1:3–16, 1992.

19. Cohen M, Fuster V, Steele PM, et al: Coarctation of the aorta: long-term follow-up and prediction of outcome after surgical correction. Circulation 80:840–845, 1989.

20. Liebman J, Sood S: Diastolic murmurs in apparently normal children. Circulation 38:755–762, 1968.

21. Steell G: The murmur of high pressure in the pulmonary artery. Med Chron (Manchester) 9: 182–188, 1888–1889.

22. Kambe T, Hibi N, Fukui Y, et al: Clinical study on the right-sided Austin Flint murmur using intracardiac phonocardiography. Am Heart J 98: 701–707, 1979.

23. Lutembacher R: De la sténose mitrale avec communication interauriculaire. Arch Mal Coeur 9: 237–260, 1916.

24. Bashi VV, Ravikumar E, Jairas PS, et al: Coexistent mitral valve disease with left-to-right shunt at the atrial level: clinical profile, hemodynamics, and surgical considerations in 67 consecutive patients. Am Heart J 114:1406–1414, 1987.

25. Flint A: On cardiac murmurs. Am J Med Sci 44: 29–54, 1862.

26. Landzberg JS, Pflugfelder PW, Cassidy MM, et al: Etiology of the Austin Flint murmur. J Am Coll Cardiol 20:408–413, 1992.

27. Rashkind WJ, Mullins CE, Hellenbrand WE, Tait MA: Nonsurgical closure of patent ductus arteriosus: clinical application of the Rashkind PDA Occluder system. Circulation 75:583–604, 1987.

28. Reidy JF, Anjos RT, Qureshi SA, et al: Transcatheter embolization in the treatment of coronary artery fistulas. J Am Coll Cardiol 18:187–192, 1991.

29. White RI, Mitchell SE, Barth KH, et al: Angioarchitecture of pulmonary arteriovenous malformations: an important consideration before embolotherapy. AJR 140:681–686, 1983.

9

THE OLDER CHILD AND ADOLESCENT WITH CHEST PAIN, MITRAL VALVE PROLAPSE, SYNCOPE

Welton M. Gersony

Chest pain, mitral valve prolapse, and syncope are three of the more perplexing problems faced by physicians caring for children and adolescents. Each represents a broad spectrum of disease ranging from totally benign to severe, even life-threatening, illness. Most cases that fall under these headings call for minimal observation and avoidance of excessive laboratory testing; the patients and their families require reassurance. Within each category, however, lurk a few patients whose devastating illnesses are the underlying cause for a common medical complaint or physical finding. Among the thousands of children with benign chest pain is the rare individual with a coronary artery abnormality. Among the plethora of individuals with trivial mitral valve prolapse, there exists a rare child with a connective tissue disease such as Marfan syndrome in whom associated aortic disease represents a future threat. From among the many adolescents who "faint in church," a patient with a serious rhythm disturbance or autonomic nervous system disorder emerges. As a result of these dire possibilities, primary physicians can find themselves in a position in which they feel obliged to refer probable benign cases to specialists, despite the anxiety and cost involved, in order to protect against missing the rare patient with serious disease.

The purpose of this chapter is not to dwell on the specifics of uncommon illnesses but to guide physicians toward making reasonable decisions regarding diagnosis and management of children or adolescents with chest pain, mitral valve prolapse, or syncope. The problem addressed in this chapter is how to accomplish primary evaluation of these patients so that selection of those for referral to subspecialists for more intensive investigation and treatment can be made on a rational basis.

CHEST PAIN

Chest pain is a common complaint among older children and adolescents, and it often creates a dilemma for the responsible physician in terms of extent of evaluation (Fig. 9–1). In most cases, there is no organic basis for chest pain. Because of either parental fears about the possibility of heart disease, lack of understanding as to the meaning of this symptom in a child compared to the adult with coronary artery disease, or both, there is pressure placed on the physician to order multiple laboratory investigations. In most instances it is not only wasteful and nonproductive, but may be detrimental because it prolongs symptoms. Moreover, the child becomes aware of the concern of the

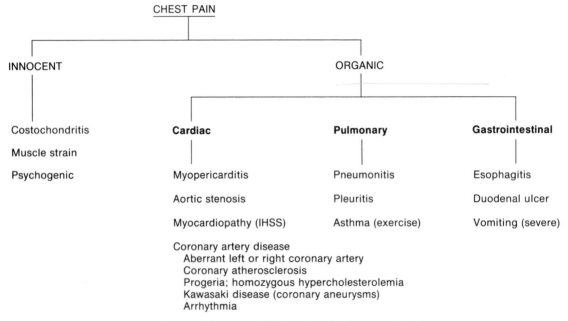

CHEST PAIN

INNOCENT

Costochondritis

Muscle strain

Psychogenic

ORGANIC

Cardiac

Myopericarditis

Aortic stenosis

Myocardiopathy (IHSS)

Coronary artery disease
   Aberrant left or right coronary artery
   Coronary atherosclerosis
   Progeria; homozygous hypercholesterolemia
   Kawasaki disease (coronary aneurysms)
   Arrhythmia

Pulmonary

Pneumonitis

Pleuritis

Asthma (exercise)

Gastrointestinal

Esophagitis

Duodenal ulcer

Vomiting (severe)

FIGURE 9–1. Evaluation of chest pain. IHSS = idiopathic hypertrophic subaortic stenosis.

physician which, together with parental fears, may create further symptoms and psychological "secondary gain" (i.e., more attention for the patient). The physician must walk a fine line between reassurance and appropriate investigation if an organic cause is suspected. Nonspecific chest pain in children tends to become more "locked in" as the numbers of consulting physicians and laboratory tests increase.

Most organic chest pain in pediatric patients occurs during or after an acute illness. Pericardial or pleural pain results from inflammation secondary to bacterial or viral infections. Severe muscular pain occurs with rasping cough, which may be either acute or chronic. Unusual physical exercise involving the muscles of the thorax, such as weight lifting, heavy labor, or other sources of acute muscle strain, may not be identified by patients as causing their chest discomfort. The most common type of chest pain is chronic with no known predisposing event or potential organic etiology. As is true in the adult, in whom the possibility of organic disease is much higher than in the child, the most important tools for evaluating chest pain are the history and physical examination.

History and Physical Examination

The child or adolescent often has mentioned chest pain intermittently in the past, although the parents may have ignored the complaint. Finally, when a saturation point is reached, help is sought. Upon questioning the child directly, it is found that the symptoms go back years but without progression. Sometimes a severe illness or death in the family, especially if cardiac in origin, or another traumatic event such as a divorce will exacerbate and exaggerate the youngster's complaints of chest pain. A simple rhythm disturbance may produce chest sensations that are not easily described by the patient. They may have been caused by short bursts of tachycardia or be the effects of premature beats. Hence the child reports a "funny feeling," and the parent assumes that it is pain.

The older child or adolescent with chest discomfort often articulates these symptoms rather well and is aware of the parents' response as questions are asked, glancing frequently in their direction. The mother or father often intervenes to "correct" some answers. The parents occasionally express verbally or nonverbally some impatience or even anger toward the child. They may feel instinctively that there is probably no disease, but they are fearful, even guilty, that prolonged symptoms of this type may have been important and that somehow they were negligent as parents for not seeking medical attention earlier. Confused parents are easier to counsel than are those who absolutely are convinced that their child has an organic explanation for the symptoms and who repeatedly have been seeking medical opinions despite previous negative physical examinations and laboratory studies. Once a history of well-defined acute or chronic respiratory, cardiac, or gastrointestinal disease has been excluded, the most useful line of questioning includes the following.

1. Accurate description of the pain. The physician must persist in attempting to discover whether the pain is sharp (e.g., stabbing, knife-like, pinching) or dull (e.g., pressure, pressing, nagging, heavy).

2. Location of the pain: substernal, left or right anterior chest, posterior thorax.

3. Radiation of pain. The pain of cardiac ischemia radiates to the left shoulder and arm.

4. Relation to respiration. This question is one of the most important in that musculoskeletal pain often is exaggerated by a deep breath.

5. Changes with body position, suggesting musculoskeletal pain.

6. Relation to exercise. Most innocent pain does not occur with exercise but is noticed when the patient is at rest and not engaged in any specific activity.

When pain is associated with strenuous activity, details as to when the pain begins and ends are important. Does the pain relent within seconds after exercise has been discontinued, or does it last many minutes or even an hour or two? The most common innocent chest pain comprises short, stabbing pains that are related to respiration or body position and that occur at rest. Pain tends to be noticed often for a few weeks and then disappears for a significant period, only to recur occasionally. The physician must be alert to the child who describes pain that is more typical of angina: deep substernal discomfort that disappears within a minute after exercise. Other patients complain of multiple types of pain that are difficult to assess but that are usually benign.

Physical examination should emphasize careful examination of the cardiopulmonary system, and findings should be correlated with positive aspects of the history. In children with nonorganic chest pain there is usually no sign of cardiac or pulmonary disease, and the child appears healthy. Occasionally the pain can be elicited by sternal or costal pressure, but most often there is no tenderness. When pain can be brought out in this manner, it is virtually diagnostic of a musculoskeletal etiology, such as costochondritis.

It is useful to ask the child and parents their opinion regarding the cause of the pain. The patient often states that the pain is coming "from my heart" or characterizes the complaint as "heart pains." It is not unusual for the child and even the parents to answer the question with, "I don't know. You are the doctor. You tell me!" This is not necessarily an inappropriate response but usually reflects a lack of insight by both the child and the parents regarding potential family dynamics influencing responses to the chest pain and the possibility of nonorganic causes.

It is especially important that time is taken to ask questions seriously, consider the answers, and carry out a full physical examination. Both the parent and child are far more reassured when the complaints are thoughtfully considered than when they are given a blanket reassurance about "growing pains" after a cursory evaluation.

Management

Innocent Pain (Musculoskeletal)

When it is almost certain that the patient's chest pain is not based on a significant organic abnormality but represents simple musculoskeletal pain or is related to psychological factors, it is best to avoid further studies. Excessive laboratory investigation may create the impression that heart disease is still a significant consideration and may make it more difficult for the child to give up "a problem" that may be resulting in secondary gains in terms of parental attention and concern.

If the physician is convinced that there is no organic disease, the best approach is to sit back in a calm manner, maintain direct eye contact with the child, and explain that you have carefully evaluated the problem and you have good news. The pain is not coming from the heart, as had been feared, but is arising from the chest wall. Therefore the pain is not important, is not dangerous, and will not result in illness or death. A statement indicating that you expect longevity is important. The physician must be cognizant of the context of the child's fears related to chest pain. The child may have become aware recently of personal mortality and may have seen people with chest pain on television who either die or are taken to a hospital eventually to have heart surgery. The child's main concern is not the pain itself, but that this symptom somehow presages death at an early age, not at some hazy, indefinite time during old age. Chest pain brings the issue of mortality close to the child at a time when such thoughts inspire massive fear. In most cases the patient likes nothing better than to be fully reassured, and obvious signs of relief are apparent in facial expressions and reactions. The parents also experience relief that they no longer have to worry about their son or daughter and are unburdened of misdirected guilt if they had attempted to ignore symptoms. It is important that reassurance be complete and that the physician's anxieties do not interfere with the process. Leaving a "doubt" so that at some remote time in the future, if the patient is found to have cardiac disease, it can be said that the door had been left open is devastating to the reassuring process. A "hedge" here may mean that more doctors will be consulted and does not represent effective "defensive" medicine. Furthermore, if reassurance is combined with ordering an excessive number of tests or consultations, anxiety is increased rather than relieved. Of course, if there are aspects to the history and physical examination suggesting that a real diagnostic question remains, further studies should be ordered and consultation with a pediatric cardiologist or other subspecialist sought.

The interview can be concluded with a statement such as, "I know that these pains are very real, and it is possible that you may continue to have them once in a while. However, I can tell you that they will not harm you, and you should pay as little attention to them as possible. No treatment is needed. Going to your parents and receiving a pain pill or being told to 'rest' is not necessary, and you do not have to limit your activities in any way. If the pains become worse or change, I will be here to help you, and we will think about this problem further. However, I am sure that this will not be necessary." Using this approach, it is remarkable how quickly complaints of chest pain in children and adolescents disappear.

Organic Chest Pain

Cardiac, pulmonary, and gastrointestinal disease may cause symptoms of chest discomfort (Fig. 9–1). As with nonorganic chest pain, the history and physical examination are most helpful for elucidating the etiology of organic pain. A history indicative of either anginal pain, fever, cough, other respiratory symptoms, chest trauma, or gastrointestinal symptoms should lead to a specific diagnosis. The physical examination is confirmatory in most instances.

It is rare that a patient with myocarditis or pericarditis presents with isolated chest pain. Individuals with inflammatory heart disease usually have fever, fatigue, and other signs of infection. A history of a recent respiratory infection is often obtained. Chest pain due to pericarditis is almost always relieved significantly when the patient is in a sitting, leaning forward position. The child or adolescent may sleep in this position. Such a history is virtually diagnostic of pericardial disease, particularly viral pericarditis. The physical examination often reveals a pericardial rub, but it may be a late finding. When myocarditis is the major component or a large pericardial effusion is present, a rub may not develop. Heart sounds may be somewhat diminished in intensity with either condition. A paradoxical pulse indicating early tamponade can be elicited by obtaining a systolic pressure with a more than 10 mm Hg fall during inspiration. Tachycardia out of proportion to either fever or activity can be present in a patient with either impending tamponade or myocarditis.

Patients with noninflammatory cardiomyopathy most often have a history of exercise intolerance. Physical examination may indicate left ventricular outflow tract obstruction or mitral insufficiency, both of which are associated with significant cardiac murmurs (see Chapter 12). The family history may be positive for instances of cardiomyopathy. Children with severe aortic stenosis at either the valvar, supravalvar, or subvalvar level can have chest pain related to decreased coronary artery perfusion during exercise. Such patients usually have a striking cardiac murmur at the left mid or upper right sternal border. It would be unusual to encounter a child or adolescent with chest pain due to severe left ventricular outflow obstruction who has not been previously evaluated.

Perhaps the most subtle cardiac cause of chest pain in children is coronary artery disease. Progeria and homozygous hypercholesterolemia associated with premature atherosclerosis have numerous other findings that would bring the patient to a physician's attention long before isolated chest pain. Kawasaki disease with coronary involvement usually is distinguished by a history of a characteristic acute illness. An older patient who had undiagnosed Kawasaki disease presenting with aneurysm formation and late stenosis causing anginal pain would be distinctly unusual and outside the experience of most cardiologists. The child with coronary anomalies, most often an aberrant left or right coronary artery, may present during childhood or adolescence with anginal chest pain. There is a history of chest pain during exercise with rapid improvement after rest and recrudescence with resumption of activity. Further evaluation of a patient with such symptoms for a possible coronary abnormality is mandatory. Helpful studies for determining the specific cause and severity of a cardiac condition associated with chest pain include electrocardiogram, echocardiogram, exercise study, stress thallium study, and, when required, cardiac catheterization with angiography.

Pneumonia or pleuritis may be associated with chest pain; these causes are usually clear on the basis of the history and physical examination. Pain may be due to muscle strain caused by coughing, or it may be direct pleuritic pain further aggravated by deep breathing or coughing. Cases of pericarditis with pleuritis may result in a mixed picture in terms of the history and physical examination.

Gastrointestinal disease may result in apparent chest pain due to misinterpretation of epigastric discomfort as anterior chest pain. Children with esophagitis may complain of chest pain that is more characteristic of esophageal distension and hyperacidity. Frequent vomiting for any reason can result in chest muscle strain and complaints related to respiratory effort. Similar symptoms can occur with flu-like illness, as generalized muscle pain may include the chest wall.

MITRAL VALVE PROLAPSE

Mitral valve prolapse (MVP) refers to a condition in which the leaflets of the mitral valve billow posteriorly toward the left atrium during ventricular systole. If the prolapse is of sufficient severity, mitral valve insufficiency occurs late during systole. In mild cases only a characteristic mid-systolic click is noted; this sign may originate from tensing of the chordae tendineae as the mitral leaflet recoils toward the left atrium, or it may emanate from a redundant valve cusp snapping backward, similar to a sail that fills rapidly from a sudden wind. Characteristically, MVP is clinically identified during auscultation on the basis of the mid-systolic click and late systolic murmur. Both click and murmur occur earlier during systole when the patient sits up. Echocardiography provides visual evidence of mitral prolapse, and Doppler studies illustrate late mitral insufficiency. The condition is most often idiopathic but can be associated with other forms of congenital heart diseases and connective tissue disorders. The prevalence of MVP in the general population has been estimated to be 4 to 21 per cent depending on the strictness of the definition,[1] and 13 per cent of normal children have prolapse of the posterior leaflet of the mitral valve on echocardiography.[2] Indeed, whether this common finding represents a normal variant is a legitimate question.

When clear-cut mitral valve prolapse is diagnosed by identification of characteristic physical findings, evaluation by a pediatric cardiologist is recommended. Unlike mitral valve disease related to congenital heart diseases such as atrioventricular canal, parachute mitral valve, and congenital mitral insufficiency, children with classic mitral valve prolapse rarely have severe regurgitation and almost never require surgical intervention. Infective endocarditis is a risk, especially when mitral insufficiency is present, and appropriate antibiotic prophylaxis is indicated. When associated with a connective tissue disease such as Marfan syndrome, mitral insufficiency may be severe and surgery may be required to repair or replace the valve. Often, however, the aortic valve and ascending aorta pose a more severe threat; progressive dilatation of the aortic root can lead to dissection and sudden death in Marfan syndrome patients, whereas the more common MVP tends to remain stable (see Chapter 17).

Many symptoms have been attributed to the presence of MVP. Rhythm disturbances, anxiety attacks, nonexertional chest pain, dizziness, syncope, fatigue, and panic attacks have been linked to MVP. Virtually no data are available, however, that confirm these associations in the pediatric population, and differentiating myth from reality in a child with MVP is difficult. The problem becomes more complicated when parents or other family members also have been diagnosed with this condition and attribute various symptoms to its presence.

Whether ectopic rhythms are associated with mitral valve prolapse, these manifestations may require attention if they result in clinical symptoms of palpitations or sequential ectopic beats that produce a tachyarrhythmia.[3] It is probably advisable not to dwell on associations between MVP and rhythm disorders but to respond to symptoms of palpitations appropriately as for any patient; planning electrocardiograms, exercise studies, 24-hour electrocardiograms, or electrophysiologic studies depends on the potential seriousness of the rhythm disorder.

In this era of more frequent use of imaging technology, MVP is being diagnosed at an increasing rate, even among patients who have no physical findings. If a patient with normal physical findings has an echocardiogram and the diagnosis of mild MVP is reported, the physician must decide whether to present it to the patient and parents as a cardiac abnormality or simply as a normal variant. If MVP is considered to be a congenital heart defect, albeit mild, there are implications as to effects on the patient's self-image, willingness to exercise and take part in sports activities, and requirements for antibiotic prophylaxis. Perhaps most important at the present time is the question as to whether the patient with MVP can obtain adequate health insurance at reasonable rates. In the judgment of most pediatric cardiologists it is best not to consider echocardiographic MVP as a disease entity if, on careful physical examination, no physical signs of MVP are found. A patient with a clear-cut click but no murmur and with MVP indicated on the echocardiogram represents an intermediate situation, in which individual medical judgments must be made with wisdom. The apparent severity of the echocardiographic abnormality may be helpful in this regard. The admonition that echocardiography is not the major consideration for the evaluation of MVP is well worth considering.

As with noncardiac chest pain, reassurance is important to avoid undue patient anxiety. Although occasional checkups are necessary for the individual with auscultatory evidence of MVP, the patient and parents must be made aware that isolated MVP, when recognized in the pediatric patient, almost never progresses in severity.

SYNCOPE

Syncope is a common event in otherwise healthy children and adolescents, but it is important to rule out certain potential etiologies. Simple syncope results from vasovagal stimulation and often recurs secondary to an obvious event such as sudden pain, anxiety, or high emotion. Syncope as a result of standing erect and rigid for a long period, especially while perspiring, in a warm environment is related to venous pooling in the lower extremities. When systemic hypotension is suspected to have occurred on a secondary basis, however, due to either a cardiac arrhythmia, an abnormal sympathetic nervous system discharge, or a metabolic disorder, more serious concerns must be raised, and more specific evaluation is required. A family history of syncope may be helpful for supporting a benign diagnosis of vasovagal fainting; but a family history of syncope associated with sudden death is important. Genetic cardiomyopathies, long QT syndrome, and severe autonomic disease are being recognized with increasing frequency.

Syncope in a child or adolescent requires a careful history. Several key questions must be asked.

1. Was the child totally conscious, or was the event more in keeping with dizziness or light-headedness?

2. Was the event sudden, or was there a prodromal period allowing the patient to sit or lie down?

3. Was the fainting episode so sudden that the patient was injured as he or she fell?

4. How long was the patient unconscious?

5. Did anyone measure the child's pulse; and if the heart rate was not recorded, as is often the case, was the pulse considered to be normal, fast, slow, or absent?

6. Was there a history of palpitations, or did the patient complain of an abnormal heartbeat prior to the syncopal event?

7. Did syncope occur during exercise?

8. If seizure activity is noted, did it occur prior to the period of unresponsiveness or afterward?

Answers to these questions almost always allow the physician to determine the difference between simple vasovagal syncope and other specific entities.

Cardiac syncope is usually associated with virtually no prodromal symptoms and often occurs during or just after exercise. Most often the patient is not aware of a cardiac irregularity. The loss of muscle tone is almost always immediate and complete. A history of falling abruptly, occasionally striking the head on the floor or furniture, is often obtained. Upon examination after the event the cardiovascular system appears to be normal. Cardiac syncope can occur with any one of a number of possible etiologies.

1. *Congenital heart disease.* As is true with chest pain, syncope secondary to severe congenital heart disease (e.g., aortic stenosis) as a first diagnostic event is rare; the cardiac examination would have long since indicated that a cardiac abnormality was present.

2. *Cardiomyopathy.* Cardiomyopathy, particularly of the hypertrophic type, may cause syncope on a hemodynamic or dysrhythmia basis. In a family with a history of cardiomyopathy and sudden death the prognosis is particularly poor; immediate, complete specialist examination is required.

3. *Rhythm disorders* (Fig. 9–2).
   a. *Tachycardia* may cause syncope on the basis of sudden low cardiac output. It is important to determine the type of dysrhythmia—atrial, junctional, or ventricular—and if a bypass tract is present (Wolff-Parkinson-White syndrome) so that appropriate treatment can be instituted (see Chapter 11).
   b. In a patient with syncope and a familial history of sudden death, the *long QT syndrome* also must be considered. Such patients are prone to life-threatening cardiac arrhythmias, including ventricular tachycardia and fibrillation. Long QT syndrome may be accompanied by deafness.
   c. *Bradycardia* can produce syncope by one of several mechanisms. Sick sinus syndrome characterizes patients whose sinus node is sluggish and prone to significant bradycardia. This finding is most often associated with patients who have undergone cardiac surgery.
   The patient with *heart block* usually is well known to the primary physician because of chronic bradycardia. Congenital heart block is apparent in the infant and in this age group rarely causes syncope. Acquired heart block is caused most commonly by surgery although the complication now is infrequent. Sudden onset of heart block can occur as a consequence of an active disease or progression of an unrecognized less severe conduction disturbance. In such a patient sudden loss of consciousness (Adam-Stokes event) is a distinct possibility; risk of syncope is less in the patient with long-standing heart block (e.g., congenital heart block).

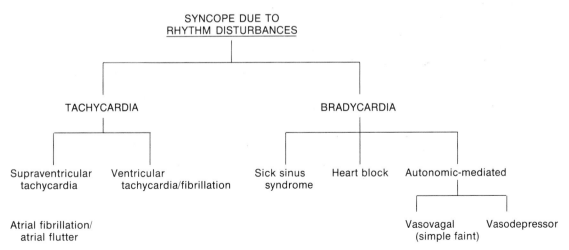

FIGURE 9–2. Evaluation of syncope due to rhythm disturbances.

d. In recent years, there has been increasing recognition of the patient with recurrent *autonomic-mediated syncope*. In contrast to children and adolescents who have single or occasional simple syncopal (vasovagal) episodes, these patients have recurrent episodes that may be associated with prolonged, marked hypotension and bradycardia. Some of these individuals have intrinsic abnormalities of their conduction systems, but most are related to unusual vagal sensitivity.

All patients with suspicious syncope require complete evaluation. Cardiovascular causes of syncope are being recognized with increasing frequency as testing and monitoring methodology have become more sophisticated. The standard electrocardiogram can reveal the diagnosis of abnormalities of atrioventricular conduction (e.g., Wolff-Parkinson-White syndrome) and long QT syndromes. Exercise studies may induce syncope, and electrocardiographic monitoring during a stress test often establishes a diagnosis. Twenty-four hour electrocardiograms can determine if an arrhythmia was noted at the time of syncope. Among patients in whom events are infrequent, however, these studies may not provide an answer. An event recorder may be more helpful because it allows the patient or parent to record an electrocardiogram either when symptoms are first noted or during or immediately after unconsciousness. Echocardiography is indicated if there is suspicion of cardiomyopathy or congenital heart disease. When a severe, life-threatening arrhythmia appears to be the cause of syncope, an electrophysiologic study may be indicated not only to make a diagnosis but to assess the effect of pharmacologic agents and in some cases to ablate an abnormal conduction pathway. Tilt-table examinations have become a useful tool for the diagnosis of recurrent autonomic-mediated fainting episodes.[4] Syncope-prone individuals may lose consciousness when tilted to an upright position, and various subtypes of syncope can be identified upon analysis of blood pressure and electrocardiographic responses (Fig. 9–2). Children and

adolescents with borderline or negative tilt-table responses may have a typical episode when isoproterenol is infused during the study.

Treatment

Treatment of syncope secondary to a cardiac abnormality depends on the specific nature of the problem. Patients with symptomatic second (Mobitz II) or third degree heart block, severe sick sinus syndrome, or certain types of autonomic-mediated syncope are best treated with implantation of a permanent pacemaker. Individuals with unexplained ventricular tachycardia or fibrillation, especially with a family history of sudden death, are managed with an automated internal cardiac defibrillator (AICD). Other types of arrhythmia are managed with pharmacologic, catheter ablation, or surgical therapy. Individuals with long QT syndrome are treated with β-blockade. β-Blockers, steroid treatment, or both are used for management of individuals with recurrent autonomic-mediated syncope demonstrated by tilt-table examination.

It is important to refer any patient with unexplained or recurrent syncope to an appropriate subspecialist for complete evaluation. "Fainting in church" certainly occurs, and it is important not to overreact to clear-cut simple syncope that can be diagnosed by history. In view of the potential life-threatening aspects of cardiac/central nervous system syncope, however, it is prudent to refer patients for further evaluation if there are significant doubts regarding etiology.

REFERENCES

1. Levy D, Savage D: Prevalence of mitral valve prolapse. Am Heart J *113*:1281–1290, 1987.
2. Warth DC, King ME, Cohen JM, et al: Prevalence of mitral valve prolapse in normal children. J Am Coll Cardiol 5:1173–1177, 1985.
3. Kavey REW, Blackman M, Sondheimer HM, Byrum CJ: Ventricular arrhythmias and mitral valve prolapse in childhood. J Pediatr *105*: 885–890, 1984.
4. Almquist A, Goldenberg IF, Milstein S, et al: Provocation of bradycardia and hypotension by isoproterenol and upright posture in patients with unexplained syncope. N Engl J Med *320*:346–351, 1989.

10

RHEUMATIC FEVER

Elia M. Ayoub

Rheumatic fever is a multisystem collagen vascular disease that follows group A streptococcal infection in some individuals who have a genetic predisposition to this disease. The underlying pathologic process is a diffuse inflammation of connective tissue, a characteristic that is shared with other collagen vascular diseases. Rheumatic fever, however, differs from other collagen vascular diseases in three major aspects. First, the agent that initiates the disease process has been recognized and is well defined. Second, cardiac involvement is much more commonly associated with rheumatic fever than with other collagen diseases. Worldwide, rheumatic fever is still the most common cause of acquired heart disease in children and young adults. Third, and possibly most compelling, rheumatic fever is a preventable disease.

A marked decline in the incidence of rheumatic fever was noted in the United States and western Europe during the second half of the twentieth century. This decline may have been responsible for the premature belief that rheumatic fever might disappear totally in these countries, which in turn led to a diminished concern about this disease in the areas of medical education and clinical practice. An unexpected resurgence of the disease in several locations in the United States,[1-7] however, has rekindled interest in rheumatic fever and emphasized the need for continued awareness of the potential damage that could result if we ignore this preventable disease. In addition, data garnered during the recent outbreaks have provided new and important information regarding bacterial and host factors that may play a role in the pathogenesis of rheumatic fever.

EPIDEMIOLOGY

Because of the causal relation between group A streptococcal infections and rheumatic fever, the epidemiology of the two illnesses is closely related. All group A streptococcal infections do not lead to rheumatic fever, however. Epidemiologic studies have shown that rheumatic fever follows infection of the upper respiratory tract but rarely, if ever, follows infection of the skin (impetigo).[8] The epidemiology of rheumatic fever therefore is more intimately related to that of group A streptococcal pharyngitis. In turn, not all cases of streptococcal pharyngitis lead to rheumatic fever. Only 2 to 3 per cent of such patients, *if untreated*, acquire this complication, and appropriate treatment of streptococcal pharyngitis can prevent rheumatic fever in almost all individuals.

The age incidence of rheumatic fever parallels that of streptococcal pharyngitis; it is most common between the ages of 6 and 16 years. Both sexes are affected equally. Racial differences are illustrated by the high incidence of rheumatic fever in the Maori population of New Zealand, in whom this high incidence transcends socioeconomic factors.[9] Socioeconomic factors, however, such as crowded living conditions and lack of accessibility to health care do play a role in the incidence of rheumatic fever. The role, which has been documented previously in the United States, is currently reflected by the high incidence of the disease in developing countries in which the incidence of rheumatic fever is 10 times higher than that in industrialized countries. Current estimates indicate that the incidence of rheumatic fever in the United States is less than 1 per 100,000, whereas in India the incidence of the disease is 100 to 150 per 100,000; about 6 million Indian school-age children are affected by the disease, and 30 to 50 per cent of cardiac disease in children and adolescents is of rheumatic etiology.[10,11]

PATHOGENESIS

Etiologic Agent

β-Hemolytic streptococci characteristically cause complete hemolysis of red blood cells surrounding colonies when cultured on sheep-blood agar medium. The individual bacterial cell, or coccus, consists of an enveloped protoplasm surrounded by a cell wall. The cell wall contains three major structures: a polysaccharide, a protein, and a peptidoglycan moiety. Some strains form a hyaluronic acid capsule around the cell wall during growth. Strains that produce large capsules are recognized by the mucoid appearance of the bacterial colonies on the agar culture medium. Based on differences in the composition of the cell-wall polysaccharide, β-hemolytic streptococci were divided into 20 groups (A to T) using sera from rabbits immunized with the different groups. Group A streptococci were subsequently separated into about 80 types (serotypes M1 to M80) based on differences in the structure of their M protein. Group A streptococci produce a number of extracellular products while growing. These products include strepolysins O and S, which are responsible for lysis of red blood cells, and a number of other enzymes such as streptokinase, hyaluronidase, four deoxyribonuclease isozymes (A, B, C, and D, of which the B isozyme is the most commonly produced), and a nicotinamide adenine dinucleotidase.

The role of β-hemolytic streptococci in the pathogenesis of rheumatic fever has been documented by clinical and microbiologic studies. The association of rheumatic fever with pharyngitis and scarlet fever outbreaks provided initial evidence for this association. Subsequent studies by several investigators defined the specific role of the group A streptococcus in this association. Until recently, it was believed that all group A streptococci could induce rheumatic fever. Evidence procured during the recent outbreaks of rheumatic fever, however, appears to confirm earlier observations that certain strains have a greater potential for inducing rheu-

matic fever than others. These rheumatogenic strains belong to the M1, M3, M5, M6, and M18 serotypes; many are highly encapsulated and form mucoid colonies in culture.[12]

Host

The concept of genetic predisposition to rheumatic fever was suggested by observations indicating that only 2 to 3 per cent of individuals develop rheumatic fever following group A streptococcal pharyngitis, whereas recurrences develop in as many as 50 per cent of patients with inactive rheumatic fever who experience another episode of streptococcal pharyngitis.[13] Family studies of patients with rheumatic fever suggested that susceptibility to the disease involves a single recessive gene.[14] Data supporting the role of heredity in susceptibility to rheumatic fever were provided by the finding of an allotypic marker on B lymphocytes, recognized by a monoclonal antibody (D8/17) that was present on the lymphocytes of almost all patients with rheumatic fever but only a small proportion (14 per cent) of normal controls.[15] Further evidence for a genetic influence was garnered from studies on the frequency of HLA antigens in patients with rheumatic fever.[16-20] Several of these studies have now shown a significantly higher prevalence of certain class II or HLA-DR antigens (HLA-DR4, DR2, DR1, and DR3) in individuals with rheumatic fever than in normal controls. The association of the various HLA-DR antigens appears to be racially related.

Mechanism of Tissue Injury

The exact mechanism by which infection with the group A streptococcus leads to organ injury in the susceptible host remains unclear. Initial theories regarding damage to the tissue by the streptococcus or by some of its toxic products have been replaced by a theory suggesting the potential involvement of an "autoimmune" mechanism in inducing the tissue damage that occurs with rheumatic fever.[21] Immunization of animals with group A streptococci has yielded antisera that bind to mammalian tissues, including cardiac, joint, and brain tissues. In addition, serum from patients with rheumatic fever contains antibodies that bind to these tissues. These observations, together with the finding of common antigenic determinants between components of the group A streptococcal cell and these mammalian tissues, support the concept of immune cross reactivity as a likely mechanism that would account for the involvement of various organs in the inflammatory process of rheumatic fever.

Streptococcal components that appear to possess common antigenic determinants with human tissues include the M protein, protoplast membrane, cell-wall polysaccharide, and capsular hyaluronate.[21–26] Both M protein and protoplast membrane have cross-reactive antigens found in cardiac sarcolemma and myosin as well as the caudate nucleus of the brain. Immunologic cross reactivity between the cell-wall polysaccharide and valvar glycoproteins has also been described. Other observations describing the presence of these circulating antibodies in the serum of patients who do not have rheumatic fever, however, raise doubt about the pathogenetic role of these cross-reactive antibodies. An alternative explanation proposes that cell-mediated immunity may play a more pertinent role in the pathogenesis of tissue injury in rheumatic fever. Studies have demonstrated that peripheral blood lymphocytes from patients with acute rheumatic fever are cytotoxic to cardiac cells grown in tissue culture.[27,28] Some of these studies also indicate that this cytotoxicity is abrogated by the addition of autologous serum, suggesting a protective role for the circulating cross-reactive antibody.[28]

These findings do not provide an explanation for the inherent susceptibility of certain individuals to rheumatic fever. The possibility that such individuals have a genetically determined abnormal immune response to a streptococcal antigen is one that has been explored. The finding of an exaggerated immune response to one of the streptococcal antigens, the group-specific polysaccharide, in patients with rheumatic mitral valve disease could support this possibility. An alternate explanation would invoke the interaction of superantigens, either the M protein(s) or the erythrogenic toxin(s), with HLA antigens of lymphocytes as a potential mediator of the hyperimmune response to the putative streptococcal antigen.[29]

PATHOLOGY

Inflammation of connective tissue is the primary pathologic process in acute rheumatic fever. Underlying this process is a diffuse vasculitis that leads to involvement of several organs, such as the heart and the brain. This vasculitis, however, is most evident clinically in the skin, where the rash that is characteristic of this disease, erythema marginatum, is seen. Most commonly involved are smaller vessels that on histologic examination show proliferation of endothelial cells.

Cardiac involvement is characterized by inflammation of the endocardium and myocardium. Severe inflammation leads to involvement of the pericardium. Unlike other collagen vascular diseases, such as systemic lupus erythematosus or rheumatoid arthritis, in which serositis is not uncommon, isolated pericarditis without myocarditis is rarely encountered in rheumatic fever. Histologic changes are not seen during the early stage of myocarditis but become evident at later stages of the inflammatory process. The changes include edema of the tissue and a cellular infiltrate consisting of lymphocytes and plasma cells but little polymorphonuclear participation. Degeneration of collagen is associated with appearance of eosinophilic deposits called fibrinoid.

The pathognomonic lesion of rheumatic myocarditis is the Aschoff cell or body. This body consists of large cells with a basophilic cytoplasm and a polymorphous nucleus, arranged in a rosette formation around an avascular center of fibrinoid. The Aschoff body is usually seen in tissue of the left atrial appendage but may be encountered in any part of the myocardium. Characteristically, this lesion is seen in subacute or chronic myocarditis but is occasionally present in patients with acute myocarditis and in those without a history of rheumatic fever.[30]

Valvulitis, the hallmark of rheumatic carditis, most commonly affects the mitral valve (Table 10–1). Isolated aortic involvement occurs less frequently. Simultaneous involvement of mitral and aortic valves is due to rheumatic fever in 97 per cent of cases.[31] Endocardial inflammation produces essentially the same histologic changes seen with myocarditis. Gross changes include hyaline degeneration with formation of verrucae at the edge of the affected valve. This lesion prevents complete valvar closure, thereby causing regurgitation. Healing may eventually occur with reversal of the inflammatory process. Progression of the process in the mitral valve may lead to fibrosis and calcification resulting in stenosis.

TABLE 10–1. ETIOLOGY OF VALVAR HEART DISEASE BASED ON PATHOLOGY EXAMINATION OF VALVES FROM PATIENTS OVER 14 YEARS OF AGE

Valve Involved	Rheumatic Etiology (%)
Only mitral	76
Only aortic	13
Mitral and aortic	97

Source: Adapted from Roberts.[31]

CLINICAL MANIFESTATIONS

Manifestations of acute rheumatic fever lag behind the acute pharyngitis by about 20 days. During this latency period, the patient is asymptomatic. Onset of the disease is marked by the appearance of fever along with a variety of symptoms that reflect inflammation of certain organs. The most common of these symptoms is migratory arthritis, involving the large joints. This manifestation is seen in about 70 per cent of patients with acute rheumatic fever. Carditis, however, occurring in about half the patients, is the most serious of the various manifestations. Sydenham chorea occurs in 10 to 15 per cent of patients. Unlike the other major manifestations of acute rheumatic fever, the symptoms of Sydenham chorea appear 2 to 12 months after the inciting pharyngitis. Other major manifestations of acute rheumatic fever include the highly specific rash of erythema marginatum and subcutaneous nodules; these manifestations are seen in about 5 per cent of patients. Any one of the major manifestations may be seen alone or in association with one or more of the other manifestations during the acute phase of the disease. The minor manifestations are less specific and are encountered frequently in association with a number of other illnesses, particularly other collagen vascular diseases.

The frequency with which major manifestations have been encountered in the United States has remained relatively the same, although a higher incidence of chorea was reported from some locations during the recent outbreaks[1,7] (Table 10–2). An exceptionally high frequency of carditis was reported in the outbreak in Utah. It may have been related to the use of Doppler echocardiography, as exclusion of patients who did not have a murmur detected by auscultation reduced the frequency of carditis to that encountered in other studies. Doppler echocardiography may identify minimal mitral regurgitation in normal individuals, so one must remain cautious about making a diagnosis based solely on echocardiographic findings. Reports from developing countries describe a high frequency of cardiac involvement, particularly mitral stenosis, which may reflect either a bias related to the collection of data from patients who are hospitalized only when severe cardiac disease is present or severe carditis resulting from recurrences of the disease because of the lack of prophylactic measures.

Major Manifestations

Arthritis is the most common yet the least specific of the major manifestations. The large joints are most commonly affected. In most instances there is evidence of inflammation of the joint with redness, warmth, and marked pain. The pain in some cases is so severe that the patient refuses to use the affected limb, leading to the appearance of pseudoparalysis. One of the characteristics of arthritis is that it is migratory in nature, with rapid resolution of the arthritis of an affected joint prior to the appearance of arthritis in a different joint. Another character-

TABLE 10–2. FREQUENCY OF MAJOR MANIFESTATIONS IN RECENTLY REPORTED OUTBREAKS OF RHEUMATIC FEVER

Outbreak	Patients with Manifestations (%)				
	Arthritis	Carditis	Sydenham Chorea	Erythema Marginatum	Subcutaneous Nodules
Veasy et al.[1] (Utah)	56	91	32	3	8
Wald et al.[2] (Pennsylvania)	47	59	30	0	0
Hosier et al.[3] (Columbus, Ohio)	65	50	18	10	3
Congeni et al.[4] (Akron, Ohio)	78	30	9	13	0
Westlake et al.[7] (Tennessee)	58	73	31	4	0

istic of the arthritis of rheumatic fever is its exquisite response to salicylates. Patients often experience rapid and total resolution of arthritis following the administration of their initial dose of aspirin. The arthritis of rheumatic fever rarely persists beyond 48 to 72 hours after initiation of salicylate therapy.

Carditis represents the most serious aspect of the morbidity in this disease and accounts for most of the mortality associated with it. Cardiac inflammation during the acute disease involves most commonly the endocardium and myocardium and, on occasion, the pericardium. Involvement of all three layers of the heart represents pancarditis, the most serious form of carditis. Carditis may occur as the only manifestation or may be associated with one or more of the other major manifestations of acute rheumatic fever. Carditis may follow arthritis in some patients, usually within 1 week after the onset of arthritis. The relative severity of concomitant arthritis and carditis are usually reciprocal: The more severe one is, the less severe is the other. Patients in whom the initially recognized major manifestation is Sydenham chorea may harbor carditis that is clinically mild and subtle; the murmur of mild mitral regurgitation may be easily missed.

Acute carditis is manifested clinically by tachycardia and almost always is associated with murmurs of valvar disease. Transient abnormalities in cardiac rhythm can occur during myocardial inflammation, including varying degrees of conduction delay, such as prolongation of the PR interval on the electrocardiogram. This finding does not establish the diagnosis of rheumatic fever, however. Severe myocarditis can result in myocardial failure manifested by cardiac enlargement on chest radiography and decreased ventricular contractility on echocardiography. Enlargement of the left atrial appendage on the chest radiograph (see Fig. 2–18) is almost pathognomonic of rheumatic mitral regurgitation. Clinical evidence of valvulitis is reflected by the presence of characteristic murmurs. The murmur of mitral regurgitation is a high-pitched, blowing systolic murmur that begins with S_1. It is heard best at the apex and radiates clearly to the left axilla. The murmur of acute mitral regurgitation tends to be decrescendo in shape, whereas the murmur of chronic mitral regurgitation is more constant in intensity. An apical mid-diastolic murmur due to increased rapid phase filling of the left ventricle may be heard in patients with significant mitral regurgitation. The high-pitched, decrescendo diastolic murmur of aortic insufficiency begins immediately after the aortic component of S_2 and is best heard in the third left intercostal space at the sternal edge. The presence of pericarditis is indicated by chest pain and a friction rub. The presence of a pericardial effusion, rarely substantial in size, can be determined by echocardiography.

Chorea (Sydenham chorea, St. Vitus dance) reflects involvement of the central nervous system in rheumatic fever. The onset of chorea may lag behind that of arthritis or carditis by several months (average 3 to 4 months). The manifestations include involuntary, purposeless movements of muscles of the extremities, muscular incoordination, fasciculations of the muscles of the tongue (wormian tongue) when protruded, irregular contractions of the muscles of the hands when the examiner's fingers are squeezed by the patient (milkmaid's grip), and spooning with pronation of the hands when the patient's arms are extended horizontally or vertically. These findings are often associated with emotional lability.

Erythema marginatum is a rash that is characteristic of rheumatic fever. It consists of erythematous, serpiginous macular lesions with pale centers seen mainly on the trunk, arms, buttocks, and thighs (never on the face). It is accentuated by the application of warmth and is not pruritic.

Subcutaneous nodules are rarely seen in the absence of chronic carditis. They are firm, painless, and mobile, with normal overlying skin. Nodules are usually present on the extensor surfaces of large joints, in the occipital region, and over the spinous processes of the vertebrae.

Minor Manifestations

Fever and arthralgia are two nonspecific *clinical manifestations* that are associated also with a number of other diseases. Fever occurs early in the course of acute rheumatic fever. Arthralgia denotes pain in the joints without objective changes.

Laboratory changes associated with acute rheumatic fever include elevated acute-phase reactants—erythrocyte sedimentation rate (ESR) and C-reactive protein (CRP)—in most patients with acute arthritis or carditis. The abnormal acute-phase reactants are reliable indices of acute disease activity. A prolonged PR interval on the electrocardiogram is seen frequently but may occur with other inflammatory processes and is not by itself a criterion for the diagnosis of carditis.

DIAGNOSIS

The diagnosis of rheumatic fever is based primarily on clinical findings. Because there is no specific test at present that allows for the definitive diagnosis of acute rheumatic fever, the Jones Criteria[32] (Table 10–3) have been established to guide the physician to confirm this diagnosis and to avoid the over-diagnosis of rheumatic fever. The finding of two of the major manifestations or, alternately, one of the major manifestations plus two of the minor manifestations described above supports this diagnosis. In view of the fact that acute rheumatic fever is a consequence of group A streptococcal pharyngitis, *establishing the diagnosis requires evidence of a recent group A streptococcal infection.* Because clinical evidence for streptococcal pharyngitis is tenuous, laboratory evidence for such an infection is considered more reliable. A positive throat culture or rapid antigen test could be used as evidence

TABLE 10–3. JONES CRITERIA (REVISED) FOR GUIDANCE IN THE DIAGNOSIS OF RHEUMATIC FEVER

The presence of two major criteria or of one major and two minor criteria indicates a high probability of acute rheumatic fever, if supported by evidence of a preceding group A streptococcal infection.

Major Manifestations	Minor Manifestations
Carditis	Clinical
Polyarthritis	Arthralgia
Chorea	Fever
Erythema marginatum	Laboratory
Subcutaneous nodules	Acute-phase reactants
	Erythrocyte sedimentation rate
	C-reactive protein
	Prolonged PR interval on ECG

Supporting Evidence of Antecedent Streptococcal Infection

Elevated or rising streptococcal antibody titer(s)
Positive throat culture or rapid antigen test for group A streptococcus

Source: Adapted from Special Writing Group of the Committee on Rheumatic Fever, Endocarditis, and Kawasaki Disease of the Council on Cardiovascular Disease in the Young of the American Heart Association 1992.[32] JAMA 268: 2069–2073, 1992. Copyright 1992, American Medical Association.

TABLE 10–4. GROUP A STREPTOCOCCAL ANTIGENS AND CORRESPONDING ANTIBODY TESTS

Antigen	Antibody Test
Extracellular product	
Streptolysin O	ASO
Streptokinase	ASK
Hyaluronidase	ASH
Deoxyribonuclease B	Anti-DNase B
Nicotinamide adenine dinucleotidase	Anti-NADase Streptozyme
Multiple antigens	
Cellular component	
Group A carbohydrate	Anti-A-CHO

for infection, although the high rate of chronic carriage of group A streptococcus at that site diminishes the reliability of these tests for diagnosing an antecedent infection. Serologic evidence for group A streptococcal infection, using the streptococcal antibody tests, is more reliable.

Infection by the group A streptococcus elicits an immune response to a number of its antigens. Several tests that assay the level of serum antibodies to the extracellular products now are available for the diagnosis of group A streptococcal infection (Table 10–4). Of these tests, the ASO is the best standardized, reliable, and most widely available. It is considered the primary streptococcal antibody test. Because antibody response to streptolysin O occurs in only about 85 per cent of patients with rheumatic fever (Table 10–5), one or more of the other tests should be utilized in patients who have a suspiciously normal ASO titer. Anti-DNase

TABLE 10–5. PATIENTS WITH ACUTE RHEUMATIC FEVER SHOWING AN ELEVATED ANTIBODY WITH ASO, ANTI-DNASE B, OR BOTH

Subjects	% Patients with Elevated Antibody Titer		
	ASO	Anti-DNase B	ASO and Anti-DNase B
Normal controls	19	19	30
Acute rheumatic fever	83	82	92
Sydenham chorea (isolated)	67	40	80

Source: Adapted from Ayoub, Wannamaker.[40,41] Reproduced by permission of Pediatrics.

B now is considered more reliable than the other tests and is available commercially. Other tests are less reproducible, but they may be used if available. It should be pointed out that the streptozyme test is the least specific of these tests and should not be relied on as a primary test for the diagnosis of antecedent streptococcal infection.[33]

Antibody response to streptococcal antigens peaks 2 to 3 weeks after the inciting infection. Except for chorea, symptoms of acute rheumatic fever appear during this interval. Performance of antibody tests on serum obtained at the time of presentation of the patient therefore is adequate. One rarely needs convalescent antibody titers on patients with acute rheumatic fever to confirm the occurrence of a recent streptococcal infection. The ASO test should be performed initially. If negative, one of the other tests is done, preferably the anti-DNase B. Despite the long period of latency for chorea, about 80 per cent of patients who present with isolated chorea show an antibody response to one of two streptococcal antigens (Table 10–5).

No established criteria are available for the diagnosis of chronic rheumatic heart disease; most antibody tests are normal in such patients. Persistence of elevated levels of antibody to the streptococcal group A carbohydrate has been found in most patients with chronic rheumatic mitral valve disease.[34–36] This test, available in certain laboratories, may help distinguish rheumatic from nonrheumatic mitral valve insufficiency in patients without a history of acute rheumatic fever. Remember that none of the streptococcal antibody tests, by itself, is diagnostic of rheumatic fever. These tests serve only to provide evidence for group A streptococcal infection and to supplement the Jones Criteria for the diagnosis of acute rheumatic fever. Enlargement of the left atrial appendage (see Fig. 2–18) in a patient with mitral regurgitation is strong evidence of rheumatic etiology. A pattern of left ventricular hypertrophy characterized by small or absent q waves and flat or negative T waves in leads V_6 and V_7 (Fig. 10–1) also is common with chronic rheumatic heart disease.

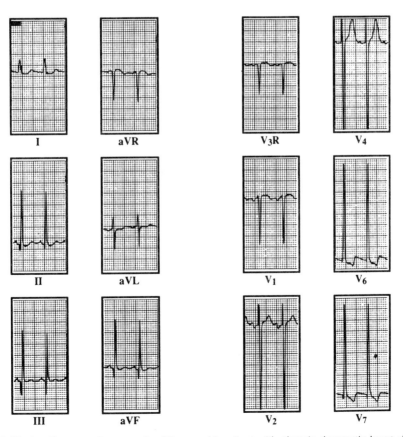

FIGURE 10–1. Electrocardiogram of a 15-year-old patient with chronic rheumatic heart disease. There is severe left ventricular hypertrophy with small q and biphasic T waves in V_6 and V_7.

DIFFERENTIAL DIAGNOSIS

Differential diagnosis of acute rheumatic fever includes primarily those diseases that present with fever and either arthritis or carditis. Collagen vascular diseases (e.g., juvenile rheumatoid arthritis, systemic lupus erythematosus, or mixed connective tissue disease) and serum sickness should be considered when a patient presents with arthritis as the only major manifestation. Postinfectious arthritis, such as gonococcal arthritis and Lyme disease, should also be considered. Unlike the migratory arthritis of rheumatic fever, rheumatoid arthritis is symmetric, and the affected joints are not erythematous but are pale and warm. Juvenile rheumatoid arthritis usually begins in children younger than 6 years of age, and in most cases the response of the arthritis to salicylates is not dramatic. Evidence for an antecedent streptococcal infection generally is lacking in nonrheumatic patients, and antinuclear antibody tests usually are negative in patients with acute rheumatic fever. The murmur of mitral regurgitation due to rheumatic heart disease should be differentiated from that due to mitral valve prolapse or other congenital heart disease. Rheumatic fever has been suggested to be a cause of mitral valve prolapse, but this possibility is unlikely. Myocarditis or pericarditis of viral etiology should be considered in the absence of evidence for antecedent streptococcal infection. Isolated pericarditis rarely is seen with rheumatic fever without evidence of concomitant myocarditis.

TREATMENT

Comprehensive management of patients with rheumatic fever includes the prevention of primary episodes of rheumatic fever in patients with group A streptococcal pharyngitis, treatment of acute manifestations of the disease, prevention of recurrences in patients who have had rheumatic fever, and prevention of bacterial endocarditis in those who have valvar disease.

Prevention of a first attack of rheumatic fever is achieved by proper diagnosis and treatment of streptococcal pharyngitis. A throat culture or a "rapid" test is accepted as a reliable method for establishing the diagnosis of streptococcal pharyngitis. A negative rapid test, however, should be confirmed by throat culture.[37] Once the etiology of a sore throat is determined to be due to the group A streptococcus by either of these methods, proper treatment should be started. A delay of 1 day in initiating antibiotic therapy is of little or no consequence in preventing rheumatic fever. More important is the duration of therapy. Antibiotics should be administered in doses that ensure adequate levels in the host for at least 10 days. Approved antibiotic regimens for treatment of streptococcal pharyngitis are shown in Table 10–6. Penicillin remains the mainstay of treatment; to date, resistance of group A streptococci to penicillin has not been encountered. Although intramuscular administration of a long-acting penicillin may be more effective, the pain associated with the injection makes oral therapy preferable to the patient. Patients allergic to penicillin can be treated with erythromycin. The use of broad-spectrum antibiotics should be discouraged, as they have no advantage over penicillin. Sulfa drugs or their derivatives, such as trimethoprim-sulfamethoxazole, do not prevent primary episodes of rheumatic fever and should not be used to treat streptococcal pharyngitis.

Treatment of a patient with acute rheumatic fever starts with eradicating the streptococcus from the site of infection. This goal is achieved by administering one of the antibiotic regimens listed in Table 10–6. Further management is directed at the individual manifestations of the disease. Arthritis associated with rheumatic fever is self-limited and responds promptly to salicylate

TABLE 10–6. PRIMARY PREVENTION OF RHEUMATIC FEVER: STREPTOCOCCAL ERADICATING ANTIBIOTIC THERAPY

Agent	Dose	Route	Duration
Benzathine penicillin G	1,200,000 U	Intramuscular	Once
Penicillin V	250 mg tid	Oral	10 Days
Erythromycin	50 mg/kg/day (maximum 1 gm/day) in 3–4 divided doses	Oral	10 Days

therapy, even in moderate doses. One should anticipate resolution of the arthritis within 72 hours after initiating salicylate treatment. Salicylate dosage is 75 to 80 mg/kg/day four divided doses for 2 weeks; this dose is then tapered and discontinued over the next 2 weeks. Steroids should not be used to treat patients with isolated arthritis.

Treatment of carditis depends on the severity of cardiac involvement. Mild carditis without cardiac failure is treated with salicylates at a dose of 80 to 100 mg/kg/day for 2 to 4 weeks depending on the clinical response. This dose is then gradually tapered and discontinued over 4 to 6 weeks while monitoring clinical and laboratory parameters, such as the ESR and CRP. As with arthritis, gradual reduction of the dose of salicylates avoids rebound of the clinical and laboratory abnormalities that occurs sometimes with abrupt discontinuation of therapy. Rebound requires reinstitution of therapeutic doses of salicylates followed by gradual withdrawal.

Severe carditis with heart failure, particularly pancarditis, requires steroid therapy. This therapy literally may be life-saving because of the rapidity with which it turns off the inflammatory response. Prednisone is given in a dose of 2 mg/kg/day, maximum 60 mg daily, for 2 to 3 weeks. It is then tapered over an additional 2 to 3 weeks. Salicylates contribute adversely to sodium load in patients with cardiac failure but should be started in the above regimen when steroids are tapered so as to avoid a rebound phenomenon. Do not misinterpret the action of these drugs. Neither salicylates nor steroids alter the subsequent outcome with respect to residual valvar disease. Supportive therapy in patients with severe carditis includes oxygen, digitalis, fluid and salt restriction, and diuretics. Because myocarditis renders the tissue sensitive to digitalis and increases cardiac irritability, digitalization should be performed carefully, using doses at the lower end of those recommended for treating heart failure (see Chapter 7). Bed rest is limited to the acute stage. The patient should be gradually ambulated once signs of active carditis resolve and cardiac status is stable. An increase in resting heart rate is directly related to the degree of carditis and is therefore a useful guide. Prolonged confinement to bed of a child with stable heart disease is unnecessary.

Sydenham chorea is self-limited in its duration, rarely lasting more than a few weeks. Occasionally, chorea persists for months or recurs over several years. Patients with severe chorea should be confined to a padded bed and placed in a quiet room. Sedation using phenobarbital at a dose of 15 to 30 mg every 6 to 8 hours or haloperidol starting at 0.5 mg and increasing to 0.8 mg every 8 hours may help control the symptoms. Valproate has also been reported to be effective.[38] Response to these sedatives is variable. Salicylates and steroids are not useful for management of isolated chorea.

CONTINUING CARE

Individuals who have had an attack of rheumatic fever are at high risk for recurrence of the disease if allowed to acquire another episode of streptococcal pharyngitis. Recurrence of the disease carries with it the potential for new cardiac involvement in individuals who had escaped this complication on a previous attack and for additional cardiac damage in individuals who had prior cardiac residua. Secondary prophylaxis aims at preventing recurrences of rheumatic fever by preventing recurrent streptococcal infections. Secondary prophylaxis has proved to be a highly effective method for preventing recurrences of rheumatic fever and for reducing the incidence of severe cardiac disease in the countries that have adopted such programs.

Regimens approved for the *secondary prophylaxis of rheumatic fever* are outlined in Table 10–7. Monthly injections of long-acting benzathine penicillin are the most effective. Oral sulfadiazine is ineffective and should not be used to treat streptococcal pharyngitis for primary prevention of rheumatic fever, but it is effective for secondary prophylaxis of this disease. It is recommended for use in patients who are allergic

TABLE 10–7. SECONDARY PREVENTION OF RHEUMATIC FEVER

Agent	Dose	Route
Benzathine penicillin G	1,200,000 U q4wk	Intramuscular
Penicillin V	250 mg bid	Oral
Sulfadiazine	1.0 gm once daily	Oral
Erythromycin ethyl succinate	250 mg bid	Oral

to penicillin. For those who do not tolerate sulfadiazine, erythromycin is the recommended alternative. Other antibiotics, such as cephalosporins, are theoretically effective but have not undergone clinical trials to prove their efficacy in primary or secondary prevention of rheumatic fever.

The risk of a recurrence of rheumatic fever decreases as the interval from the previous episode of rheumatic fever increases. This risk is highest during the 5-year interval following the last attack. Therefore secondary prophylaxis should be instituted immediately after the diagnosis of rheumatic fever is established. The duration of prophylaxis is related to the presence of cardiac involvement and the risk of acquiring streptococcal pharyngitis. Patients with cardiac involvement, particularly those with severe residua, should receive intramuscular benzathine penicillin for the first 5 years and then should continue either this or an alternative regimen for their lifetime. Patients who are receiving warfarin (Coumadin) because of the presence of an artificial valve should not be given intramuscular injections and therefore must receive oral prophylaxis. Prophylaxis may be discontinued in only selected patients with arthritis who have completed at least 5 years of prophylaxis and who have reached the age of 20 years. It is preferable to maintain on continuous prophylaxis individuals with rheumatic fever who live or work in an environment whose population density, particularly of children and youth, creates a significant risk of exposure to streptococcal infection.

In addition to using secondary prophylaxis to prevent recurrences of rheumatic fever by preventing streptococcal pharyngitis, patients with residual valvar disease also must receive routine *prophylaxis to prevent bacterial endocarditis* (see Chapter 15). Patients must be seen for follow-up evaluation at regular intervals after the acute episode. The purposes of these clinic visits are to assess the status of the disease and ensure compliance with prophylaxis. Education of the patient regarding the reasons for and the value of prophylaxis is the most effective way to ensure that a patient who may otherwise feel well adheres to the prophylaxis that has been prescribed. The most compelling reason for prophylaxis is the knowledge that resolution of cardiac residua occurs in 70 to 80 per cent of patients with rheumatic heart disease who adhere to prophylaxis after their initial episode.[39]

REFERENCES

1. Veasy LG, Wiedmeier SE, Orsmond GS: Resurgence of acute rheumatic fever in the intermountain area of the United States. N Engl J Med *316*: 421–427, 1987.
2. Wald ER, Dashefsky B, Feidt C: Acute rheumatic fever in western Pennsylvania and the tristate area. Pediatrics *80*:371–374, 1987.
3. Hosier DM, Craenen JM, Teske DW: Resurgence of rheumatic fever. Am J Dis Child *141*:730–733, 1987.
4. Congeni B, Rizzo C, Congeni J: Outbreak of rheumatic fever in northeast Ohio. J Pediatr *111*: 176–179, 1987.
5. Papadinos T, Escanmilla J, Garst P: Acute rheumatic fever at a navy training center—San Diego, California. MMWR *37*:101–104, 1988.
6. Sampson GL, Williams RG, House MD: Acute rheumatic fever among army trainees—Fort Leonard Wood, Missouri, 1987–1988. MMWR *37*: 519–522, 1988.
7. Westlake RM, Edwards KM, Graham TP: Adult rheumatic fever: resurgence in Tennessee. Pediatr Res *25*:106A, 1989.
8. Wannamaker LW: Differences between streptococcal infections of the throat and of the skin. N Engl J Med *282*:23–31, 1970.
9. Wannamaker LW: Changes and changing concepts in the biology of group A streptococci and in the epidemiology of streptococcal infections. Rev Infect Dis *1*:967–975, 1979.
10. Markowitz M: The decline of rheumatic fever: role of medical intervention. Pediatrics *106*: 545–550, 1966.
11. Agarwal BL: Rheumatic heart disease unabated in developing countries. Lancet *11*:910–911, 1981.
12. Kaplan EL, Johnson DR, Cleary PP: Group A streptococcal serotypes isolated from patient and sibling contacts during the resurgence of rheumatic fever in the United States in the mid-1980's. J Infect Dis *159*:101–103, 1989.
13. Rammelkamp Jr CH: Epidemiology of streptococcal infections. Harvey Lect Ser *51*:113–142, 1956.
14. Wilson MG, Schweitzer M: Pattern of hereditary susceptibility in rheumatic fever. Circulation *10*: 699–704, 1954.
15. Khanna AK, Buskirk DR, Williams RC: Presence of a non-HLA B cell antigen in rheumatic fever patients and their families as defined by a monoclonal antibody. J Clin Invest *83*:1710–1716, 1989.
16. Anastasiou-Nana MI, Anderson JL, Carlquist JF: HLA-DR typing and lymphocyte subset evaluation in rheumatic heart disease: a search for immune response factors. Am Heart J *112*:992–997, 1986.
17. Jhingham B, Henra NK, Reddy KS: HLA, blood groups and secretor status in patients with established rheumatic fever and rheumatic heart disease. Tissue Antigens *267*:172–178, 1986.
18. Maharaj B, Hammond MG, Appadoo B: HLA-A, B, DR, and DQ antigens in black patients with severe chronic rheumatic heart disease. Circulation *76*:259–261, 1987.
19. Taneja V, Mehra NK, Reddy KS, et al: HLA-DR/DQ and reactivity to B cell alloantigen D8/17 in Indian patients with rheumatic heart disease. Circulation *80*:335–340, 1989.
20. Ayoub EM, Barrett DJ, Maclaren NK, Krischer JP:

Association of class II human histocompatibility leukocyte antigens with rheumatic fever. J Clin Invest 77:2019–2025, 1986.

21. Kaplan MH: Rheumatic fever, rheumatic heart disease, and the streptococcal connection: the role of streptococcal antigens cross reactive with heart tissue. Rev Infect Dis *1*:988–996, 1979.

22. Zabriskie JB, Freimer EH: An immunological relationship between group A streptococci and mammalian muscle. J Exp Med *124*:661–668, 1966.

23. Dale JB, Beachey EH: Multiple heart-cross-reactive epitopes of streptococcal M proteins. J Exp Med *161*:113–122, 1985.

24. Husby G, Van de Rijn I, Zabriskie JB, et al: Antibodies reacting with cytoplasm of the subthalamic and caudate nuclei neurons in chorea and acute rheumatic fever. J Exp Med *144*:1094–1110, 1976.

25. Goldstein I, Reybeyrotte P, Parlebas J, et al: Isolation from heart valves of glycopeptides which share immunological properties with streptococcus hemolyticus group A polysaccharides. Nature *219*:866–868, 1968.

26. Sandson J, Hamerman D, Janis R, et al: Immunologic and chemical similarities between the streptococcus and human connective tissue. Trans Assoc Am Physicians *81*:249–257, 1968.

27. Yang LC, Soprey PR, Wittner MK, et al: Streptococcal induced cell mediated immune destruction of cardiac myofibers in vitro. J Exp Med *146*: 344–360, 1977.

28. Hutto J, Ayoub EM: Cytotoxicity of lymphocytes from patients with rheumatic carditis to cardiac cells in vitro. *In* Streptococcal Disease and Immune Response. Orlando, FL, Academic Press, 1980, pp. 733–738.

29. Tomai M, Kolb M, Majundar G, Beachey EH: Superantigenicity of streptococcal M protein. J Exp Med *172*:359–362, 1990.

30. Murphy GE: Nature of rheumatic heart disease: with special reference to myocardial disease and heart failure. Medicine (Baltimore) *39*:289–340, 1960.

31. Roberts WC: Anatomically isolated aortic valvular disease; the case against it being of rheumatic etiology. Am J Med *49*:151–159, 1970.

32. Special Writing Group of the Committee on Rheumatic Fever, Endocarditis and Kawasaki Disease of the Council on Cardiovascular Disease in the Young of the American Heart Association 1992: Guidelines for the diagnosis of rheumatic fever (Jones criteria, 1992, update). JAMA *268*: 2069–2073, 1992.

33. Gerber MA, Wright LL, Randolph MF: Streptozyme test for antibodies to group A streptococcal antigens. Pediatr Infect Dis J 6:36–40, 1987.

34. Dudding BA, Ayoub EM: Persistence of streptococcal antibody in patients with rheumatic valvular disease. J Exp Med *128*:1081–1098, 1968.

35. Shulman ST, Ayoub EM, Victorica BE: Differences in antibody response to streptococcal antigens in children with rheumatic and non-rheumatic mitral valve disease. Circulation 50: 1244–1251, 1974.

36. Appleton RS, Victorica BE, Ayoub EM: Specificity of persistence of antibody to the streptococcal Group A carbohydrate in rheumatic valvular heart disease. J Lab Clin Med *105*:1:114–119, 1985.

37. Lewey S, White CB, Lieberman MM, Morales E: Evaluation of the throat culture as a follow-up for an initially negative enzyme immunosorbent assay rapid streptococcal antigen detection test. Pediatr Infect Dis J 7:765–769, 1988.

38. Daoud AS, Zaki M, Shaki R, Al-Saleh Q: Effectiveness of sodium valproate in the treatment of Sydenham's chorea. Neurology *40*:1140–1141, 1990.

39. Tompkins DG, Boxerbaum B, Liebman J: Long-term prognosis of rheumatic fever patients receiving regular intramuscular benzathine penicillin. Circulation 45:543–551, 1973.

40. Ayoub EM, Wannamaker LW: Evaluation of the streptococcal deoxyribonuclease B and diphosphopyridine nucleotidase antibody tests in acute rheumatic fever and acute glomerulonephritis. Pediatrics 29:527–538, 1959.

41. Ayoub EM, Wannamaker LW: Streptococcal antibody titers in Sydenham's chorea. Pediatrics 28: 946–956, 1958.

11

DISTURBANCES OF CARDIAC RHYTHM

Michael L. Epstein

Many kinds of cardiac rhythm disturbances occur in infants and children, the incidence depending on how extensive an investigation is undertaken. For the most part, these arrhythmias are of no clinical significance. Recurrent or sustained arrhythmias may require thorough evaluation and treatment; those causing symptoms mandate complete evaluation and aggressive management. The incidence of arrhythmias in infants and children with heart disease is increased because of changes that follow cardiac surgery. As more knowledge about the mechanism of these arrhythmias is gained, however, progress can be made in minimizing and possibly eliminating serious rhythm disturbances. Fortunately, the long-term prognosis for most of these children is excellent.

Disturbances of cardiac rhythm are characterized in this chapter as abnormalities of impulse initiation, abnormalities of impulse conduction, or a combination of the two. No attempt is made to present a detailed discussion of all arrhythmias. Common arrhythmias are discussed with primary emphasis on diagnosis and appropriate management by the primary care physician.

When evaluating a patient suspected to have an arrhythmia, one must keep in mind that many variations in sinus rhythm (initial cardiac impulse originating from the sinus node with subsequent conduction through the normal conduction system) are considered normal. These variations affect both regularity and rate. Careful attention to this phenomenon may eliminate the need for referral to a specialist.

Evaluation by the primary care physician of a patient with a suspected arrhythmia need not be complex. Careful history taking is important particularly in regard to complaints of "palpitations" or "tachycardia." How fast is the heart rate? Under what circumstances do symptoms appear? How anxious is the child? The parent? Physical examination may reveal occasional premature beats, but most likely the examination is normal. Depending on the complaint, an electrocardiogram, which should be a standard 12-lead tracing, may be useful. A so-called rhythm strip generally is of no additional benefit for a patient whose physical examination did not reveal a rhythm disturbance.

If the history is convincing for the possibility of rhythm disturbance, or if symptoms are more substantial, additional evaluation may be indicated. It probably is best accomplished by specialist referral.

Additional simple procedures that can be accomplished for rhythm analysis are ambulatory electrocardiographic monitoring (Holter monitoring) and event monitoring. Ambulatory monitoring is continuous two-channel electrocardiographic recording for 24 hours. This technique allows recording during sleep and normal activity. A patient diary permits correlation of symptoms with rhythm changes. Symptoms may not occur during a particular 24-hour interval, in which case an event monitor is useful. This monitor is a hand-held instrument that can be applied to the chest immediately upon noting a symptom. It allows electrocardiographic recording for 30 to 60 seconds. Several events can be recorded, after which the instrument is down-loaded via an ordinary telephone to the monitoring heart station where a permanent paper recording is made. This process erases the tape, allowing the event monitor to be used again.

Evaluation of chest pain and syncope or near-syncope is discussed in Chapter 9.

ANATOMY OF THE CARDIAC CONDUCTION SYSTEM

The initial electrical impulse normally arises from the sinus node, a specialized collection of anatomically distinct cells located on the high lateral right atrium just below its junction with the superior vena cava (Fig. 11–1). The rate of impulse generation from the sinus node varies with autonomic tone, circulating catecholamines, and a variety of medications. The impulse activates atrial musculature and travels along broad pathways that are not anatomically distinct from the rest of the atrial tissue.[1] The impulse enters the ventricles through the atrioventricular node, a second collection of specialized myocardial cells located on the right side of the central fibrous body between the orifice of the coronary sinus and the annulus of the medial leaflet of the tricuspid valve. The ventricular end of the atrioventricular node continues as a compact "tail," known as the bundle of His, that penetrates the ventricular septum. The bundle of His divides into right and left bundle branches. The left bundle branch bifurcates into anterior and posterior fascicles. The right and two left bundles terminate in the myocardium as networks of Purkinje fibers resulting in activation of ventricular myocardium. Knowledge of these major components of the cardiac conduction system is helpful as one thinks about mechanisms of various disturbances in cardiac rhythm.

DISORDERS OF IMPULSE FORMATION

Variations in Sinus Rhythm

Sinus rhythm is defined as a continued series of heartbeats characterized by the presence of a P wave that has a normal frontal plane axis followed, after an appropriate interval (PR), by a QRS complex. The normal sinus P wave axis is directed to the left and inferiorly. (It is directed to the right and inferiorly in individuals with mirror-image situs inversus.) Sinus arrhythmia, a normal finding in children, is characterized by repetitive variation in the P to P (and therefore R to R) interval with otherwise normal sinus rhythm characteristics. Variation in rate coincides with respiration and is modulated by a variety of reflexes. The rate increases with inspiration and slows with expiration. Sinus bradycardia is considered by many to be an arrhythmia, although it simply is sinus rhythm at a rate below accepted normal standards.[2,3] Similarly, sinus tachycardia is normal sinus rhythm at a rate higher than the accepted standard for the patient's age.[2,3]

Premature Beats

Premature atrial contractions (PACs: premature atrial beats, atrial extrasystoles) are

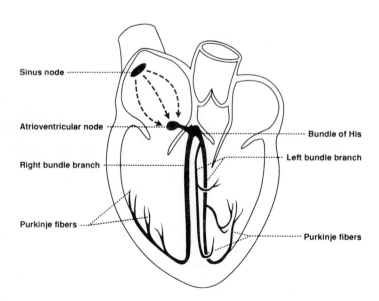

Sinus node

Atrioventricular node

Right bundle branch

Purkinje fibers

Bundle of His

Left bundle branch

Purkinje fibers

FIGURE 11–1. Cardiac conduction system.

complexes that arise in atrial tissue and that occur early in relation to the prevailing rhythm. PACs typically have a P wave whose morphology is different from that of the sinus P wave (Fig. 11–2). If the premature beat occurs late following the previous normal impulse or arises low in the atrium relatively close to the atrioventricular node, the PR interval may be shortened. If the interval from the last normal P wave to the premature beat is short, the succeeding PR interval may be mildly prolonged compared to the normal interval. When the PAC is even earlier, it may not be conducted into the ventricles because the conduction system is still refractory. In this case there is no QRS, and a pause appears in the ventricular rhythm. The most common cause of a pause in ventricular rhythm is a nonconducted PAC. Occasionally, the impulse from a PAC is conducted through the atrioventricular (AV) specialized conduction system (AV node, bundle of His, and Purkinje system) at a time when only a portion of the bundle branches remain refractory. It results in aberrant conduction to the ventricular myocardium, manifested as change in configuration, usually widening, of the QRS complex (Fig. 11–2).

Premature junctional contractions (PJCs: junctional extrasystoles) behave much like the PACs. The typical electrocardiographic pattern of a PJC is a QRS complex that occurs prematurely in relation to the prevailing rhythm but that does not have an identifiable P wave preceding it. A PJC may occur

at a time when a portion of the bundle branches is refractory and therefore may demonstrate aberrant ventricular conduction as just described with PACs. The pause that follows a PAC or a PJC usually is noncompensatory, meaning that the interval from the last normal QRS complex to the first normal QRS complex following the premature complex is less than two times the normal R to R interval. This phenomenon occurs because, in most cases, the premature impulse penetrates the sinus node, resetting it. The next sinus node impulse occurs at the normal interval after this premature depolarization of the sinus node, which creates a total interval that includes a single atrial cycle length and the premature interval, the sum of which is less than twice the normal R to R interval. It may be impossible to distinguish by standard electrocardiogram between a PJC and a PAC that arises so low in the atrium that its P wave is hidden by the QRS.

Premature ventricular contractions (PVCs: premature ventricular beats, ventricular extrasystoles) are impulses arising from a site somewhere in the ventricles; they occur early in relation to the prevailing rhythm. The electrocardiographic pattern typically is that of an abnormal QRS complex, usually widened, that has little or no resemblance to the normal QRS complex (Fig. 11–3). There is no P wave associated with the early QRS complex. The T wave, representing ventricular repolarization, that follows the abnormal QRS demonstrates di-

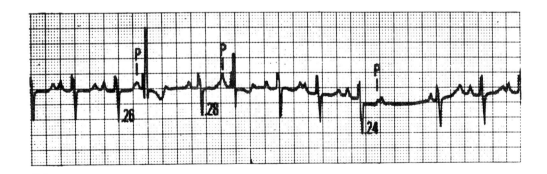

II

FIGURE 11–2. Single-lead electrocardiogram from a patient with frequent premature atrial contractions. P waves occur prematurely (labeled P) in relation to the prevailing rhythm with morphology different from that of the sinus P waves. The QRS complexes following the first and second premature atrial contractions are conducted aberrantly, resulting in morphology that differs slightly from that of the normally conducted beats. The third premature atrial contraction is not conducted into the ventricles because it is even more premature (note numbers indicating time from QRS to premature P wave), falling during the absolute refractory period.

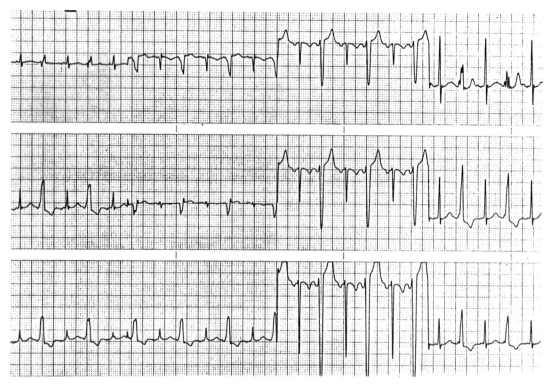

FIGURE 11–3. Twelve-lead electrocardiogram demonstrating premature ventricular contractions occurring in a bigeminal pattern. QRS complexes of the abnormal beats are widened with repolarization (T wave) occurring in a direction opposite to that of the ventricular depolarization (QRS). Although in many leads a P wave is seen immediately preceding the abnormal QRS complex, the atrial depolarization has not had time to be conducted to the ventricle, hence the absence of an appropriate PR interval. Note the uniform morphology of the PVCs and the constant coupling interval to the previous normal ventricular depolarization. This tracing illustrates the 12 leads in three simultaneously recorded strips reading in columns from top to bottom and from left to right: Leads I, II, III; aVR, aVL, aVF; V_3R, V_1, V_2; V_4, V_6, V_7. (For reference see Fig. 5–3.)

rection opposite to that of the major QRS deflection. A compensatory pause commonly follows a PVC, in which case the interval from the last normal QRS complex preceding the PVC to the first normal post-PVC complex is approximately twice the normal inter-QRS interval. This pattern occurs because the premature beat arising from the ventricle is not conducted in a retrograde manner back through the atrioventricular specialized conduction system into the atrium and therefore does not reset the sinus node. The atrial rate is not altered, thus producing a compensatory pause. It is true, however, that a PVC can be conducted in a retrograde manner to the atria thereby resetting the sinus node. Hence the absence of a compensatory pause does not prove that an early QRS is not ventricular in origin.

The presence of a single premature atrial, junctional, or ventricular contraction is common in infants and children. Prevalence var-

ies from 15 per cent to 30 per cent depending on the method used to detect its presence.[4–6] These and other arrhythmias are much more likely to be noted when a patient is monitored with a 24-hour Holter recording device than when evaluated with a standard electrocardiogram that can be completed in less than 30 seconds. The presence of single premature contractions usually is of no clinical significance, even when they occur in a bigeminal pattern (i.e., after each normal beat) for long periods. Unlike circumstances in adult patients, the number of premature beats during a given period of time (i.e., PACs or PVCs per 24 hours) is of little importance and may vary widely from one recording to another. Treatment designed simply to diminish the number of premature beats per day is therefore not warranted. Treatment indications depend on whether symptoms are present that are related to the etiology of the arrhythmia, if there is associated cardiac disease (i.e., myocarditis), or whether the patient is receiving a medication or has an electrolyte imbalance that may predispose to the development of arrhythmias.

Single premature contractions are especially common in two circumstances. First, newborns frequently have premature contractions, usually atrial, but they do not cause symptoms.[4,5] Typically these premature beats resolve by 2 to 3 weeks of age and require no treatment. Second, healthy adolescents can have frequent PVCs. If monitored for an extended period, the number of PVCs per day can be in the thousands, and long patterns of ventricular bigeminy may be recorded. This arrhythmia is almost always benign. Clinical and electrocardiographic findings that support a benign clinical condition include[6]:

1. Absence of underlying heart disease

2. Uniform QRS morphology

3. Suppression of the PVCs by exercise-induced increase in sinus rate

4. Constant coupling interval (interval from the onset of the last normal QRS complex to onset of the PVC)

5. Normal resting corrected QT interval

The presence of two or three consecutive PVCs was considered in the past to be an ominous sign. More recent studies, however, have indicated that couplets and triplets are benign if the clinical conditions are the same as outlined above for single PVCs.[7,8]

Supraventricular Tachycardia

There are a variety of mechanisms that explain a sustained supraventricular tachycardia, the most common of which is reentry involving one or more cardiac structures. Reentry describes excitation around a fixed obstacle (Fig. 11–4). During normal conduction, excitation progresses down both pathways, each of which may have different conduction velocities. If both pathways cause excitation of the distal tissue, the resulting complex may be a fusion beat with a portion of myocardium activated through each pathway. The most characteristic example of this dual activation is the ventricular preexcitation characteristic of Wolff-Parkinson-White syndrome. Reentrant tachycardia occurs when excitation is blocked in one of the

Mechanism of Re-entry

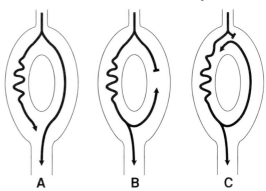

FIGURE 11–4. Reentry around an anatomic or physiologic obstruction. (*A*) During normal rhythm, excitation proceeds down both pathways, one with slowed conduction. Resulting activation of the distal tissue may be from a single pathway or a fusion of activation from both pathways. (*B*) Interruption of conduction down one pathway (usually the rapidly conducting branch) allows conduction entirely down the other pathway. (*C*) Delayed conduction in the slow pathway allows recovery of excitability in the pathway. The impulse travels in a retrograde direction through the fast pathway, initiating a sustained tachycardia through the reentry circuit.

pathways but can conduct through the other pathway. If the intact conduction is slow enough, excitation can progress around the obstruction and pass in a retrograde fashion through the previously blocked pathway. A sustained reentry excitation may then commence.

Several conditions must exist for a sustained tachyarrhythmia to occur:

1. Two or more anatomically or functionally distinct pathways that are in electrical continuity

2. Transient or permanent unidirectional block in one of the pathways

3. Sufficiently slow conduction in the conducting pathway to allow previously excited tissue to recover excitability

The most frequent sustained tachyarrhythmia requiring intervention or treatment is known commonly as paroxysmal atrial tachycardia (PAT). The usual mechanism of this arrhythmia is reentry involving one or more cardiac structures. The term PAT therefore is not totally descriptive of the mechanism of the arrhythmia. Similarly, the term supraventricular tachycardia (SVT) is not accurate because in most instances the ventricles participate in the reentry circuit. SVT is nevertheless widely used as a general term. The typical electrocardiographic pattern is QRS complexes of normal width occurring at a rapid rate (usually 220 to 300 beats/minute) (Fig. 11–5). In many instances, identifiable P waves are present, appearing as negative deflections more closely related to the preceding QRS complex than to the succeeding one. With this common form of tachycardia, the anterograde limb of the reentry circuit is the normal atrioventricular specialized conduction system—hence the normal QRS complexes. The retrograde limb of the circuit is an accessory pathway with more rapid conduction than that present in the anterograde limb of the circuit. It is for this reason that the P waves are more closely related to the preceding QRS complex.

This form of SVT is the most common arrhythmia associated with Wolff-Parkinson-White (WPW) syndrome.[9] The WPW syndrome requires a standard electrocardiogram for diagnosis. It is caused by the presence of a strand of myocardium (bypass fiber) connecting epicardially an atrium to a ventricle over the fibrous annulus that ordinarily separates atrial from ventricular myocardium.[10] The bypass fiber usually is single but can be multiple and can occur anywhere around the tricuspid valve ring or posteriorly or laterally around the mitral valve ring. The electrocardiographic hallmarks of WPW syndrome are a short PR interval and a delta wave (slurring of the upstroke of the QRS complex) that widens the QRS (Fig. 11–6). Total time from the onset of P to the conclusion of QRS is approximately normal. The QRS is a fusion beat resulting from simultaneous activation of the ventricles through both the normal atrioventricular specialized conduction system and the accessory myocardial tissue strand. As the portion of ventricular myocardium that is activated via the accessory strand increases, there is a greater degree of ventricular preexcitation (delta wave) recorded on the electrocardiogram.

The mechanism of tachycardia in patients with WPW syndrome usually is anterograde activation of the ventricular myocardium via the normal atrioventricular specialized conduction system, thereby producing normal QRS complexes.[11,12] The accessory pathway forms the retrograde limb of the reentry circuit; thus in most cases of WPW syndrome, the delta wave is not present during tachy-

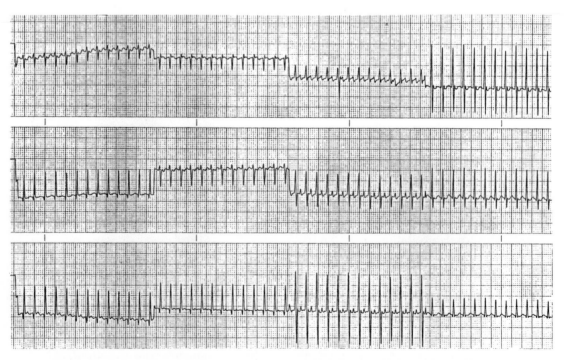

FIGURE 11–5. Twelve-lead electrocardiogram demonstrating tachycardia with a narrow QRS complex at a rate of 300 beats/minute. The P wave is noted with retrograde activation more closely related to the preceding QRS complex than the succeeding one. The mechanism of this tachycardia was subsequently determined to be atrioventricular reentry utilizing a concealed left-sided accessory connection. Leads are described in the legend of Figure 11–3.

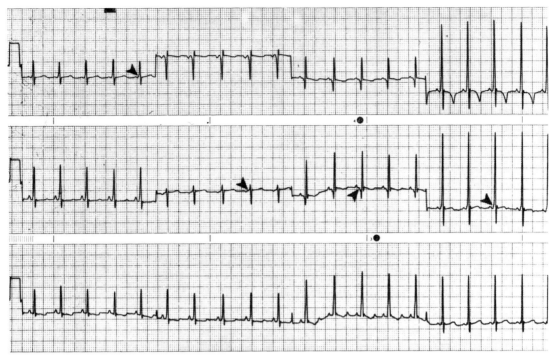

FIGURE 11–6. Twelve-lead electrocardiogram from a patient with typical electrocardiographic findings of Wolff-Parkinson-White syndrome. Note the slurring of the upstroke of each QRS complex (delta wave) denoted in some of the leads by the solid arrow. Leads are described in the legend of Figure 11–3.

cardia. Much less commonly, the antero-grade limb of a tachycardia circuit is the accessory pathway, and the retrograde limb of the circuit is either the atrioventricular specialized conduction system or a second pathway. In this event, all ventricular myocardium is activated via the accessory pathway, causing QRS complexes that resemble PVCs. These complexes have been termed maximally preexcited. This arrhythmia, known as antidromic reciprocating tachycardia, can resemble ventricular tachycardia because of the wide, bizarre QRS complexes.

An individual may have an accessory connection that is "concealed," thus producing an electrocardiogram that has normal QRS complexes both at normal rate and during tachycardia.[13] In this circumstance, the accessory pathway either conducts only in the retrograde direction or the refractory period of the accessory pathway in the anterograde direction is so long that in usual circumstances the heart rate is fast enough that atrioventricular conduction through the accessory pathway (manifesting as the delta wave on the surface electrocardiogram) cannot become apparent. In most instances of a concealed pathway, only sophisticated invasive electrophysiologic study can prove its presence and determine with certainty the mechanism of a tachycardia.

It is possible for an individual to manifest WPW syndrome on a standard electrocardiogram but never to experience tachycardia. Such an individual may not be able to conduct in retrograde direction through the accessory pathway. The absence of tachycardia in individuals with WPW syndrome, however, is uncommon. Episodes may not occur or may not be recognized during childhood but likely do occur at some time.

Acute treatment of supraventricular tachycardia usually attempts to heighten the vagal tone to the AV node using straining, gagging, or sudden application of ice water to the face.[14] Eyeball massage never should be used because of potential injury to the eye itself, including retinal detachment. If vagal maneuvers are unsuccessful, administration of intravenous medication usually is necessary. Intravenous digoxin takes some time to become effective, so it ordinarily is not used for acute treatment of SVT. Intravenous verapamil has been successful[15,16] but has the potential complication of secondary hypotension and cardiac collapse, especially when administered to infants under 3 months of age.[17] This complication is rare beyond early infancy. Intravenous adenosine has, for the most part, supplanted the need to consider use of verapamil. A reasonable starting dose is 50 µg/kg IV bolus. This dose can be increased every 1 to 2 minutes by 50 µg/kg increments to a maximum of 200 µg/kg. Adenosine is effective in interrupting tachycardia. It does so by blocking conduction through the AV node.[18,19] The half-life of adenosine is less than 10 seconds, it has little direct effect on the myocardium, and complications are uncommon. Adenosine, however, should not be used in patients with asthma. Older children should be alerted that they may experience brief breathlessness and a warm sensation. If administration of adenosine either is ineffective or is not feasible because of a patient's deteriorating clinical condition, synchronized direct-current (DC) cardioversion should be used. A small amount of energy ordinarily is sufficient for successful cardioversion; for example, a newborn may require no more than 1 to 2 joules (watt-seconds) per kilogram body weight.

Subsequent medical management of the patient who has had an episode of SVT is directed at causing delay of conduction through one limb of the tachycardia circuit. Most often an attempt is made to delay conduction through the atrioventricular node using digoxin, β-adrenergic blocking agents (e.g., propranolol), or calcium channel blocking agents (e.g., verapamil). More aggressive medical management sometimes is necessary, either instead of or in addition to these medications. It may include a variety of antiarrhythmic agents, including quinidine, flecainide, and amiodarone.

Patients who have frequent episodes of tachycardia, especially those who may be resistant to drug treatment, should be considered for electrophysiologic study to determine the exact mechanism of the tachycardia. During that study such a patient may be determined to be a candidate either for radiofrequency catheter ablation of an accessory pathway or for surgical division of the pathway. These methods interrupt the tachycardia circuit, eliminating the arrhythmia.[20,21]

Ectopic atrial tachycardia is a true supraventricular arrhythmia caused by enhanced automaticity of a focus somewhere within the atria.[22] Such a focus may be provoked by catecholamines, drugs, or other stimuli resulting in activation of the atria at rapid rates. The typical electrocardiographic pattern of such an arrhythmia includes abnormal P wave morphology and an increase in heart rate that is gradual and progressive until it reaches a steady rapid rate. Typically, cessation of this arrhythmia is also gradual. The ventricular rate resulting from this tachycardia depends on the actual atrial rate and the degree of delay through the AV node. Treatment can be directed at increasing delay through the AV node, thereby decreasing ventricular rate, using agents such as digoxin, propranolol, or verapamil. Medications directed at the ectopic focus itself include propranolol, quinidine, flecainide, and amiodarone. It is not unusual, however, for such an ectopic focus to be resistant to medical management. In such a case, transcatheter radio-frequency ablation or surgical removal of the focus can be considered. Fortunately, this arrhythmia is not common.

Atrial flutter is an arrhythmia that is uncommon in patients who have not previously undergone cardiac surgery. Atrial flutter is characterized on the electrocardiogram by a typical "sawtooth" pattern of atrial activation and some degree of atrioventricular block (Fig. 11–7). The atrial rate usually is greater than 300 beats/minute, and the ventricular response can be variable. The mechanism of atrial flutter is thought to be a form of intraatrial reentry tachycardia. A surgical scar provides a focus around which atrial reentry can occur, suggesting a reason for the increased incidence of atrial flutter postoperatively. Treatment for atrial flutter is similar to that described for ectopic atrial tachycardia despite the differing mechanisms of these arrhythmias.

Atrial flutter can be seen in otherwise healthy newborns. It has been considered to be an ominous finding,[23] but more recent studies suggest that in the absence of underlying cardiac disease (i.e., myocarditis, cardiomyopathy) atrial flutter in the newborn usually is benign.[24] If the infant is stable, digoxin administration usually results in conversion to normal sinus rhythm, which is maintained even if the medication is stopped. An infant who either is hemodynamically unstable or does not respond to medication should have DC cardioversion. It is almost always successful.

Atrial fibrillation in the pediatric patient is even less common than atrial flutter. It occurs in patients who have had cardiac sur-

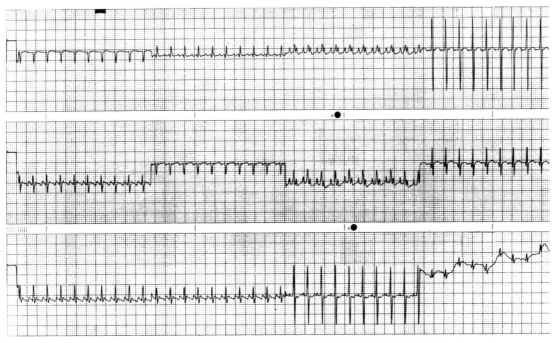

FIGURE 11–7. Twelve-lead electrocardiogram from a newborn demonstrating atrial flutter with 2 : 1 atrioventricular block; atrial rate is 430 beats/minute, and ventricular rate is 215 beats/minute. Note the characteristic "sawtooth" pattern created by atrial activity best seen in leads II, III, and aVF. P waves are most readily identified in leads V₃R and V₁. Leads are described in the legend of Figure 11–3.

gery[25] or in patients with a markedly dilated atrium. Paroxysmal atrial fibrillation has been observed in otherwise healthy children and adolescents, and its etiology is unclear. In the adolescent and young adult one should keep in mind that drug abuse or acute alcoholism can cause this arrhythmia. Depending on the clinical findings, DC cardioversion may be necessary. Recurrence is unusual, especially in a normal individual. The typical electrocardiographic pattern of atrial fibrillation includes a disorganized undulation of the baseline with varying irregular QRS complexes, some of which may be aberrantly conducted (Fig. 11–8). Medical treatment is similar to that outlined for ectopic atrial tachycardia and atrial flutter.

Ventricular Tachycardia

Ventricular arrhythmias in the healthy pediatric patient almost always take the form of PVCs occurring singly or, less commonly, in couplets or triplets.[6–8] Longer salvos of ventricular rhythm can occur in otherwise healthy patients. Sustained ventricular rhythm can be benign depending on the clinical situation. Ventricular tachycardia can occur in an otherwise healthy child or

adolescent.[26] These patients usually present with palpitations but are otherwise asymptomatic. The underlying arrhythmia may be discovered incidentally on a Holter monitor or less commonly on a routine electrocardiogram. Findings of normal cardiac examination, normal chest radiograph, and arrhythmia suppression by exercise point to the absence of a serious underlying condition.[6] These patients have normal cardiac structure and function on echocardiography and seldom require treatment. Association of this arrhythmia with either symptoms, especially syncope, or the presence of some other cardiac abnormality creates ominous implications and mandates further, more aggressive evaluation and treatment.[26–28]

Ventricular tachycardia in children occurs most commonly in the postoperative cardiac patient, especially those who have undergone a ventriculotomy.[29] It is not entirely clear which patients are at risk, although there is evidence to suggest, for example, that residual hemodynamic abnormalities, such as right ventricular dysfunction and residual right ventricular outflow tract obstruction in patients who have had repair of tetralogy of Fallot,[30] contribute to the occurrence of this tachyarrhythmia. In all likelihood, the extent of surgery, degree of myo-

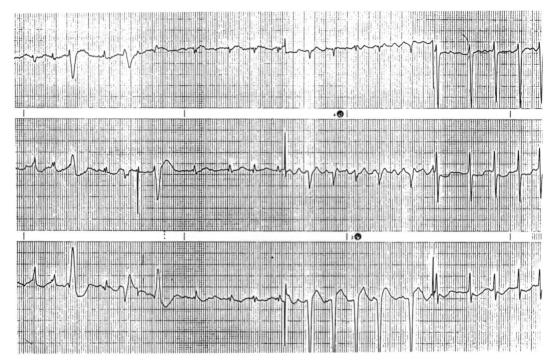

FIGURE 11–8. Twelve-lead electrocardiogram from a 21-year-old patient with a prosthetic mitral valve and chronic atrial fibrillation. A continuously undulating baseline without distinct atrial contractions (P wave) is seen with a variable ventricular response. Occasional aberrant ventricular conduction is manifested by widened abnormal-appearing QRS complexes. Leads are described in the legend of Figure 11–3.

cardial protection during surgery, and other factors contribute to the incidence of ventricular tachycardia as well. Treatment of ventricular tachycardia in postoperative patients has been successful using antiarrhythmic agents (e.g., quinidine, mexilitine, flecainide), β-blockers, and amiodarone among others. More aggressive management, such as ablation of a tachycardia focus with or without alleviation of the residual hemodynamic abnormality, sometimes is necessary.

Two additional specific circumstances in infants and children deserve mention. First, ventricular tachycardia is rare in infants; therefore one must be aware of conditions, such as a cardiac tumor, that can make the individual susceptible.[31] The presence of a tumor or another underlying cause for this life-threatening arrhythmia may be difficult to determine in infants and usually requires aggressive evaluation.

Second, the presence of ventricular tachycardia in more than one member of a family is rare except when the long QT interval syndrome is present. This condition, believed due to an imbalance of autonomic nervous system input into the heart,[32] may occur in association with[33] or without[34] congenital deafness. Delayed ventricular repolarization, manifesting as a prolonged QT interval on the surface electrocardiogram, predisposes these patients to development of a form of ventricular tachycardia that has a characteristic electrocardiographic pattern. This pattern, called *torsades de pointes*, or twisting of the points, also may be seen in patients with prolongation of the QT interval for other reasons, such as drug treatment (e.g., imipramine, quinidine). Management of the idiopathic form of long QT interval syndrome is difficult and may involve use of medication (propranolol, phenytoin), stellate ganglion ablation, or permanent pacemaker implantation.[35,36]

DISORDERS OF IMPULSE CONDUCTION

This section discusses arrhythmias resulting from impaired atrioventricular conduction rather than disorders that include enhanced conduction (see discussion regarding WPW syndrome, above). Abnormalities of conduction of the electrical impulse from the atria to the ventricles may occur spontaneously or may be secondary to an operative procedure. The significance of the conduction abnormality depends on the associated symptoms, although occasionally the clinical condition or the site of the conduction abnormality is important even in the absence of symptoms.

Abnormalities of atrioventricular conduction can be divided into three forms.

1. First degree heart block—manifesting as prolongation of the PR interval (Fig. 11–9)

2. Second degree heart block—manifesting either as nonconduction of an atrial impulse following progressive prolongation of the PR interval (Wenckebach phenomenon, Mobitz type I second degree block) or sudden nonconduction of an atrial impulse without previous PR interval prolongation (Mobitz type II second degree block)

3. Third degree, or complete, heart block—manifesting as total lack of relation between the regular, usually more rapid, atrial contractions and the slower ventricular contractions (Fig. 11–10)

If the site of impulse block is on the atrial side of the bundle of His and the subsequent ventricular activation occurs through the normal atrioventricular specialized conduction system, the QRS complex appears normal on the electrocardiogram. If, however, the site of block is more distal in the conduction system, a rare finding, the QRS complexes are widened and have an abnormal frontal plane axis.

Congenital complete heart block is the most common spontaneous abnormality of conduction. This condition often is detected in utero because of a slow fetal heart rate. Diagnosis of complete heart block can be made with fetal cardiac ultrasonography by noting contraction of the atria at normal or increased rates and a much lower rate of contraction of the ventricles. The fetus usually develops normally and most commonly has no structural cardiac abnormality. When structural heart disease is present, it most commonly is ventricular inversion ("corrected transposition of the great arteries")

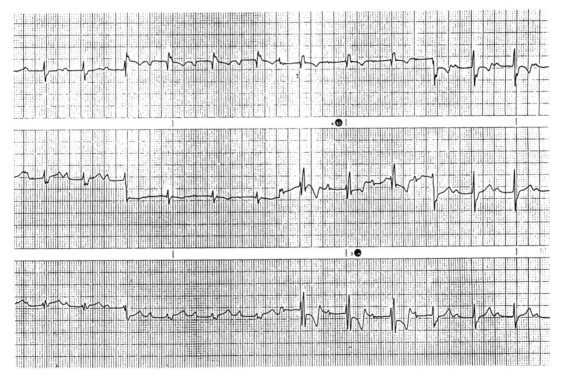

FIGURE 11–9. Twelve-lead electrocardiogram from a patient having undergone repair of a ventricular septal defect. Intact atrioventricular conduction is noted, but the PR interval is prolonged (0.32 second). QRS complexes demonstrate right bundle branch block morphology secondary to a ventriculotomy. The QRS abnormality is not due to the prolonged PR interval. Leads are described in the legend of Figure 11–3.

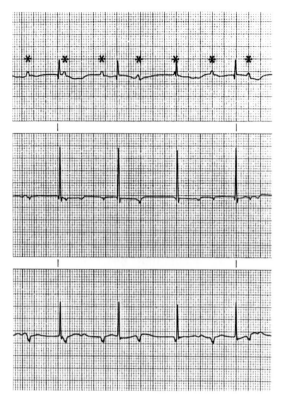

FIGURE 11–10. Rhythm strip electrocardiogram with three simultaneously recorded leads demonstrating complete atrioventricular block. The asterisks denote atrial activity occurring at a rate of 100 beats/minute. QRS complexes also are regular but at a rate of 62 beats/minute.

or one of its variations.[37] Pathology studies have demonstrated a high incidence of abnormal development of the conduction system associated with this cardiac lesion.

Infants born with congenital complete heart block and structurally normal hearts have a high incidence of maternal lupus erythematosus.[38] Indeed, the presence of lupus erythematosus is found occasionally by careful investigation of an otherwise asymptomatic mother who has given birth to an infant with congenital complete heart block. Although the process leading to heart block in the neonate is undetermined, it is presumed that maternal antibody crosses the placenta and in some way interrupts normal fetal atrioventricular conduction.

The significance of congenital complete heart block and the indications for treatment depend on the presence of symptoms, which in turn relate primarily to the slow ventricular rate. In a natural history study it was found that infants with congenital complete heart block generally do well if the ventricular rate is more than 55 beats/minute and the atrial rate is less than 140 beats/minute.[37] If an infant either has evidence of congestive cardiac failure or fails to thrive for no other discernible reason, treatment is indicated and almost always takes the form of placement of a permanent electronic pacemaker.

Complete heart block can occur in an older child or adolescent as a result of an acute disease process such as myocarditis or rheumatic fever. This complication is uncommon even in children who are otherwise quite ill. Temporary pacing may be accomplished by transvenous or external methods. If the child's clinical condition does not warrant placement of a permanent pacemaker, intact atrioventricular conduction likely will recur when the acute illness subsides.

The most common cause for acquired complete heart block is cardiac surgery. The incidence of postoperative complete heart block has fallen dramatically compared to the early years of surgical repair for congenital cardiac disease. Occasionally, however, a particular surgical procedure is necessary despite the patient having a known high risk of damage to the cardiac conduction system, and this risk is acceptable in order to treat the underlying hemodynamic abnormality. Treatment of surgically induced complete heart block almost always includes placement of a permanent electronic pacemaker.

Lesser degrees of conduction abnormality occur but usually are of little clinical significance. Abnormalities of function of the AV node, without complete interruption of conduction, may occur as a result of either a disease process (e.g., rheumatic fever) or a surgical procedure. Although intact atrioventricular conduction may continue, conduction time from the atria to the ventricles can be prolonged and manifests as an increased PR interval on the surface electrocardiogram. In a patient who either has recovered from an acute illness or has undergone a surgical procedure, stable PR interval prolongation is of no clinical significance. Similarly, a patient having undergone a ventriculotomy for repair of congenital cardiac disease often has the pattern of right bundle branch block but remains asymptomatic.

ELECTRONIC PACEMAKERS

An electronic pacemaker is the only reliable treatment for patients with symptoms caused by diminished cardiac output (e.g., congestive cardiac failure, exercise intolerance, syncope) due to slow ventricular rate. Most pediatric patients requiring pacemaker implantation are children born with congenital heart disease who have undergone a surgical procedure that has resulted in either disruption of the atrioventricular conduction system (surgically induced heart block) or damage to the sinus node with inadequate junctional (or lower) pacemaker response (sinus node dysfunction). Other patients requiring pacemaker implantation are infants born with congenital complete heart block in whom the lower pacemaker rhythm is exceptionally slow, causing inadequate cardiac output. The most important indication for pacemaker implantation is the presence of symptoms, not the absolute ventricular rate, underlying heart disease, or the presence of pauses noted on electrocardiographic monitoring.[39]

Pacemakers have become sophisticated over the 35 to 40 years of their development. Pacemaker generators have been made smaller, and lead systems have improved so that, for all practical purposes, patient size from infancy to adulthood no longer presents a technical problem for pacemaker implantation. The decision to implant a pacemaker, however, should be made only after careful consideration of all factors, as it obligates the patient to lifelong pacemaker therapy. It necessitates, at the least, pacemaker generator changes at intervals varying usually between 3 and 9 years.

Furthermore, the pediatric patient is at risk of lead fracture due to body growth and the need to replace lead systems because of exit block, especially epicardial leads.[40] The pediatric physician and the patient's family unit should be aware that a pacemaker is likely to affect the individual's socioeconomic status and life style by affecting physical activity, employability, and access to medical and life insurance, among other things.

Advancements in the design of modern pacemakers has improved their capabilities substantially. A standard code has been developed to describe the method of pacemaker function.[41] The original three-letter code now has been expanded to five letters to include a notation for pacemaker programmability and antitachycardia function, but the initial three-letter code is still used most commonly.[42] The first letter of the code describes the cardiac chamber being paced

(V = ventricle; A = atrium; D = dual, or both chambers). The second letter of the code describes the chamber being sensed (V = ventricle; A = atrium; D = dual). Finally, the third letter of the code describes the mode of action (I = inhibited; T = triggered; D = dual function). A pacemaker with the capability for dual chamber pacing requires a lead on the atrium and a separate lead attached to the ventricle. An O in the code indicates no function for that code designation. The simplest pacemaker, therefore, would be VOO, which indicates that the ventricle is paced, there is no sensing function, and the pacemaker is neither inhibited or triggered by spontaneous cardiac activity.

The most common pacemaker in use today, especially in adults, is a VVI unit: The ventricle is paced, but the pacemaker also has the capability to sense electrical activity from the ventricle and is inhibited by spontaneous ventricular activity. A pacemaker that senses atrial activity and is triggered by that activity to pace the ventricle would be coded VAT.

Pacemakers that have the capability of pacing the atrium, ventricle, or both and of sensing spontaneous activity from either chamber, which then dictates the mode of action, are among the most sophisticated and are coded DDD.

Most pacemakers require regular evaluation at centers capable of thorough electronic evaluation. Noninvasive communication with the pacemaker generator by means of radiofrequency transmissions permits measurement of heart rate, sensitivity, and electrical output (either voltage or pulse duration); pacemaker functions also can be programmed and reprogrammed. The goals of regular evaluation and pacemaker programming are to ensure the longest possible generator life and to detect impending generator or lead failure.

Current pacemaker generators can vary heart rate by means of several kinds of sensor. These pacemakers possess the capability of increasing and decreasing heart rate in response to activity, body temperature, respiratory impedance, intracardiac pressure, and so on, even though they require only a single lead attached to the ventricle. Detailed discussion of the advantages and disadvantages of these various systems is beyond the scope of this chapter. Suffice it to say that at the present time few pediatric patients have this generation of pacemaker in place; therefore long-term experience for young pediatric patients is unknown.

Development of the electronic pacemaker, and especially its recent innovations, has provided a marked decrease in morbidity and mortality for patients with many forms of congenital heart disease who require heart rate support in order to maintain cardiac output.

The primary care physician should be familiar with the patient's pacemaker function to the extent that findings suggesting pacemaker malfunction are recognized; such knowledge includes type of pacemaker, minimum ventricular rate, and electrocardiographic pattern.

REFERENCES

1. Spach MS, Miller WT III, Barr RC, Geselowitz DB: Electrophysiology of the internodal pathways: determining the difference between anisotropic cardiac muscle and a specialized tract system. *In* Little RC (ed): Physiology of Atrial Pacemakers and Conductive Tissues. 1st Ed. Mount Kisco, NY, Futura Publishing, 1980, pp. 367–380.
2. Southall DP, Richards J, Mitchell P, et al: Study of cardiac rhythm in healthy newborn infants. Br Heart J 43:14–20, 1980.
3. Southall DP, Johnston F, Shinebourne EA, Johnston PGB: 24-Hour electrocardiographic study of heart rate and rhythm patterns in population of healthy children. Br Heart J 45:281–291, 1981.
4. Morgan BC, Guntheroth WG: Cardia arrhythmias in normal newborn infants. J Pediatr 67:1199–1202, 1965.
5. Southall DP, Richards J, Brown DJ, et al: 24-Hour tape recordings of ECG and respiration in the newborn infant with findings related to sudden death and unexplained brain damage in infancy. Arch Dis Child 55:7–16, 1980.
6. Jacobsen J, Garson A Jr, Gillette PC, McNamara DG: Premature ventricular contractions in normal children. J Pediatr 92:36–38, 1978.
7. Schubert CJ, Epstein ML: Significance of ventricular couplets and triplets in children and young adults. Pediatr Cardiol 5:259, 1984.
8. Paul T, Marchal C, Garson A Jr: Ventricular couplets in the young: prognosis related to underlying substrate. Am Heart J 119:577–582, 1990.
9. Wolff L, Parkinson J, White PD: Bundle branch block with short PR interval in healthy young people prone to paroxysmal tachycardia. Am Heart J 5:685–704, 1930.
10. Truex RC, Bishof JK, Hoffman EL: Accessory atrioventricular muscle bundles of the developing human heart. Anat Rec 13:45–60, 1958.
11. Mantakas ME, McCue CM, Miller WW: Natural history of Wolff-Parkinson-White syndrome discovered in infancy. Am J Cardiol 41:1097–1103, 1978.
12. Gillette PC: Advances in the diagnosis and treatment of tachydysrhythmias in children. Am Heart J 102:111–119, 1981.
13. Gillette PC: Concealed anomalous cardiac conduction pathways: a frequent cause of supraventricular tachycardia. Am J Cardiol 40:848–852, 1977.
14. Waxman MB, Wald RW, Sharma AD, et al: Vagal techniques for termination of paroxysmal supraventricular tachycardia. Am J Cardiol 46:655–664, 1980.
15. Soler-Soler J, Sagrista-Sauleda J, Cabrera A, et al: Effect of verapamil in infants with paroxysmal supraventricular tachycardia. Circulation 59:876–879, 1979.
16. Porter CJ, Gillette PC, Garson A Jr, et al: Effects of verapamil on supraventricular tachycardia in children. Am J Cardiol 48:487–491, 1981.
17. Epstein ML, Kiel EA, Victorica BE: Cardiac decompensation following verapamil therapy in infants with supraventricular tachycardia. Pediatrics 75:737–740, 1985.
18. Overholt ED, Rheuban KS, Gutgesell HP, et al: Usefulness of adenosine for arrhythmias in infants and children. Am J Cardiol 61:336–340, 1988.
19. Till J, Shinebourne EA, Rigby ML, et al: Efficacy and safety of adenosine in the treatment of supraventricular tachycardia in infants and children. Br Heart J 62:204–211, 1989.
20. Gallagher JJ, Gilbert M, Svenson RH, et al: Wolff-Parkinson-White syndrome: the problem, evaluation and surgical correction. Circulation 51:767–785, 1975.
21. Schlüter M, Kuck K-H: Radio frequency current for catheter ablation of accessory atrioventricular connections in children and adolescents: emphasis on the single-catheter technique. Pediatrics 89:930–935, 1992.
22. Keane J, Plauth WH Jr, Nadas AS: Chronic ectopic tachycardia of infancy and children. Am Heart J 84:748–757, 1972.
23. Moller JH, Davachi F, Anderson RC: Atrial flutter in infancy. J Pediatr 75:643–651, 1969.
24. Dunnigan A, Benson DW Jr, Benditt DG: Atrial flutter in infancy: diagnosis, clinical features, and treatment. Pediatrics 75:725–729, 1985.
25. Radford DJ, Izukawa T: Atrial fibrillation in children. Pediatrics 59:250–256, 1977.
26. Deal BJ, Miller SM, Scagliotti D, et al: Ventricular tachycardia in a young population without overt heart disease. Circulation 73:1111–1118, 1986.
27. Vetter VL, Josephson ME, Horowitz LN: Idiopathic recurrent sustained ventricular tachycardia in children and adolescents. Am J Cardiol 47:315–322, 1981.
28. Rocchini AP, Chun PO, Dick M: Ventricular tachycardia in children. Am J Cardiol 47:1091–1097, 1981.
29. Kavey RW, Blackman MS, Sondheimer HM: Phenytoin therapy for ventricular arrhythmias occurring late after surgery for congenital heart disease. Am Heart J 104:794–798, 1984.
30. Garson A Jr, Randall DC, Gillette PC, et al: Prevention of sudden death after repair of tetralogy of Fallot: treatment of ventricular arrhythmias. J Am Coll Cardiol 6:221–227, 1985.
31. Garson A Jr, Gillette PC, Titus JL, et al: Surgical treatment of ventricular tachycardia in infants. N Engl J Med 310:1443–1445, 1984.
32. Schwartz PJ, Locati E: The idiopathic long Q-T syndrome: pathogenetic mechanisms and therapy. Eur Heart J 6(Suppl D):103–114, 1985.
33. Jervell A, Lange-Nielsen F: Congenital deaf mutism, functional heart disease with prolongation

of the QT interval, and sudden death. Am Heart J *54*:59–68, 1957.

34. Romano C, Gemme G, Pongiglione R: Aritmie cardiache rare dell'eta pediatrica. Clin Pediatr (Bologna) *45*:656–664, 1963.

35. Schwartz PJ, Locati EH, Moss AJ, et al: Left cardiac sympathetic denervation in the therapy of congenital long QT syndrome: a world wide report. Circulation *84*:503–511, 1991.

36. Moss AJ, Liu JE, Gottlieb S, et al: Efficacy of permanent pacing in the management of high risk patients with long QT syndrome. Circulation *84*: 1524–1529, 1991.

37. Michaëlsson M, Engle MA: Congenital complete heart block: an international study of the natural history. Cardiovasc Clin *4*:85–101, 1972.

38. Chameides L, Truex RC, Vetter V, et al: Association of maternal systemic lupus erythematosus with congenital complete heart block. N Engl J Med *297*:1204–1207, 1977.

39. Dreifus LS, Fisch C, Griffin JC, et al: Guidelines for implantation of cardiac pacemakers and antiarrhythmia devices. J Am Coll Cardiol *18*:1–13, 1991.

40. Epstein ML, Knauf DG, Alexander JA: Long-term follow-up of transvenous cardiac pacing in children. Am J Cardiol *57*:889–890, 1986.

41. Parsonnet V, Furman S, Smyth NPD: Implantable cardiac pacemakers—status report and resource guideline. Am J Cardiol *34*:487–500, 1974.

42. Parsonnet V, Furman S, Smyth NPD: A revised code for pacemaker identification. PACE *4*: 400–403, 1981.

12
CARDIOMYOPATHY

Benjamin E. Victorica

The problem addressed in this chapter is the child or adolescent who presents in heart failure with no history of heart disease but in whom you suspect a cardiomyopathy. "Cardiomyopathies are heart muscle diseases of unknown causes."[1] Diseases of heart muscle appear to be more prevalent now than in the past perhaps because either they have increased in incidence or, more likely, they are being recognized more frequently. They have also become more frequent causes of morbidity, disability, and mortality.[2]

The World Health Organization (WHO)[1] has classified cardiomyopathies on a functional basis as dilated, hypertrophic, or restrictive. Heart muscle diseases of known cause or associated with disorders of other systems are grouped as "specific heart muscle disease"; more than 75 have been described.[2] The WHO has classified these problems as infective, metabolic, or general system diseases, hereditary or familial disorders, and sensitivity or toxic reactions.[1] Cardiomyopathies are not rare in infants and children. The most common types are idiopathic dilated cardiomyopathy, hypertrophic cardiomyopathy, and a dilated cardiomyopathy secondary to cardiotoxicity of anthracycline drugs.

DILATED CARDIOMYOPATHY

It should be with considerable humility that cardiologists view their ability to determine the etiology of most cases of dilated cardiomyopathy; they should have even less pride in their therapeutic regimens. It is good to see a forthright admission that apart from the most obvious indicators of severity, we do not even know how to predict the outcome of most forms of dilated cardiomyopathy.—Warren Guntheroth, M.D.[3]

Dilated cardiomyopathy (DCM) is a disease of the myocardium characterized by impaired systolic function of the ventricles, particularly the left, leading to congestive heart failure. DCM comprises more than 90 per cent of all cardiomyopathies. At necropsy, both ventricles are dilated, but the thickness of the septum and left ventricular free wall is normal. Histologic findings are nonspecific.

Etiology and Pathogenesis

Little is known about the etiology and pathogenesis of the disease. A positive family history is present in 6 per cent of cases and in some families appears to be genetically transmitted.[4,5] In some instances there appears to be a nutritional factor associated with the process. Selenium deficiency was found to be the probable cause of a childhood epidemic of DCM that occurred in a limited region in China (Keshan disease).[6] It has been reported in association with a low serum level of carnitine with clinical response to treatment with L-carnitine.[7] The anthracycline antibiotics continue to be among the most valuable anticancer agents in use today. Among them, doxorubicin (Adriamycin) has broad activity in the treatment of carcinomas, sarcomas, and lymphomas. Its use can be complicated, however, by the development of chronic cardiotoxicity resulting in a DCM. Frequency and severity of this cardiotoxicity are related to the cumulative dose. It is unusual at doses below 450 mg/sq meter but increases in frequency at cumulative doses in excess of 450 to 550 mg/sq meter. The risk of clinical congestive heart failure exceeds 50 per cent at cumulative doxorubicin doses of 1000 mg/sq meter.[8] Once congestive heart failure has developed, the mortality rate is

30 to 60 per cent. Chronic doxorubicin cardiotoxicity can become clinically apparent days, months, or even years after the last dose.[9]

Many cases of idiopathic dilated cardiomyopathy probably are due to a previous episode of viral myocarditis. The most common agents in infants and children are coxsackie B virus, echovirus, and influenza virus. Diagnosis is confirmed by isolating the virus from culture and by the increased antibody titers between the acute and convalescent phases of the disease. Many newborns and young infants recover completely. In others chronic myocardial damage may be due to a persistent subclinical viral infection.[10,11] There is increasing evidence to support the theory that DCM is a sequel of previous viral myocarditis.[12,13] Not all viruses are myotropic, and not all patients infected with myotropic viruses develop either myocarditis or DCM. On the other hand, DCM is seen with increasing frequency in patients with acquired immunodeficiency syndrome (AIDS).[14] Isolation of cardiomyotropic viruses from myocardium is rarely possible later than 2 weeks after onset of an infection. For this reason subacute and chronic myocarditis as well as noninflammatory DCM have been considered to have an immune or autoimmune origin.[15,16] Cardiac-specific antibodies have been detected in patients with DCM using indirect immunofluorescence and absorption techniques.[17] The viral and autoimmune hypotheses are not necessarily exclusive; infection may be an initiating or precipitating stimulus for an autoimmune response.[10]

Clinical Findings

Dilated cardiomyopathy is characterized by the presence of a large, dilated heart with reduced systolic and abnormal diastolic function that usually presents with the clinical findings of congestive heart failure.[18] Infants manifest tachypnea, cough, wheezes, difficulty feeding, sweating, and irritability. Occasionally, the diagnosis is made after a chest radiograph is obtained because of "cold symptoms," and unexpected cardiomegaly is found. Older infants and children present with fatigue or decreased exercise tolerance. Peripheral edema, hepatomegaly, and ascites occur later as a result of right heart failure. In a series of 24 patients the median age of presentation was 2 years of age. It is of interest that 50 per cent had onset of symptoms within 3 months of an acute febrile illness.[19]

Physical examination reveals signs of decreased peripheral perfusion with cold, clammy skin, weak pulses, and delayed capillary filling. The apical impulse is displaced to the left and inferiorly. There is persistent tachycardia and prominent apical mid-diastolic filling sounds. An S_4 may be heard at the apex. The S_2 is usually narrowly split. A high-frequency systolic murmur of mitral regurgitation is often present. Hepatomegaly is a frequent finding, particularly in infants, but peripheral edema is rare.

The chest radiograph always shows cardiomegaly, sometimes marked. Signs of pulmonary venous obstruction with redistribution of flow are usually present (Fig. 12–1). In the presence of severe congestive heart failure, signs of pulmonary edema may be present (see Fig. 2–31). The electrocardiogram shows persistent sinus tachycardia, prolonged PR interval, and left atrial enlargement. Left ventricular hypertrophy is usually present (Fig. 12–2). Occasionally, the child presents with palpitations or rhythm disturbances. In contrast to the adult population, atrial arrhythmias in children are more frequent than ventricular arrhythmias.[20] Two-dimensional echocardiography is diagnostic, showing a dilated left ventricle with poor contractility. Left ventricular thrombus is present in approximately 20 per cent of cases.

Differential Diagnosis

The differential diagnosis is particularly important in infants who present with cardiomegaly and signs of left ventricular dysfunction. Two specific diagnostic possibilities should be considered. The first is anomalous origin of the left coronary from the pulmonary artery. Before birth the left coronary artery receives blood flow from the pulmonic trunk, which has the same pressure as the aorta. Pulmonary artery pressure drops after birth, forward blood flow through the anomalous left coronary artery diminishes, and flow may reverse, resulting in ischemia and infarction of the left ventricular anterolateral wall. The infant may have symptoms of myocardial ischemia manifested by crying spells due to angina. After infarction there is clinical evidence of mitral valve regurgitation and congestive heart failure. A chest radiograph demonstrates

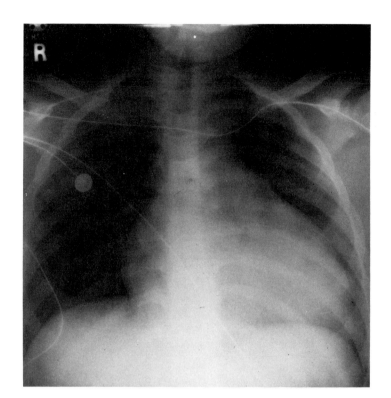

FIGURE 12–1. Portable chest radiograph of a girl with severe dilated cardiomyopathy. Note the marked cardiomegaly associated with pulmonary venous congestion.

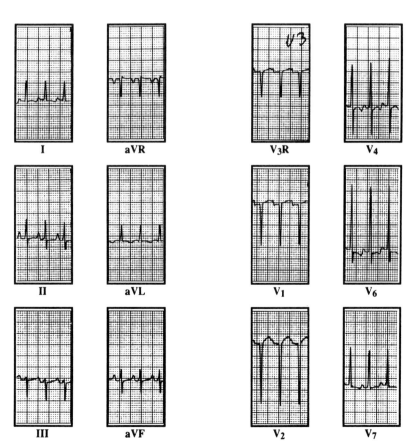

| I | aVR | V₃R | V₄ |

| II | aVL | V₁ | V₆ |

| III | aVF | V₂ | V₇ |

FIGURE 12–2. Electrocardiogram in a patient with dilated cardiomyopathy showing right and left atrial enlargement and left ventricular hypertrophy with ST and T wave abnormalities, suggesting myocardial impairment.

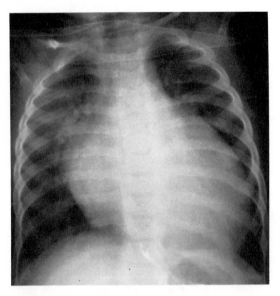

FIGURE 12–3. Chest radiograph of an infant with anomalous origin of the left coronary artery from the pulmonary artery. As a result of an anterolateral myocardial infarct, there is cardiomegaly and a pattern of pulmonary venous obstruction (redistribution of the flow toward the upper lobes).

cardiomegaly and evidence of pulmonary venous congestion (Fig. 12–3). The electrocardiogram is of great diagnostic value when it demonstrates the characteristic pattern of an anterolateral infarct (Fig. 12–4).

The second consideration is acute myocarditis. The clinical presentation is variable, and most patients are identified because of sudden onset of congestive heart failure. Physical examination demonstrates significant tachycardia, out of proportion to the fever, muffled heart sounds, and an S_3-S_4 apical summation sound. Mitral valve regurgitation may be present as well as a pericardial friction rub. The chest radiograph shows cardiomegaly and pulmonary congestion. A large pericardial effusion is rare. The electrocardiogram typically shows low-voltage conduction disturbances and atrial or ventricular arrhythmias. Characteristically, there are ST-T changes that occasionally are dramatic.[21]

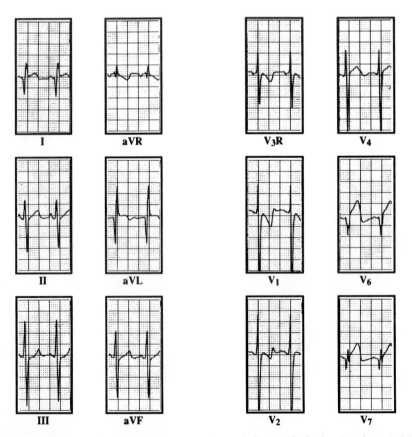

FIGURE 12–4. Electrocardiogram on the same patient as in Figure 12–3, showing characteristic and diagnostic features of an anterolateral infarct. Note the deep q waves in I and aVL and the abnormal R wave progression in the precordial QRS complexes with sudden shift to a qR (sometimes by lead V4).

Prognosis and Management

The overall long-term prognosis of DCM in children is usually grim, although some children live a long time in a relatively stable clinical condition. Patients with progressive myocardial dysfunction associated with symptoms of congestive heart failure, serious rhythm disturbances, or both have a poor prognosis.[22] In several series the 5-year survival was reported to be between 35 and 55 per cent.[19,23]

Treatment is symptomatic. The goal is to make the patient feel better and live longer. The treatment approach can be divided into preload reduction (e.g., diuretics), inotropic therapy (e.g., digitalis), and afterload reduction (e.g., vasodilators). Some centers follow a protocol and select therapeutic agents depending on the functional status of the patient according to the New York Heart Association classification.[24] Class I or II patients are usually treated as outpatients. A diuretic commonly used in children is furosemide at a dose of 1 mg/kg twice a day. Electrolytes should be monitored, particularly serum potassium. Excessive volume depletion can decrease ventricular filling pressures below the optimal level, resulting in a further decrease in cardiac output. Digoxin, despite having a relatively weak positive inotropic effect, is of value for chronic treatment of these patients. It is particularly useful when atrial arrhythmias are present.

Introduction of vasodilators has been a major therapeutic advance in the management of DCM. Vasodilation reduces the load of the failing heart. Angiotensin-converting enzyme (ACE) inhibitors (captopril, enalapril) have been shown to improve symptoms, improve exercise tolerance, and even reduce mortality.[25] Enalapril lowers peripheral resistance by reducing arterial vasoconstriction induced by angiotensin II.[26] These drugs can cause significant hypotension when first administered and so should be started as low doses with the patient in bed. Because of the risk of systemic emboli, anticoagulant therapy should be considered, particularly in the presence of severely depressed left ventricular function.[27]

Patients with severe congestive heart failure and in functional class III or IV require hospitalization to initiate therapy. They also require maximal diuretic therapy. Dopamine at low doses (2 to 3 μg/kg/min IV) increases renal flow and urine output. Use of a potent inotropic agent usually is necessary.

Dobutamine is a synthetic catecholamine that stimulates β_1-, β_2-, and α-receptors. Unlike dopamine, it does not cause the release of endogenous norepinephrine, so it does not produce significant hypertension or rhythm disturbances. The cardiac output is increased using 5 to 10 μg/kg/min IV. This effect can last for days or weeks after a short infusion course.[28,29] Patients who do not respond well to catecholamines and who are in severe congestive heart failure often improve with amrinone.[30] Amrinone, a nonsympathomimetic drug, produces both positive inotropic effect and vasodilation. An intravenous loading dose is used followed by an infusion at 5 to 10 μg/kg/min. Thrombocytopenia is a frequent side effect. The combined effect of dobutamine and amrinone has maintained terminally ill patients awaiting cardiac transplantation. Most children undergoing cardiac transplant have suffered from DCM. Timing of cardiac transplant remains a challenge.[31]

HYPERTROPHIC CARDIOMYOPATHY

Hypertrophic cardiomyopathy (HCM) is an important cause of disability and death in young adults; fortunately, it is rare in children. It is a primary disease of cardiac muscle characterized by a hypertrophied, nondilated left ventricle.[32]

Pathophysiology

The ventricular septum is usually thicker than the left ventricular free wall. In contrast to previous thought, many patients with HCM either have no or only mild left ventricular outflow tract obstruction at rest. Obstruction occurs as a result of abnormal systolic anterior motion of the mitral valve apparatus, particularly of the anterior leaflet, against the thick septum.[33] It has been postulated that much of this motion is due to a Venturi effect produced by the blood as it is ejected through a narrow left ventricular outflow tract.[34] A characteristic phenomenon of this lesion is rapid ejection of most of the left ventricular stroke volume early during systole.[35] The onset of mitral apparatus–septal contact correlates with the onset of the systolic gradient and rapid deceleration of aortic flow.[36] Based on the degree of left ventricular outflow tract obstruction, HCM has been classified as nonobstructive or obstructive. This classification is somewhat artificial, as patients who are followed clinically for some time may move from one group to the other. The markedly hypertrophic, stiff left ventricle with low compliance produces an "inflow obstruction,"[37] causing impaired diastolic filling.[38]

Etiology

Hypertrophic cardiomyopathy appears to be familial in approximately 60 per cent of cases; in 75 per cent of pedigrees the pattern of inheritance is consistent with autosomal dominant transmission.[39] (See Chapter 17.) The overall percentage of affected relatives in a group of families, however, is only 20 per cent, and most have "subclinical" manifestations of the disease detected only by echocardiogram. HCM also has been described in patients with Noonan syndrome.[40]

Clinical Findings

This disorder occurs more commonly in male individuals. The clinical presentation and course can be variable. Infants, rarely affected, may have clinical findings that mimic other congenital anomalies.[41] Older children and adolescents usually are asymptomatic but may present with a heart murmur or have exercise intolerance, chest pain, dizziness, syncope, or palpitations. These symptoms occur in patients with either the nonobstructive or the obstructive form of the disease. There is a significant incidence of sudden cardiac death in children and young adults, which may be the initial presentation. Findings on physical examination depend on the hemodynamic status. Without obstruction, cardiac findings reflect the dynamic systolic phase and poor left ventricular compliance. The apical impulse is prominent, there is no significant systolic murmur, and there are apical mid-diastolic filling sounds. Patients with obstruction have a medium-frequency systolic ejection murmur best heard between the apex and the third left intercostal space. The intensity of the murmur correlates with the degree of outflow tract obstruction. This murmur is louder during the Valsalva maneuver and is diminished by squatting. A high-frequency apical murmur of mitral valve regurgitation also can be present. Peripheral pulses are easily palpable and unusually brisk, particularly in the presence of obstruction. A bifid pulse (pulsus bisferiens) may be noted, particularly in the carotid artery. The chest radiograph is normal or may show some degree of cardiomegaly with a left ventricular configuration. Pulmonary vascularity may be normal or may show a pattern of pulmonary venous obstruction. The electrocardiogram is abnormal in most patients. Left atrial enlargement and left ventricular hypertrophy with ST-T changes of "strain" are common (Fig. 12–5). Abnormal left precordial q waves may be seen. A two-dimensional echocardiogram is diagnostic, showing left ventricular hypertrophy but with a much thicker septum (asymmetric septal hypertrophy). Systolic anterior motion of the anterior mitral valve leaflet against the thick septum is present in patients with outflow obstruction.

Prognosis and Management

Approximately 50 per cent of infants and young patients with HCM either die suddenly or show progressive clinical deterioration.[34,42] A family history of sudden death indicates a poor prognosis. Unsustained ventricular tachycardia on Holter monitoring does not indicate increased risk unless the patient either has a history of impaired consciousness (e.g., syncope or cardiac arrest) or manifests inducible sustained ventricular tachycardia during electrophysiologic studies. The presence of both symptoms—impaired consciousness and inducible sustained ventricular tachycardia—identifies patients at high risk.[43]

Treatment of HCM is directed at alleviating symptoms and preventing sudden death. Propranolol has been used for many years and may produce clinical improvement. There are no definite data, however, to show that propranolol alters the natural history of the disease or prevents sudden death.[44] Because sudden death often occurs during severe exertion children should be advised against competitive sports. Calcium channel blockers (verapamil) also may result in long-term clinical improvement perhaps by improving left ventricular diastolic relaxation. In some patients, however, verapamil can increase outflow tract obstruction, causing pulmonary edema. Patients with severe, symptomatic outflow tract obstruction unresponsive to medical therapy may require surgical treatment.[44]

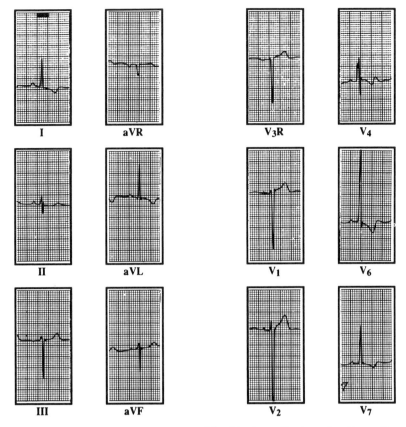

FIGURE 12–5. Electrocardiogram in a young adult with obstructive hypertrophic cardiomyopathy. There is severe left ventricular hypertrophy with negative T waves in V_6 and V_7.

REFERENCES

1. WHO, ISFC Task Force: Report of the WHO/ISFC task force on the definition and classification of cardiomyopathies. Br Heart J 44:672–673, 1980.
2. Abelmann WH, Lorell BH: The challenge of cardiomyopathy. J Am Coll Cardiol 13:1219–1239, 1989.
3. Guntheroth WG: Congestive cardiomyopathy in children [Editorial Comment]. J Am Coll Cardiol 15:194–195, 1990.
4. Berko BA, Swift M: X-linked dilated cardiomyopathy. N Engl J Med 316:1186–1191, 1987.
5. Ross RS, Bulkley BH, Hutchins GM, et al: Idiopathic familial myocardiopathy in three generations: a clinical and pathological study. Am Heart J 96:170–179, 1978.
6. Yang GQ, Chen JS, Wen ZE, et al: The role of selenium in Keshan disease. Adv Nutr Res 6:203–231, 1984.
7. Tripp ME, Katcher ML, Peters HA, et al: Systemic carnitine deficiency presenting as familial endocardial fibroelastosis: a treatable cardiomyopathy. N Engl J Med 305:385–390, 1981.
8. Von Hoff DD, Layard MW, Basa P, et al: Risk factors for doxorubicin-induced congestive heart failure. Ann Intern Med 91:710–717, 1979.
9. Lipshultz SE, Colan SD, Gelber RD: Late cardiac effects of doxorubicin therapy for acute lymphoblastic leukemia in childhood. N Engl J Med 324:808–815, 1991.
10. Caforio AL, Goodwin JF: Current insights into the pathogenesis and treatment of dilated cardiomyopathy. Prim Cardiol 18:37, 1992.
11. Bowles NE, Richardson PJ, Olsen GJ, et al: Detection of Coxsackie B virus-specific RNA sequences in myocardial biopsy samples from patients with myocarditis and dilated cardiomyopathy. Lancet 1:1120–1122, 1986.
12. Abelmann WH: Myocarditis as a cause of dilated cardiomyopathy. In Engelmeier RS, O'Connell JB (eds): Therapy of Dilated Cardiomyopathy and Myocarditis. New York, Marcel Deckker, 1988, p. 221.
13. Cambridge G, MacArthur CGE, Waterson AP, et al: Antibodies to Coxsackie B viruses in congestive cardiomyopathy. Br Heart J 41:692–696, 1979.
14. Cohen IS, Anderson DW, Virmani R, et al: Congested cardiomyopathy in association with the acquired immunodeficiency syndrome. N Engl J Med 315:628–630, 1986.
15. McManus BM, Gauntt CJ, Cassling RS: Immunopathologic basis of myocardial injury. Cardiovasc Clin 18:163–184, 1988.
16. Yokoyama A: Natural killer cells in dilated cardiomyopathy. Tohoku J Exp Med 154:335–344, 1988.
17. Caforio ALP, Bonifacio E, Stewart JT, et al: Novel

organ-specific circulating cardiac autoantibodies in dilated cardiomyopathy. J Am Coll Cardiol 15: 1527–1534, 1990.

18. Rezkalla S, Kloner RA: The guide to cardiology: myocarditis and cardiomyopathy. Cardiovascular Reviews and Reports, February 1991, pp. 48–66.

19. Taliercio CP, Seward JB, Driscoll DJ, et al: Idiopathic dilated cardiomyopathy in the young: clinical profile and natural history. J Am Coll Cardiol 6:1126–1131, 1985.

20. Friedman RA, Moak JP, Garson A Jr: Clinical course of idiopathic dilated cardiomyopathy in children. J Am Coll Cardiol 18:152–156, 1991.

21. Hoyer MH, Fischer DR: Acute myocarditis simulating myocardial infarction in a child. Pediatrics 87:250–253, 1991.

22. Gersony WM: The child with dilated cardiomyopathy: prognostic consideration and management decisions [Editorial Comment]. J Am Coll Cardiol 18:157–158, 1991.

23. Chen SC, Nouri S, Balfour I, et al: Clinical profile of congestive cardiomyopathy in children. J Am Coll Cardiol 15:189–193, 1990.

24. Massin EK: Current treatment of dilated cardiomyopathy. Tex Heart Inst J 18:41–49, 1991.

25. CONSENSUS Trial Study Group: Effects of enalapril on mortality in severe congestive heart failure. N Engl J Med 316:1429–1434, 1987.

26. Todd PA, Heel RC: Enalapril: a review of its pharmacodynamic and pharmacokinetic properties and therapeutic use in hypertension and congestive heart failure. Drugs 31:198–248, 1986.

27. Fuster V, Gersh BJ, Giuliani ER, et al: The natural history of idiopathic dilated cardiomyopathy. Am J Cardiol 47:525–531, 1981.

28. Liang CS, Sherman LG, Dohert JV: Sustained improvement of cardiac function in patients with congestive heart failure after short-term infusion of dobutamine. Circulation 69:113–119, 1984.

29. Applefeld MM, Newman KA, Sutton FJ, et al: Outpatient dobutamine and dopamine infusions in the management of chronic heart failure: clinical experience in 21 patients. Am Heart J 114: 589–595, 1987.

30. Bottorff MB, Rutledge DR, Pieper JA: Evaluation of intravenous amrinone: the first of a new class of positive inotropic agents with vasodilator properties. Pharmacotherapy 5:227–237, 1985.

31. Keogh A, Freund J, Baron DW, et al: Timing of cardiac transplantation in idiopathic dilated cardiomyopathy. Am J Cardiol 61:418–422, 1988.

32. Frank S, Braunwald E: Idiopathic hypertrophic subaortic stenosis: clinical analysis of 126 patients with emphasis on the natural history. Circulation 37:759–788, 1968.

33. Henry WL, Clark CE, Griffith JM, et al: Mechanism of left ventricular outflow obstruction in patients with obstructive asymmetric septal hypertrophy (idiopathic hypertrophic subaortic stenosis). Am J Cardiol 35:337–345, 1975.

34. Maron BJ: Cardiomyopathies. In Adams FH, Emmanouilides, Riemenschneider TA (eds): Moss' Heart Disease in Infants, Children and Adolescents. 4th Ed. Baltimore, Williams & Wilkins, 1989, pp. 940–964.

35. Braunwald E, Lambrew CT, Rockoff SD, et al: Idiopathic hypertrophic subaortic stenosis: I. A description of the disease based upon an analysis of 64 patients. Circulation 30(Suppl IV):3–119, 1964.

36. Shah PM, Gramiak R, Kramer DH: Ultrasound localization of left ventricular outflow obstruction in hypertrophic obstructive cardiomyopathy. Circulation 40:3–11, 1969.

37. Goodwin JF, Hollman A, Cleland WP, et al: Obstructive cardiomyopathy simulating aortic stenosis. Br Heart J 22:403–414, 1960.

38. Hanrath P, Mathey DG, Siegert R, et al: Left ventricular relaxation and filling pattern in different forms of left ventricular hypertrophy: an echocardiographic study. Am J Cardiol 45:15–23, 1980.

39. Maron BJ: The genetics of hypertrophic cardiomyopathy. Ann Intern Med 105:610–613, 1986.

40. Ehlers KH, Engle MA, Levin AR, et al: Eccentric ventricular hypertrophy in familial and sporadic instances of 46XX,XY Turner phenotype. Circulation 45:639–652, 1972.

41. Maron BJ, Tajik AJ, Ruttenberg HD, et al: Hypertrophic cardiomyopathy in infants: clinical features and natural history. Circulation 65:7–17, 1982.

42. Fiddler GL, Tajik AJ, Weidman WH, et al: Idiopathic hypertrophic subaortic stenosis in the young. Am J Cardiol 42:793–799, 1978.

43. Fananapazir L, Chang AC, Epstein SE, McAreavey D: Prognostic determinants in hypertrophic cardiomyopathy: prospective evaluation of a therapeutic strategy based on clinical, Holter, hemodynamic and electrophysiologic findings. Circulation 86:730–740, 1992.

44. Blanchard DG, Ross J Jr: Hypertrophic cardiomyopathy: prognosis with medical or surgical therapy. Clin Cardiol 14:11–19, 1991.

13

KAWASAKI SYNDROME

Anne H. Rowley and Stanford T. Shulman

Kawasaki syndrome was first described in 1967 by Tomisaku Kawasaki, when he reported his experience with 50 children who manifested a distinctive clinical illness.[1] Kawasaki syndrome was originally named mucocutaneous lymph node syndrome by Kawasaki and was thought to be a benign childhood illness. By late 1970, however, it was clear that as many as 10 fatal cases of this illness had occurred in Japan, all in children under 2 years of age who appeared either to have recovered or to have been improving. Kawasaki's original report in the English-language literature in 1974[2] was followed in 1976 by that of Melish and coworkers,[3] who described the same illness in 16 children in Hawaii. Melish independently had developed the same diagnostic criteria for Kawasaki syndrome during the early 1970s prior to learning of the Japanese experience with the same illness. The availability of echocardiography since about 1979 has shown that approximately 20 per cent of untreated patients with Kawasaki syndrome develop cardiovascular sequelae, with a range of severity from asymptomatic coronary artery ectasia or aneurysm formation to giant coronary artery aneurysms with thrombosis, myocardial infarction, and sudden death. Kawasaki syndrome appears now to have replaced acute rheumatic fever as the leading cause of identifiable acquired heart disease in children in the United States.[4]

CLINICAL FEATURES

In the absence of a specific diagnostic test for Kawasaki syndrome, the diagnosis is established by the presence of fever and at least four of five other principal clinical criteria without other explanation for the illness (Table 13–1).[5]

Fever in the patient with Kawasaki syndrome is generally high spiking (usually to 104°F or higher), remittent, and prolonged. The duration of fever is usually 1 to 2 weeks in untreated patients.

Conjunctival injection is unique in the patient with Kawasaki syndrome; it involves the bulbar conjunctivae much more severely than the palpebral or tarsal conjunctivae and is not associated with exudate. It usually begins shortly after the onset of fever and persists for 1 to 2 weeks in patients not treated with γ-globulin.

Changes in the mouth are characterized by dryness, fissuring, peeling, and bleeding of the lips; erythema of the oropharyngeal mucosa; strawberry tongue with diffuse erythema and prominent papillae; and the lack of oral or lingual ulcerations.

Findings on the hands and feet are distinctive. Erythema of the palms and soles occurs, sometimes with firm, indurated hands and feet. The latter limits fine motor movements and may be painful enough to result in refusal to bear weight. Desquamation of the fingers and toes begins in the periungual region and may extend to involve the palms and soles as well. It is not seen during the first week of illness but characteristically is noted 10 to 20 days after the onset of fever. Approximately 1 to 2 months after the onset of illness, deep transverse grooves across the nails (Beau's lines) may appear that subsequently grow out with the nail. Occasionally a nail is shed.

The *rash* of Kawasaki syndrome usually appears within 5 days after onset of fever and may take many forms: an urticarial exanthem with large erythematous plaques, a morbilliform maculopapular rash that may be multiforme-like with target lesions, a scarlatiniform erythroderma, or rarely a fine micropustular form. There is usually wide

TABLE 13–1. DIAGNOSTIC CRITERIA FOR KAWASAKI SYNDROME

Fever of at least 5 days' duration[a]

Presence of four of the following five conditions
Bilateral conjunctival injection
Changes of the mucosa of the oropharynx, including injected pharynx, injected and/or dry fissured lips, strawberry tongue
Changes of the peripheral extremities, such as edema and/or erythema of hands and/or feet, desquamation usually beginning periungually
Rash, primarily truncal; polymorphous but nonvesicular
Cervical lymphadenopathy

Illness not explained by other known disease process

[a] In the presence of classic features, experienced observers usually can make the diagnosis of Kawasaki syndrome prior to the fifth day of fever.

involvement of the trunk and extremities. Perineal accentuation may be present. Bullae and vesicles are not seen, and pustular lesions rarely are seen. Desquamation occurs in areas other than the palms and soles in about 10 per cent of patients, particularly in the perineal region.

The final diagnostic criterion, *cervical lymphadenopathy*, is seen in 50 to 75 per cent of patients, whereas the other five criteria are each observed in more than 90 per cent of patients. At least one lymph node greater than 1.5 cm in diameter is necessary to fulfill this criterion. The nodes are usually unilateral but may be bilateral and are firm and somewhat tender. They are nonfluctuant, do not yield pus when aspirated, and typically do not yield bacterial growth when cultured. An occasional patient, usually over 3 years of age, may demonstrate cervical lymphadenopathy as the most striking clinical symptom of Kawasaki syndrome. Such patients may have impressive, tender, erythematous cervical node swelling that fails to improve with antibiotic therapy. Conjunctival injection, extremity changes, erythematous lips, and rash may be overlooked in the face of severe cervical adenitis. The clinician therefore should look carefully for other clinical signs of Kawasaki syndrome in patients with cervical adenitis, particularly if the adenitis is not responding to antibiotic therapy.

Associated features of Kawasaki syndrome include *arthralgia* and *arthritis*, seen in up to 30 per cent of patients. Arthritis can occur during the first week of illness and is usually polyarticular, involving the knees, ankles,

and hands. Evidence of *aseptic meningitis* is seen in at least one fourth of patients who undergo lumbar puncture. Cerebrospinal fluid in these patients contains an average of 25 to 100 white blood cells (WBCs)/cu mm, with lymphocyte predominance, and normal glucose and protein values. *Cardiac disease* occurs in about 20 per cent of patients and is discussed later in the chapter. *Hepatic dysfunction* with mild obstructive jaundice and mildly to moderately elevated levels of serum transaminases occurs occasionally. Acute noncalculous distension of the gallbladder (*hydrops*) is seen in Kawasaki syndrome patients and presents with a right upper quadrant mass and guarding during the first 2 weeks of illness. It resolves without surgical intervention. Ultrasonography is useful for diagnosis.[6] Other associated features include *diarrhea, pneumonitis*, and *sterile otitis media* (Table 13–2).

The course of Kawasaki syndrome can be divided into three clinical phases. The *acute febrile phase*, usually lasting 7 to 14 days, is characterized by fever, conjunctival injection, mouth and lip changes, swelling and erythema of the hands and feet, rash, lymphadenopathy, aseptic meningitis, diarrhea, and hepatic dysfunction. During the *subacute phase*, fever, rash, and lymphadenopathy resolve, but irritability, anorexia, and conjunctival injection persist. Desquamation of the fingers and toes, arthritis and arthralgia, myocardial dysfunction, and thrombocytosis are seen during this phase, which typically lasts approximately from day 10 to day 25 after the onset of illness. The *convalescent stage* begins when all clinical signs of illness have disappeared and continues until the erythrocyte sedimentation rate (ESR) returns to normal, usually 6 to 8 weeks after the onset of illness.

Occasionally a patient experiences clinical rebound, with recurrence of fever and

TABLE 13–2. ASSOCIATED NONCARDIAC FEATURES OF KAWASAKI SYNDROME

Extreme irritability, especially in infants
Arthralgia, arthritis
Aseptic meningitis
Hepatic dysfunction
Hydrops of the gallbladder
Diarrhea
Otitis media
Pneumonitis, mild, radiologically but not clinically apparent
Erythema and induration at site of BCG inoculation (rare in United States, common in Japan)

other acute clinical signs, such as rash and conjunctival injection, after these signs had appeared to resolve. Rebound occurs most often within a few weeks of the onset of illness and is associated with an increased risk of coronary artery disease.[7] Second attacks or recurrences have been reported in 3 to 4 per cent of Japanese patients,[8] although the recurrence rate in the United States appears to be lower.

Atypical cases of Kawasaki syndrome have been recognized with increasing frequency.[9-11] The illness may be more severe and more difficult to diagnose in young infants, as their individual manifestations may be more subtle.[12] Coronary artery disease may follow an illness that includes some features of Kawasaki syndrome but that does not fulfill classic diagnostic criteria.[13] This point suggests that children with a prolonged unexplained febrile illness, especially when associated with subsequent peripheral desquamation, should undergo echocardiography 3 to 4 weeks after the onset of illness. The purpose is to identify those patients with illnesses characterized by incomplete Kawasaki syndrome manifestations who develop significant coronary abnormalities, so appropriate therapy and monitoring can be instituted.

The differential diagnosis of Kawasaki syndrome includes scarlet fever, staphylococcal "scalded skin" syndrome, toxic shock syndrome, Rocky Mountain spotted fever, leptospirosis, Stevens-Johnson syndrome, drug reactions, and juvenile rheumatoid arthritis. The recent upsurge in cases of measles (rubeola) in large urban areas of the United States has allowed comparison of the clinical features of measles and Kawasaki syndrome. There are striking similarities between the clinical presentation of these two illnesses that emphasize the difficulty of identifying cases of Kawasaki syndrome in countries where measles remains common. There are some important differences, however. Conjunctivitis due to measles is generally exudative, whereas that due to Kawasaki syndrome is nonexudative. Koplik spots are diagnostic for measles, whereas discrete oral lesions are not seen with Kawasaki syndrome. The rash of measles generally begins on the face, particularly behind the ears and at the hairline, whereas the rash of Kawasaki syndrome generally begins on the extremities and trunk. Swelling of the hands and feet is commonly seen with both illnesses. The WBC count and ESR in uncomplicated measles are both low, whereas in Kawasaki syndrome a high WBC count with neutrophilia and a markedly elevated ESR are the rule. When it is difficult to differentiate the diseases by standard clinical and laboratory data, a rapid immunoglobulin M (IgM) antibody test for measles is invaluable.

LABORATORY FEATURES

Laboratory findings are nonspecific and nondiagnostic for Kawasaki syndrome. Most characteristic is a moderate to marked leukocytosis with a predominance of neutrophils during the first week of illness. Elevation of the ESR is almost universal, and high values are helpful for distinguishing Kawasaki syndrome from viral illnesses and drug reactions. The platelet count usually is normal during the first week of illness but begins to rise during the second week, peaking at about 3 weeks at a mean count of 800,000/cu mm, although it may rise to as high as 2,000,000/cu mm. Serum IgE levels are moderately elevated in most patients during the acute or subacute stages of illness.[14] Hypoalbuminemia is surprisingly common and often correlates directly with the length of illness. Hypercoagulability and platelet activation are present in Kawasaki syndrome and provide a basis for therapy.[15]

EPIDEMIOLOGY

Kawasaki syndrome is almost exclusively an illness of young children. About 80 per cent of patients are under the age of 4 years, and the syndrome is uncommon after 8 years of age. Kawasaki syndrome occurs worldwide and affects children of all races, with Asians (particularly Japanese and Koreans) at highest risk and caucasians apparently at lowest risk.[16]

A study of Japanese children with Kawasaki syndrome revealed that the overall rate of a second case of Kawasaki syndrome developing in a family within 1 year after onset of the first case was significantly higher for siblings than the rate for the general population of age-matched children. In addition, more than half of the second cases developed within 10 days after the first case occurred; and in three of four sets of twins who both developed Kawasaki syndrome, the illness appeared on the same date.[17] These findings suggest that Kawasaki syndrome develops in genetically predisposed individuals after concurrent exposure to an infectious agent.

Studies in the United States and Europe have revealed similar findings. The peak age of Kawasaki syndrome patients is 18 to 24 months, older than in Japan. Epidemics of illness occur primarily during late winter and spring at approximately 3-year intervals. Kawasaki syndrome occurs most commonly in children of middle and upper socioeconomic status. Because of racial differences in the incidence of Kawasaki syndrome, genetic factors have been investigated. HLA typing studies have yielded conflicting data that do not support an association of the disease with specific HLA types.[18-20]

ETIOLOGY

The etiology of Kawasaki syndrome remains unknown. In two outbreaks of Kawasaki syndrome in the United States, a history of an antecedent respiratory illness was obtained from significantly more patients than from controls.[16] An etiologic agent that has been investigated is a retrovirus because of striking immunoregulatory abnormalities seen in patients with Kawasaki syndrome. At the present time, however, evidence is lacking to indicate that Kawasaki syndrome is etiologically related to a retrovirus. Another group of lymphotropic agents, the herpesviruses, have been investigated and do not appear to be related to Kawasaki syndrome. This group includes human herpesvirus 6,[21] which was in fact discovered to be the causative agent of roseola infantum during studies of Kawasaki syndrome and control children.

Infrequent person-to-person transmission, data on secondary cases in siblings and twins, differences in racial incidence, and clinical findings of vasculitis and arthritis suggest that this illness may be caused by an infectious agent(s) that leads to an immune-mediated syndrome in certain genetically predisposed individuals.

CARDIOVASCULAR MANIFESTATIONS

Soon after Kawasaki's initial report, it became apparent that a few children with Kawasaki syndrome died suddenly and unexpectedly, usually during the third or fourth week after onset of illness when they appeared to be recovering. Death was usually due to massive myocardial infarction secondary to coronary artery thrombosis in areas of coronary aneurysm formation or coronary stenosis[2] (Fig. 13–1). It is now known from echocardiographic and angiocardiographic data that about 20 per cent of untreated patients with Kawasaki syndrome develop coronary artery abnormalities, including aneurysms. Data from Japan document fatality rates as low as 0.08 per cent (T. Kawasaki, personal communication, 1989), a consequence of both improved therapy and recognition of milder cases.

The earliest cardiac complications occur within the first 10 days of illness. Myocarditis, occasionally severe, probably is present to some degree in all patients. Less common features include pericarditis with effusion, mitral or aortic insufficiency (or both), and arrhythmias. Electrocardiographic changes are present in at least one third of patients and include flattening and depression of the ST segment, flattening or inversion of the T wave, decreased voltage, and conduction disturbances, such as heart block. Over the next 5 weeks, these findings generally resolve, but acute coronary arteritis during the first 2 weeks of illness may lead to coronary artery aneurysm formation. From studies employing daily echocardiograms, Kato documented coronary artery wall changes in echodensity as early as 7 days after onset of fever.[22] Hirose and colleagues demonstrated that coronary dilation is first detected at a mean of 10 days of illness and that the peak frequency of coronary dilation or aneurysms occurs within 4 weeks of onset.[23] Although ectasia may be seen earlier, saccular or fusiform coronary aneurysms usually develop between the 18th and 25th days after onset of illness. Development of echocardiographic coronary abnormalities after 4 weeks of illness is rare. Most fatalities occur during the period from 2 to 12 weeks after onset of illness, usually from thrombosis of a coronary aneurysm leading to myocardial infarction, from acute myocarditis, or, rarely, from rupture of a coronary aneurysm with resulting hemopericardium.

Aneurysmal changes of the coronary arteries may resolve or persist. The fate of coronary aneurysms in Kawasaki syndrome was well described by Kato et al.[24] At 1 to 3 months after the onset of Kawasaki syndrome, 15 per cent of all patients in this study had angiographic evidence of coronary aneurysms. Repeat angiography 5 to 18 months later in those with abnormalities

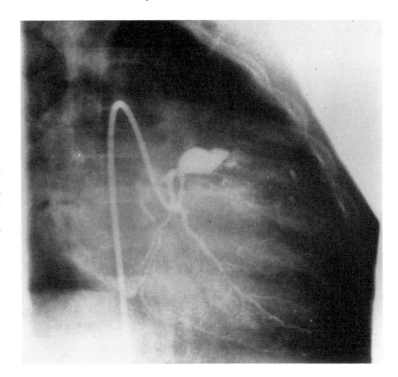

FIGURE 13–1. Left coronary angiogram in a 15-month-old caucasian girl with Kawasaki syndrome demonstrating a grossly dilated left anterior descending coronary artery with an abrupt thrombotic occlusion. It resulted in myocardial infarction of the apex of the left ventricle.

showed that in about 50 per cent of the patients the aneurysms had resolved. Of those with persistent abnormalities, one half had smaller aneurysms compared to patients in their previous study, one third had resolution of the aneurysms but developed complete obstruction or marked coronary stenosis, and the remainder had fine irregularities of the coronary arterial walls without stenosis. Thrombi that form within abnormal coronary vessels may increase in size over time or may recanalize. It is increasingly clear that resolution of coronary artery vasculitis may result in stenosis of the vessel, and that stenosis often leads to significant coronary obstruction and myocardial ischemia.

The implications of echocardiographic and angiocardiographic resolution of initially abnormal coronary artery findings are unknown. It is possible that the vessels remain abnormal, despite regaining normal caliber, and that these patients may be at risk for the development of premature atherosclerosis and myocardial infarction later in life. Studies have demonstrated that such vessels frequently lack normal elasticity, as shown by impaired ability to dilate with increased cardiac output.[25] Long-term follow-up studies are essential to determine if Kawasaki syndrome patients who do not develop detectable coronary abnormalities or who have apparent complete resolution of

coronary aneurysms are at increased risk of premature ischemic events as adults.

Two-dimensional echocardiography is used routinely in patients with Kawasaki syndrome to detect and follow coronary artery changes. Proximal portions of the coronary arteries are more easily visualized by echocardiography than are the distal portions, but aneurysms most often arise proximally, and this technique demonstrates more than 90 per cent of aneurysms detected by angiography.[23,26]

Certain clinical factors appear to be predictive of increased risk for development of coronary artery disease in Kawasaki syndrome. The absence of such risk factors, however, does not remove the need for routine echocardiography in all patients with Kawasaki syndrome, including those with a low predicted risk of developing aneurysms. Factors that are most strongly predictive of coronary disease include duration of fever for more than 16 days, recurrence of fever after an afebrile period of at least 48 hours, arrhythmias other than first-degree heart block, male sex, age less than 1 year, and cardiomegaly.[7] Male caucasians younger than 1 year are apparently at highest risk.[27] The prevalence of serious coronary abnormalities is particularly high among those less than 6 months of age. Other factors that have been associated with increased risk for development of coronary disease include the presence of a pericardial effusion and mitral regurgitation on echocardiogram obtained at the time of clinical presentation,[28] cryoprecipitates in serum,[29] and low platelet count, hematocrit, and serum albumin level at presentation.[30] Patients who develop giant coronary artery aneurysms, defined as those with a maximum internal diameter of at least 8 mm, are at greatest risk for development of coronary thrombosis, stenosis, and myocardial infarction.[31] Myocardial infarctions were asymptomatic in 37 per cent of patients and usually occurred within the first year of illness, although 27 per cent of patients developed this complication more than 1 year after onset.

THERAPY AND MANAGEMENT

Therapy for Kawasaki syndrome is aimed at reducing inflammation in the myocardium and the coronary artery wall and preventing thrombosis by inhibiting platelet aggregation (Table 13–3). More specific therapy awaits discovery of the etiologic agent of Kawasaki syndrome. A consensus statement dealing with the management of Kawasaki syndrome, prepared by the North

American participants of the Third International Kawasaki Disease Symposium held in Tokyo in December 1988, has been published.[32] Aspirin at dosages of 80 to 100 mg/kg/day (30 to 50 mg/kg/day in Japan) has been used for the acute phase of Kawasaki syndrome to reduce inflammation. It is now clear that aspirin and intravenous γ-globulin (IVGG) result in a much more rapid antiinflammatory effect than aspirin alone. High-dose aspirin usually is reduced to a lower dosage on about the 14th day of illness. Acute Kawasaki syndrome patients should be treated with a single 2000 mg/kg infusion of IVGG and high-dose aspirin (80 to 100 mg/kg/day in four doses) within the first 10 days of the onset of illness. Aspirin provides an important antithrombotic effect during the convalescent phase of the illness; the aspirin dose is reduced to 3 to 5 mg/kg/day as a single daily dose beginning on the 14th day of illness. Aspirin is discontinued if no coronary abnormalities have been detected by echocardiography by 6 to 8 weeks after the onset of illness. Aspirin therapy should be interrupted if the patient develops an illness suspected to be varicella or influenza in order to reduce the theoretic risk of Reye syndrome. Use of an alternative antiplatelet agent such as dipyridamole should be considered during this interval if the patient is deemed at particularly high risk for myocardial infarction.

Although corticosteroid therapy might seem of theoretic value for suppressing inflammation, a study comparing aspirin and steroid therapy demonstrated coronary aneurysms in 64.7 per cent of steroid-treated patients compared with 11.1 per cent of aspirin-treated patients.[33] Steroids are, therefore, contraindicated for treatment of Kawasaki syndrome.

Furusho was the first to use IVGG in the treatment of Kawasaki syndrome patients in Japan. His results suggested that IVGG 400 mg/kg/day for 5 days with aspirin (30 to 50 mg/kg/day) was superior to aspirin alone in preventing the development of echocardiographic coronary abnormalities.[34] A U.S. multicenter study used IVGG 400 mg/kg/day for 4 days with aspirin (80 to 100 mg/kg/day) and employed blinded echocardiographic readings interpreted according to a uniform, predetermined protocol.[35] This study demonstrated that: (1) coronary artery abnormalities were detected by echocardiography at 7 weeks after enrollment in 14 of 79 (18 per cent) aspirin-treated patients, but

TABLE 13–3. CURRENT RECOMMENDED THERAPY FOR KAWASAKI SYNDROME

Acute Stage
 Aspirin: 80–100 mg/kg/day in 4 divided doses until about the 14th illness day.
 Intravenous γ-globulin: 2000 mg/kg as a single dose given over 12 hours.

Convalescent Stage (after 14th illness day in afebrile patient)
 Aspirin: 3–5 mg/kg/day in single dose; discontinue 6–8 weeks after onset of illness after verifying by echocardiography that no coronary abnormalities are present.

Chronic Therapy for Patients with Coronary Abnormalities
 Aspirin 3–5 mg/kg/day in single dose; may add dipyridamole in selected patients thought to be at high risk; consider discontinuing when echocardiography verifies absence of aneurysms.
 Coumadin or heparin, together with antiplatelet therapy, may be advisable in patients with particularly severe coronary findings or with evidence of a past coronary thrombosis.

Acute Coronary Thrombosis
 Prompt fibrinolytic therapy with streptokinase, urokinase, or tissue plasminogen activator should be attempted at a tertiary care center under supervision of a cardiologist.

in only 3 of 79 (4 per cent) patients treated with IVGG and aspirin ($p = 0.005$); and (2) significantly more rapid resolution of fever and laboratory indices of inflammation occurred in the IVGG-treated group. The dramatic antiinflammatory effect of IVGG on acute Kawasaki syndrome frequently is apparent within a few hours of initiation of the infusion. At a mean of 30 months after the onset of acute Kawasaki syndrome, the prevalence of coronary artery abnormalities was 11 per cent in the aspirin group and only 2 per cent in the patients treated with IVGG and aspirin.[36] IVGG therefore also reduces the prevalence of long-term coronary artery abnormalities. Moreover, echocardiographically determined left ventricular function abnormalities normalize significantly more rapidly in patients treated with IVGG and aspirin than in patients treated with aspirin alone.[37]

A phase II trial of 549 patients comparing a regimen of a single 2000 mg/kg dose of IVGG plus aspirin (80 to 100 mg/kg/day) to treatment with IVGG 400 mg/kg/day for 4 days plus aspirin was accomplished by the U.S. Multicenter Kawasaki Study Group.[38] Two weeks after enrollment coronary artery abnormalities were present (seen by echocardiogram) in 24 of 263 children (9.1 per cent) in the 4-day group and 12 of 260 children (4.6 per cent) in the single-infusion group ($p = 0.098$). Four of the five patients who developed giant coronary aneurysms (internal diameter >8 mm) were treated with the 4-day regimen. Children treated with the single-infusion regimen had more rapid defervescence, shorter duration of fever, and more rapid return to normal of the laboratory measures of acute inflammation. The two groups had a similar incidence of adverse effects, none of which was life-threatening.

Therefore single-dose IVGG at 2000 mg/kg with aspirin (80 to 100 mg/kg/day) is the treatment of choice for acute Kawasaki syndrome patients, as it is at least as effective as the 4-day regimen, is well tolerated as a 10- to 12-hour infusion, results in more rapid resolution of fever and laboratory indices of acute inflammation, and should reduce the duration and cost of hospitalization for acute Kawasaki syndrome. It continues to be the recommendation of the U.S. Multicenter Kawasaki Study Group that all children diagnosed with Kawasaki syndrome within 10 days of onset of fever should receive high-dose IVGG as early as possible.

It is unclear whether all commercially available IVGG preparations are equally efficacious in Kawasaki syndrome. The IVGG product that has been tested most rigorously in the United States is that made by Immuno AG (Vienna, Austria), licensed in the United States under the trade name Iveegam.[35,38] Iveegam has been well tolerated as administered in the U.S. multicenter clinical trials, with virtually no serious side effects.[35,38] Anaphylaxis may occur in patients with severe IgA deficiency if the IVGG product contains IgA. Other occasional side effects, such as chills or fever, may be alleviated by slowing or temporarily interrupting the infusion. Administration of a large volume of colloid to acute Kawasaki syndrome patients with abnormalities in myocardial function might theoretically result in cardiac failure, but it was not a significant clinical problem in the U.S. multicenter trials, perhaps because of the improved cardiac function that results promptly from administration of IVGG. None of the IVGG preparations commercially available in the United States has been associated with transmission of hepatitis or human immunodeficiency viruses.

Incomplete or atypical Kawasaki syndrome poses serious diagnostic and therapeutic dilemmas. A child who presents within the first 10 days of an illness with some but not all features of Kawasaki syndrome, a markedly elevated ESR, and perhaps other features associated with Kawasaki syndrome such as sterile pyuria, irritability, or arthritis should be treated with IVGG and aspirin. The decision to treat possible atypical Kawasaki syndrome with IVGG must be made on an individual basis. Infants, particularly those under 6 months of age, frequently lack full diagnostic criteria for Kawasaki syndrome. A particularly high index of suspicion is necessary to make the diagnosis in these patients.[12] Unfortunately, these young infants with Kawasaki syndrome are also at substantially higher risk of developing coronary artery abnormalities.

A few patients with acute Kawasaki syndrome who receive IVGG have persistent fever 24 hours after completion of the infusion(s). Some patients may demonstrate an initial defervescence but then may develop recurrent fever after being afebrile for 24 hours or more. In both of these circumstances, possible retreatment with IVGG should be considered. Limited experience suggests that retreatment with IVGG is safe and appears to result in an improved antiinflammatory effect in many patients with persistent or recurrent fever. It has not been established that retreatment decreases the risk of coronary sequelae in these patients.

After treatment with IVGG, the administration of measles-mumps-rubella (MMR) vaccine should be delayed for at least 5 months (except during a measles outbreak, when it may be prudent to administer vaccine earlier and repeat the vaccination at a later time) because of the persistence of passively acquired measles antibody in serum of Kawasaki syndrome patients for the 4 to 5 months following IVGG therapy.[39] Schedules for administration of other routine childhood vaccinations do not need to be interrupted.

Dipyridamole is occasionally used in conjunction with aspirin in patients with coronary aneurysms, especially if there is a suggestion of thrombus formation. Digitalis and diuretics are used as needed in the patient with congestive heart failure. Caution in the use of digitalis is necessary if the patient has myocarditis.

Patients with Kawasaki syndrome should undergo periodic physical examinations with complete blood counts, ESR determinations, and platelet counts until these values return to normal. Liver function tests may be abnormal during the first week of illness.

A baseline electrocardiogram and echocardiogram should be obtained during the first week of illness. Echocardiography is repeated 2 to 3 weeks after onset of illness, as coronary aneurysms usually are first apparent at this time. If the echocardiogram is normal during the third week, it should be repeated about 1 month later. If this third study also fails to demonstrate an abnormality and the ESR and platelet count have returned to normal, aspirin is discontinued. Development of aneurysms more than 6 weeks after the onset of illness is unusual unless clinical evidence of inflammation persists.

If the patient has an abnormal echocardiogram during the acute or convalescent stage of illness, aspirin is continued and the abnormalities followed by repeat echocardiograms. Low-dose aspirin may be continued indefinitely even if aneurysms resolve, as the endothelial lining may remain abnormal despite return of the artery to apparently normal caliber. Not everyone agrees with this approach, however, and many authorities discontinue aspirin when the echocardiogram has normalized.

In patients with persistent small solitary aneurysms, long-term low-dose aspirin should be administered. In these patients and those in whom coronary artery abnormalities have resolved, no restriction of physical activities is needed. Stress testing should be considered for these patients, however; and additional studies, such as a myocardial perfusion scan, may be indicated if stress testing, echocardiography, or clinical data suggest myocardial ischemia. If myocardial ischemia is demonstrated, angiocardiography is indicated to evaluate coronary artery anatomy, which, in turn, may direct further management.

In patients with large or multiple coronary aneurysms without obstruction, long-term antiplatelet drugs (aspirin with or without dipyridamole) should be administered, and some recommend anticoagulant therapy in addition. The activities of these patients should be restricted.

A difficult management problem of Kawasaki syndrome is the patient who develops obstructive changes in one or more coronary arteries. Obstruction may be due to thrombosis or stenosis of the vessel secondary to intimal proliferation and fibrosis. Some patients with small thrombi can be managed with oral anticoagulant therapy alone. Intracoronary or intravenous thrombolytic therapy has been used in selected patients who have significant acute thrombosis, with varying degrees of efficacy.[40,41] At present, there is limited experience with transluminal coronary angioplasty.[41,42] Kitamura reviewed the national experience in Japan with 170 Kawasaki syndrome patients who underwent coronary bypass grafting from 1975 to 1991, most between 5 and 10 years of age.[43] The survival rate for these patients was 87 per cent at 4 years and 45 per cent at 10 years. The Japanese experience also indicates the superiority of internal mammary artery grafts over saphenous vein grafts.[43,44]

REFERENCES

1. Kawasaki T: Acute febrile mucocutaneous syndrome with lymphoid involvement with specific desquamation of the fingers and toes in children. Jpn J Allergy *16*:178–222, 1967 [in Japanese].

2. Kawasaki T, Kosaki F, Okawa S, et al: A new infantile acute febrile mucocutaneous lymph node syndrome (MLNS) prevailing in Japan. Pediatrics 54: 271–276, 1974.

3. Melish ME, Hicks RM, Larson EJ: Mucocutaneous lymph node syndrome in the United States. Am J Dis Child 130:599–607, 1976.

4. Taubert KA, Rowley AH, Shulman ST: A U.S. nationwide hospital survey of Kawasaki disease and acute rheumatic fever. J Pediatr 119:279–282, 1991.

5. Centers for Disease Control: Kawasaki disease—New York. MMWR 29:61–63, 1980.

6. Slovis TL, Hight DW, Philippart AI, et al: Sonography in the diagnosis and management of hydrops of the gallbladder in children with mucocutaneous lymph node syndrome. Pediatrics 65: 789–794, 1980.

7. Asai T: Evaluation method for the degree of seriousness in Kawasaki disease. Acta Paediatr Jpn 25:170–175, 1983.

8. Nakamura Y, Fyita Y, Jagai M, et al: Epidemiology of Kawasaki disease in Japan (1988). Presented at the Third International Kawasaki Disease Symposium, Tokyo, December 1988.

9. Fujiwara H, Fujiwara T, Kao T-C, et al: Pathology of Kawasaki disease in the healed state. Acta Pathol Jpn 36:857–867, 1986.

10. Salo E, Pelkonen P, Pettay O: Outbreak of Kawasaki syndrome in Finland. Acta Paediatr Scand 75: 75–80, 1986.

11. Canter CE, Bower RJ, Strauss AW: Atypical Kawasaki disease with aortic aneurysm. Pediatrics 68: 885–888, 1981.

12. Burns JC, Wiggins JW Jr, Toews WH, et al: Clinical spectrum of Kawasaki disease in infants younger than 6 months of age. J Pediatr 109: 759–763, 1986.

13. Rowley AH, Gonzalez-Crussi F, Gidding SS, et al: Incomplete Kawasaki disease with coronary artery involvement. J Pediatr 110:409–413, 1987.

14. Kusakawa S, Heiner DC: Elevated levels of immunoglobulin E in the acute febrile mucocutaneous lymph node syndrome. Pediatr Res 10: 108–111, 1976.

15. Burns JC, Glode MP, Clark SH, et al: Coagulopathy and platelet activation in Kawasaki syndrome: identification of patients at high risk for development of coronary artery aneurysms. J Pediatr 105: 206–211, 1984.

16. Bell DM, Rink EW, Nitzkin JL, et al: Kawasaki syndrome: description of two outbreaks in the United States. N Engl J Med 304:1568–1575, 1981.

17. Fujita Y, Nakamura Y, Sakata K, et al: Kawasaki disease in families. Pediatrics 84:666–669, 1989.

18. Kato S, Kimura M, Tsuji K, et al: HLA antigens in Kawasaki disease. Pediatrics 61:252–255, 1978.

19. Matsuda I, Hattori S, Hagata N, et al: HLA antigens in mucocutaneous lymph node syndrome. Am J Dis Child 131:1417–1418, 1977.

20. Melish M: Kawasaki syndrome. Pediatr Ann 11: 255–268, 1982.

21. Messner C, Fulton D, Sanderlin K, Pellett P: Human herpesvirus-6 and the etiology of Kawasaki disease. Presented at the Third International Kawasaki Disease Symposium, Tokyo, December 1988.

22. Kato H: Data presented at the First International Kawasaki Symposium, Hawaii, January 1984.

23. Hirose O, Misawa H, Kamiya Y, et al: Two dimensional echocardiography of coronary artery in Kawasaki disease (MCLS): detection, changes in acute phase, and follow-up observation of the aneurysm. J Cardiogr 11:89–104, 1981 [in Japanese; English abstract].

24. Kato H, Ichinose E, Yoshioka F, et al: Fate of coronary aneurysms in Kawasaki disease: serial coronary angiography and long-term follow-up study. Am J Cardiol 49:1758–1766, 1982.

25. Tomita Y, Baba K, Fukaya T, et al: Coronary arterial response to intracoronary nitroglycerin in Kawasaki disease [abstract]. In Proceedings of the Second World Congress of Pediatric Cardiology. New York, Springer-Verlag, 1985.

26. Yoshikawa J, Yanagihara K, Owaki T, et al: Cross-sectional echocardiographic diagnosis of coronary artery aneurysms in patients with the mucocutaneous lymph node syndrome. Circulation 59: 133–139, 1979.

27. Shulman ST, McAuley JB, Pachman LM, et al: Epidemiology of Kawasaki syndrome in an urban U.S. area with a small Asian population. Am J Dis Child 141:420–425, 1987.

28. Gidding SS, Duffy CE, Pajcic S, et al: Usefulness of echocardiographic evidence of pericardial effusion and mitral regurgitation during the acute state in predicting development of coronary arterial aneurysms in the late stage of Kawasaki disease. Am J Cardiol 60:76–79, 1987.

29. Herold BC, Davis AT, Arroyave CM, et al: Cryoprecipitates in Kawasaki syndrome: association with coronary artery aneurysms. Pediatr Infect Dis J 7:255–257, 1988.

30. Nakano H, Ueda K, Saito A, et al: Scoring method for identifying patients with Kawasaki disease at high-risk of coronary aneurysm. Am J Cardiol 58: 739–742, 1986.

31. Nakano H, Ueda K, Saito A, et al: Repeated quantitative angiograms in coronary arterial aneurysm in Kawasaki disease. Am J Cardiol 56:846–851, 1985.

32. Shulman ST (ed), et al: Management of Kawasaki syndrome: a consensus statement prepared by North American participants of the Third International Kawasaki Disease Symposium, Tokyo, Japan, December 1988. Pediatr Infect Dis J 8: 663–667, 1989.

33. Kato H, Koike S, Yokoyama T: Kawasaki disease: effect of treatment on coronary artery involvement. Pediatrics 63:175–179, 1979.

34. Furusho K, Kamiya T, Kaano H, et al: High-dose intravenous gammaglobulin for Kawasaki disease. Lancet 2:1055–1058, 1984.

35. Newburger JW, Takahashi M, Burns JC, et al: The treatment of Kawasaki syndrome with intravenous gammaglobulin. N Engl J Med 315:341–347, 1986.

36. Takahashi M, Newburger JW, for the Multicenter Kawasaki Syndrome Study Group: Long-term follow up of coronary artery abnormalities in Kawasaki syndrome treated with and without IV gamma globulin. Circulation 82(Suppl III):717, 1990.

37. Newburger JW, Sanders SP, Burns JC, et al: Left ventricular contractility and function in Kawasaki syndrome. Circulation 79:1237–1246, 1989.

38. Newburger JW, Takahashi M, Beiser AS, et al: A single infusion of intravenous gamma globulin compared to four daily doses in the treatment of

acute Kawasaki syndrome. N Engl J Med *324*: 1633–1639, 1991.

39. Mason WH, Takahashi M: Kinetics of intravenous gammaglobulin in Kawasaki syndrome. Presented at the Third International Kawasaki Disease Symposium, Tokyo, December 1988.

40. Terai M, Ogata M, Sugimoto K, et al: Coronary arterial thrombi in Kawasaki disease. J Pediatr *106*:76–78, 1985.

41. Sonobe T, Kataoka T, Kawasaki T: Percutaneous transluminal coronary reperfusion and intravenous coronary thrombolysis in Kawasaki Disease. Presented at the Third International Kawasaki Disease Symposium, Tokyo, December 1988.

42. Echigo S: Percutaneous transluminal coronary angioplasty for the children with coronary artery lesion due to Kawasaki disease. Presented at the Third International Kawasaki Disease Symposium, Tokyo, December 1988.

43. Kitamura S: Myocardial revascularization surgery in children with Kawasaki disease. Presented at the Fourth International Kawasaki Disease Symposium, Hawaii, 1991.

44. Suzuki A, Kamiya T, Ono Y, et al: Aortocoronary bypass surgery for coronary arterial lesions resulting from Kawasaki disease. J Pediatr *116*: 567–573, 1990.

Part III
SPECIAL CLINICAL PROBLEMS

14

INTEGRATED CARDIOVASCULAR HEALTH PROMOTION IN CHILDHOOD

*William B. Strong, Chairman; Richard J. Deckelbaum,
Samuel S. Gidding, Rae-Ellen W. Kavey,
Reginald Washington, and Jack H. Wilmore, Members;
and Cheryl L. Perry*

EDITORS' NOTE

This chapter represents the combined effort of a large group of individuals working for and with the American Heart Association; this group is ably represented by the authors of this chapter. It is unusual to present a previously published manuscript as a chapter in a book. We believe, however, as Dr. Strong suggested, that this work contains the subject matter that we sought and that rearranging the material to create a different facade would not improve on it. The American Heart Association has kindly permitted us to reproduce the work here.

The editors have added Figure 14–4, which we hope will be used in some form by our practitioner readers to call attention to patients at risk.

Coronary heart disease remains the leading cause of death in the United States, re-

This chapter is a reprint of an article published in Circulation, Vol. 84, April 1992, pp 1638–1650. Reprinted by permission of the American Heart Association, Inc.

"Integrated Cardiovascular Health Promotion in Childhood" was approved by the American Heart Association Steering Committee on October 16, 1991.

Inquiries should be sent to the Office of Scientific Affairs, American Heart Association, 7272 Greenville Avenue, Dallas, Texas 75231-4596.

sponsible for close to half a million deaths each year. Over the past two decades, convincing evidence has emerged that links defined risk factors in adults with an accelerated atherosclerotic process. Pathological data have shown that atherosclerosis begins in childhood, and that the extent of atherosclerotic change in children and young adults can be correlated with the presence of the same risk factors identified in adults. It thus seems eminently reasonable to initiate healthful life style training in childhood to promote improved cardiovascular health in adult life.

The goal of this document is to provide strategies for promotion of cardiovascular health that can be integrated into routine pediatric care. Five critical areas are reviewed: cigarette smoking, physical activity, obesity, hypertension, and levels of cholesterol.

Background information, methods of assessment, and means for intervention are discussed for each area. Brief sections on assessment of family history and interaction of risk factors are also included. A cardiovascular health schedule has been developed to help the practitioner implement these suggestions within the framework of regular pediatric care. Rather than labeling specific children as abnormal, strategies are directed toward promoting optimal cardiovascular health for all children.

CIGARETTE SMOKING

Background

In 1984 Dr. C. E. Koop called smoking "the chief single avoidable cause of death in our society and the most important public health issue of our time." It is useful to consider cigarette smoking as a behavioral and social illness that is widely prevalent and results in enormous morbidity and mortality. Because most smokers acquire their habit in the early teenage years, the solution of the problem must involve pediatricians and other health professionals who treat children.

Smoking is of great significance in a pediatric practice for four reasons: (1) If all smoking were eliminated from the United States, it is estimated that there would be 19 per cent less abruptio placenta, 22 per cent fewer infants born with low birth weights (less than 2500 gm), 33 per cent less heart disease, 41 per cent fewer childhood deaths between 1 month and 5 years of age, 50 per cent less bladder cancer, and 90 per cent less lung cancer. (2) Many children are, in effect, already smoking on a regular basis by breathing the residual smoke from cigarettes lit and inhaled by their parents. Even indirect and passive smoking incurs substantial health consequences and causes a significant percentage of minor and major illnesses among children. (3) The precursors to the adoption of cigarette smoking are evident in childhood, and smoking onset can be influenced by intervention. (4) The onset of smoking is usually in adolescence and has immediate social and medical consequences. Intervention that can prevent use, delay onset, or minimize smoking among adolescents is likely to prevent habitual use. The predictors of smoking are numerous, and a consistent antismoking message from key health-related role models may lower smoking rates in all age groups and subcultures. The message about cigarette smoking, in contrast to that of many other risk-related behaviors, is unequivocal. The physician should explicitly support the concept of not smoking. In the office this includes promotion of smoking cessation among adults and adolescents, as well as overt reinforcement for not smoking.

Assessment

Patients and their parents should be asked if they have tried cigarettes, whether they smoke, and, if they intend to quit, if they have experimented or are regular smokers. Smoking levels of children, adolescents, and their parents should be documented in the medical charts. Silence on this subject by a physician is interpreted as an indication that smoking is not a significant health risk.

What You Can Do

Physicians who treat infants, children, and adolescents deal with vastly different levels of intellectual and social maturity. Both the theory and practical details of smoking interventions differ among these groups. Behavioral prescriptions to use for each age group are summarized in Table 14–1.

Infants

With infants, intervention is not directed at the patient but at the parents. The infant whose parents smoke is exposed not only to the harmful effects of passive smoke inhalation but also observes smoking by the most powerful role models in his or her social environment.

Physicians who care for children play a unique role with a segment of the young adult population—parents. People between the ages of 18 and 35 years are less likely to visit physicians than are older people and are difficult to reach with a preventive message; yet young smokers, who have accumulated only a few pack-years of smoking, benefit most from cessation. Physicians can provide the effective intervention and counseling they need. Smokers rate physicians as providing the greatest motivation to quit smoking, ahead of urging by friends and relatives, legal restriction of smoking at work and in public places, higher taxes, and antismoking advertising.

One model of promoting smoking cessation among adults has four components: asking, motivating, setting a quit date, and reinforcing. Asking parents about smoking is the first crucial step. This should occur during each office visit. Motivating, the second component of promoting smoking cessation, occurs on two levels: The physician must motivate the parent to attempt to quit smoking, and the physician must motivate himself or herself to deliver a cessation message. When parents who smoke have been identified and then motivated to quit by discussion of the immediate health and social con-

TABLE 14–1. METHODS PHYSICIANS CAN USE TO PROMOTE NONSMOKING

Objective	Target	Strategy
To reduce the amount of passive smoking by the infant	Parents and others close to the infant	Encourage cessation of smoking among parents and/or nonsmoking near the infant. 1. Ask about parents smoking habits. 2. Motivate parents to quit smoking through immediate risks to infant. 3. Set a date on which the smoker agrees to quit. 4. Reinforce ex-smokers.
To teach children that smoking is a harmful and addictive behavior	Children in elementary school and the distal social environment	Promote nonsmoking by emphasizing: 1. Harmful physical consequences of smoking 2. Addictive nature of cigarettes 3. Advertising techniques that mask real effects of smoking 4. Smoke-free environments at home and at the doctor's office
To encourage adolescents to remain or become nonsmokers through social skills development	Adolescents in secondary schools	Promote nonsmoking by emphasizing: 1. Immediate physiological and social consequences 2. Ways to deal with pressures to smoke 3. Commitment to nonsmoking 4. Alternatives

sequences, the actual cessation attempt can be negotiated. An effective way to do this is to set a date in the near future on which the smoker agrees to quit and enter it into the child's medical chart. This third component may increase both the number of attempts to quit and the success of those attempts. The final component is reinforcement. Although smoking cessation manuals and specialized clinics can now achieve reliably high initial rates of cessation, recidivism is also frustratingly high: Fewer than three of ten smokers who quit will remain abstinent after 1 year.

Children

When children are asked from whom they learn most about health, the second most frequent response, after mothers, is doctors. Children see physicians as both medical experts and role models for appropriate health behavior. The messages delivered by physicians are interpreted as facts and translated into evidence for or against particular habits. The physician serves a special role in being able to provide information at critical times in a child's development as well as being an alternative health role model for the child.

Four strategies for discussing smoking with children are suggested. First, it should be emphasized that not starting to smoke—not even a puff—is the best way to avoid becoming a regular smoker. Because some experimentation does occur during this stage, this advice could help delay or prevent that experimentation. Certain times in which physicians are likely to see children, such as for camp physical examinations, sports, or school changes, may be particularly significant occasions for physicians to discourage smoking. School transitions, for example from elementary to junior high school, are times of marked acceleration in smoking onset rates. Second, the harmful health consequences of smoking should be pointed out, for example, cancer, emphysema, and heart disease, as well as the addictive, habit-forming qualities of nicotine. Most adults who smoke begin doing so as adolescents without the knowledge that the effects of nicotine are so pernicious and the habit so tenacious. Third, smoking advertisements should be shown to children, with an emphasis on how little is written about the well-known harmful effects of smoking and how advertising falsely portrays the smoking habit to be enjoyable. Finally, the physician should provide a nonsmoking environment in the office, one without ashtrays and with signs indicating that smoking and a physician's office are incompatible.

Adolescents

Adolescents are clearly the group most at risk for beginning to smoke. At this stage, the long-term harmful effects of smoking should be deemphasized; adolescents recognize the health consequences of smoking but see them as remote and irrelevant. Instead, smoking is seen as having more immediate positive consequences, such as becoming part of a group or being more mature. The pediatrician should concentrate on more proximal methods to discourage smoking for adolescent smokers and nonsmokers. Consequences like bad breath, smelling like smoke, and nicotine stains on the fingers are of concern to self-conscious adolescents. The effect of nicotine on heart rate, blood pressure, and steadiness are evident after a single cigarette and, once pointed out to a young smoker, can serve as a repeat warning every time a cigarette is smoked. An eco-lyzer, which measures the amount of carbon monoxide in expired air, could be used by a physician to determine whether the adolescent is smoking. The immediate harmful effects of carbon monoxide could be used to encourage nonsmoking.

Peer influences appear to be the most important proximal factor for initiation. Learning to say no to peer pressure seems critical. The physician or nurse practitioner could review types of peer pressure situations and provide opportunities for the adolescent to practice refusal. Direct reinforcement for nonsmoking or commitments to nonsmoking could be used. A contract or a statement of intention not to smoke by the adolescent could be used by the physician. A letter to the patient commending his or her positive health behavior might be a powerful reinforcer. Finally, the physician can promote alternatives to smoking. Because adolescents smoke for particular reasons, for example to fit in with a group, to lose weight, or to appear older, smoking serves important functions. Attention to the life style of the adolescent and the needs that smoking fulfills can help the physician generate alternative behavioral prescriptions for the adolescent and maintain nonsmoking as the ideal.

PHYSICAL ACTIVITY

Background

The health benefits associated with a physically active life style in children include weight control, lower blood pressure, improved psychological well-being, and a predisposition to increased physical activity in adulthood. Higher levels of physical activity in adults have been associated with a long life and decreased risk of cardiovascular disease.

A healthy level of physical activity requires regular participation in activities that increase energy expenditure above resting levels. An active child participates in physical education classes, plays sports, performs regular household chores, spends recreational time outdoors, and regularly travels by foot or bicycle. A sedentary child minimizes opportunities for play or recreation at school, spends the majority of his or her leisure time watching television, and regularly travels by car. Many socioeconomic factors contribute to the diminished physical activity of American children. Schools have redistributed funding and time commitments in favor of academic programs and away from physical education programs because of costs and the recent emphasis on poor performance by American children in standard academic disciplines. Many children have either a single parent or two working parents, and supervision after school may not be as conducive to participation in peer-based recreational activities as in the past. Recent observations in children suggest increased obesity, television viewing, and playing of computer games, indicating that they are less physically active than in the past. Positive social values, including improved interpersonal skills, diffusion of tensions, and improved high school performance associated with regular participation in physical activity and sports, are less emphasized today.

Assessment

A clinically useful assessment of a child's level of physical activity should be age related and take into account the following confounders: individual differences in physical fitness levels, physical ability, inclination to participate in various sports, and opportunity to participate. Assessment can begin as early as age 2 to 3. Asking parents to rate their child as more or less active than other children is an easy and reliable way to begin. Afterward, questions related to the physical activity standards listed below may be asked. The child's age, gender, and inclination toward activity as well as the season of the year and parental attitudes toward activity should be considered.

Healthy Physical Activity Standards. Some general guidelines for healthy physical activity are listed below.

1. Regular walking, bicycling, and backyard play; use of stairs, playgrounds, and gymnasiums; and interaction with other children

2. Less than 2 hours per day watching television or videotapes

3. Weekly participation in age-appropriate organized sports, lessons, clubs, or sandlot games

4. Daily school or day-care physical education that includes a minimum of 20 minutes of coordinated large-muscle exercise

5. Regular participation in household chores

6. Weekly family outings that involve walking, cycling, swimming, or other recreational activities

7. Positive role modeling for a physically active life style by parents, other caretakers, physicians, and school personnel

What You Can Do

Emphasis should be placed on play (rather than exercise) and on activities that are enjoyed by the child, that are consistent with the child's skill level, and that can be accomplished given the family's personal resources and interests (Table 14–2). Physical activity is important for all children, including those who are clumsy and less coordinated. Following are some general suggestions:

1. Formally address the subject of exercise in your practice.

2. Advise parents to include planned activities instead of food as part of the family's reward system for positive accomplishments.

3. Advise parents to establish time limits for sedentary activities and encourage a daily time for physical activity.

4. Emphasize the benefits of regular physical activity: an improved cardiovascular risk factor profile, increased energy expenditure, improved weight control, a general sense of physical well-being, improved interpersonal skills, and an outlet for psychological tension.

5. Do not include or exclude a child from activities because of physical or mental limitations. Tailor suggestions for exercise to the child's physical ability.

6. Encourage participation in pick-up games, noncompetitive activities, and organized sports; emphasize sports that can be enjoyed throughout life; participation in summer camp; and school physical education programs.

TABLE 14–2. METHODS PHYSICIANS CAN USE TO PROMOTE PHYSICAL ACTIVITY

Objective	Target	Strategy
Incorporate physical activity counseling into medical practice	Children, parents, and physicians	Ask about physical activity patterns, encourage parents to be more active, and recommend activities specific to the child's age, family circumstances, and environment.
Universal participation in increased physical activity	All children, including those who are clumsy, overweight, or handicapped	For older children, emphasize sports in which they can participate all their life, deemphasize the competitive and achievement-oriented nature of sports programs, and increase emphasis on participation and teamwork; encourage an active life style at a young age.
Improve children's access to physical activity programs	Schools, media, and local, state, and national government	Improve physical education programs in schools and day care; encourage the maintenance of high-quality and safe public play spaces; and promote in the media life-long participation in sports and the benefits of a physically active life style.

7. Make suggestions appropriate to the age of the child.

8. Incorporate advocacy of physical education into your role as a school health professional, if applicable. Make sure all children, including those who are less coordinated, are involved.

9. Teach parents the importance of being role models for active life styles and providing children with the opportunities for those activities.

10. Be an advocate for physical health in your community.

Changes in physical activity levels over time may be difficult to assess, but the results of increased physical activity are easily documented. A decrease in the time needed to complete the 1-mile walk/run test administered in school is an objective measure of better cardiorespiratory endurance. An improved weight-for-height ratio, the family or patient's own admission of life style change, fewer hours spent watching television, and favorable changes in blood pressure, total cholesterol level, and high density lipoprotein (HDL) cholesterol level can be related to an increasingly active life style. The long-term benefit of physical activity counseling in childhood may not be realized until adulthood, when the maintenance of a healthy life style prevents the increase in weight, sedentary activity, blood pressure, and cholesterol levels characteristic of the third and fourth decades of life.

OBESITY

Background

A preoccupation with body weight has become a characteristic of our adolescent and adult populations. This concern with weight is justified in a certain subset of both populations, because elevated body weight is a predisposing factor for hypertension, blood lipid level abnormalities, adult-onset diabetes, and coronary artery disease. Between 13 and 36 per cent of 12- to 17-year-old Americans are obese. Depending on gender and race an additional 4 to 12 per cent may be considered super-obese. These data represent a 39 per cent increase in the prevalence of obesity when compared with data collected between 1966 and 1970. Equally alarming, there has been a 54 per cent increase in the prevalence of obesity among children aged 6 to 11 years. Obese children are at an increased risk for obesity as adults. Physicians are in a position to promote desirable body weight (Table 14–3).

Assessment

It is important to discriminate between overweight and obesity. Overweight is defined as exceeding the population norm or average weight considering that person's gender, height, and frame. Obesity is defined as an excessive amount of body fat. It is possible to be obese and within the normal weight range and to be overweight and of normal body fat. With children and adolescents, it is important to consider both weight and some measure of body composition; for example, skinfold fat thicknesses at selected sites. In adults, overweight and obesity, as distinct entities, have both been identified as risk factors for various chronic diseases such as hypertension, coronary heart disease, lipid abnormalities, and diabetes. Maintaining body weight below 120 per cent of normal values and/or skinfold fat thickness less than the 85th percentile appear to be reasonable guidelines for children and adolescents who may be at increased risk for cardiovascular diseases.

TABLE 14–3. METHODS PHYSICIANS CAN USE TO PROMOTE DESIRABLE BODY WEIGHT

Objective	Target	Strategy
To identify children who are obese rather than overweight	Physicians, health promoters, physical education teachers	Use skinfold calipers or other indirect measures of body composition
To encourage a healthier selection of foods (i.e., those with reduced fat and salt content)	Child, adolescent, parent	Promote the understanding of food labels and explain how to determine the relative fat content of food
To encourage a more active life style	Child, adolescent	Promote daily school physical education, emphasizing moderate to vigorous activity, and encourage after-school and weekend outdoor activity when possible

What You Can Do

To help patients prevent overweight and obesity, physicians may recommend the following tips.

1. Selection of a healthy diet—For cardiovascular health, cancer prevention, and optimum athletic performance, a diet low in fat and high in complex carbohydrates (e.g., fruit, vegetables) is the diet of choice. This is also true of the optimum diet for either weight loss or weight maintenance. People tend to consume more calories per day on higher-fat diets. Most scientists and clinicians recommend a diet in which fat provides no more than 30 per cent of total calories.

2. Dietary moderation, not restriction—A nutrition plan sure to fail is one in which favorite foods are forbidden. It is important to practice moderation when dieting. The occasional dish of ice cream or piece of pie is all right as long as it really is occasional (e.g., not more than once or twice a week).

3. First helpings but no seconds—Advise your patients to eat as much healthy food as they want with their first plate, but to take no second helpings. This will generally reduce the overall intake of calories but not leave them feeling deprived.

4. Snack food—Snacks are acceptable, but the type of food eaten at snack time is important. The number of calories consumed during snacking add up quickly, so low-calorie, healthy snack food like fruit and vegetables should be selected. Snacking should be limited.

5. Food as an inappropriate reward—Too often high-fat and high-sugar foods are used to reward desired behavior; food should not be used as a reward.

6. Increased levels of daily physical activity—It is surprising how even a small change in daily activity helps to maintain optimum weight. Encourage your patients to walk or ride their bikes rather than taking the car, to stand up when talking on the telephone, and to take the stairs, avoiding elevators and escalators. Help them be creative, adding to this list to increase their daily activity.

7. Formal exercise program—Adding a formal exercise program to the daily schedule can help control weight. Not only are more calories expended but the number of calories consumed may even decrease. Bicycling, walking or jogging, and participation in games and sports are examples of exercise patients can do regularly.

8. An enjoyable exercise routine—Exercise should not be punishment, despite what some persons may have experienced in school physical education classes (e.g., extra laps for tardiness). However, people do not all enjoy the same activities. Thus individuals should find activities that they can enjoy and perform successfully. Aerobic activity uses calories quickly, and muscle building exercise increases the metabolically active fat-free mass.

9. Exercise time as a priority—One thing is true of almost all individuals: Everyone is busy. However, a busy schedule should never leave out time for activity. Once that starts to happen, it is difficult to get back into the habit.

10. Parents as important role models—By modeling appropriate dietary and activity habits, parents can have a significant positive influence on the health of their children.

11. Realistic expectations—The media have convinced most people that they can look like popular movie stars or athletes. Ask patients to look at their brothers and sisters, parents, uncles and aunts, and grandparents to get a realistic idea of the role genetics play in body shape or type. Remind them that there is little one can do to change that. It is also important to remember that weight gains are necessary in the growing child and adolescent, and only unusual gains should be of concern.

HYPERTENSION

Background

Elevated blood pressure accelerates the development of coronary artery disease and contributes significantly to the pathogenesis of cerebrovascular accidents, heart failure, and renal failure. Among all the risk factors cited by the landmark Framingham Study, hypertension has been identified as the most potent antecedent of cardiovascular disease. Because hypertension is usually silent, physicians have a responsibility to identify individuals at risk. Blood pressure rises with age, but hypertension begins in childhood. Physicians therefore have an important role to play in educating children and families about blood pressure and the preventive measures useful in reducing hypertension.

Assessment

The AHA's Council on Cardiovascular Disease in the Young supports the recommendation of the Second Task Force on Blood Pressure that all children 3 years of age and older should have their blood pressure measured in a physician-monitored setting. The measurement should be performed with a mercury sphygmomanometer, with the child sitting and his or her right arm resting on a supporting surface at heart level. The width of the blood pressure cuff should be at least two thirds the length of the upper arm, and the bladder should be long enough to almost encircle the arm. The recommendations of the AHA should be followed, including inflation of the cuff to a pressure of 20 to 30 mm Hg above systolic blood pressure and cuff deflation at 2 to 3 mm Hg/second. Korotkoff fourth and fifth sounds have both been suggested as being representative of diastolic blood pressure in children. Electronic instruments are convenient and accurate for measurement of systolic blood pressure. It is this committee's belief that true diastolic blood pressure is not accurately assessed by indirect methods in infants and children. Therefore caution should be used in interpretation of diastolic blood pressures in these patients.

Blood pressure measurements in noncooperative, agitated children are misleading. Attempts must be made to obtain reliable resting measurements. If the child is not quiet, his or her status should be recorded with the blood pressure. The Second Task Force developed a flow chart for identification of children with elevated blood pressure (Fig. 14–1). Elevated blood pressure in children is defined as systolic blood pressure consistently above the 95th percentile. In adults, elevation of systolic blood pres-

sure is as important as elevated diastolic blood pressure as a risk factor.

What You Can Do

Blood pressure graphs developed by the Second Task Force should be used to interpret and track blood pressure measurements. It is useful to review the blood pressure graphs with the child and parent, indicating how the child's blood pressure compares with that of his or her peers. Attention to the child's height and weight is important because blood pressure is directly related to both. Tall youths may have a blood pressure at the top of, or just above, the normal range for age but within the normal range for weight. Obese youths are more likely to be hypertensive than leaner ones. Values for the 95th percentile for height and weight for each age group are shown in Table 14–4. If resting blood pressure equals or exceeds the 95th percentile on three separate occasions and the elevation cannot be explained by height or weight, the diagnosis of hypertension should be made and an appropriate evaluation undertaken. In Table 14–4 hypertension is classified by age group. The Second Task Force report presents a succinct diagnostic evaluation for the child whose blood pressure is elevated.

The Council on Cardiovascular Disease in the Young recommends early detection of blood pressure elevation. Appropriate management includes the initiation of nonpharmacological therapies such as active dietary counseling and physical activity prescriptions. Because pharmacological agents cannot lower blood pressure without side effects, such intervention is reserved for children whose blood pressure is consistently very high and for those with significant secondary hypertension. Because obesity in childhood and the development of obesity in adolescence are strongly related to hypertension in adult life, weight control, prevention of obesity, and a physically active life style are strongly encouraged. Even in early childhood, significant differences in blood pressure can be accounted for by fitness and body fatness. Weight loss and improved cardiovascular conditioning have been demonstrated to lower blood pressure in hypertensive adolescents.

The council also believes that it is prudent to recommend moderation in the use of salt. Most studies suggest that increased salt in-

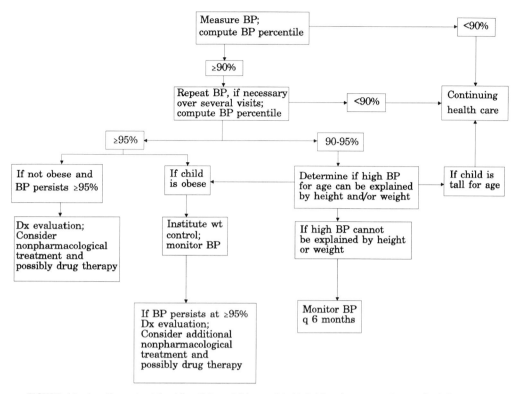

FIGURE 14–1. Flow chart for identifying children with high blood pressure in need of diagnostic evaluation and treatment. BP = blood pressure; Dx = diagnosis; q 6 months = every 6 months. (From Report of the Second Task Force on Blood Pressure Control in Children. Reprint of the Task Force Report by the National Heart, Lung, and Blood Institute. Dallas, American Heart Association, 1987. By permission.)

TABLE 14–4. CLASSIFICATION OF HYPERTENSION BY AGE GROUP

Age Group	Significant Hypertension (mm Hg)	Severe Hypertension (mm Hg)
Newborn		
7 days	Systolic BP ≥ 96	Systolic BP ≥ 106
8–30 days	Systolic BP ≥ 104	Systolic BP ≥ 110
Infants		
<2 years	Systolic BP ≥ 112	Systolic BP ≥ 118
	Diastolic BP ≥ 74	Diastolic BP ≥ 82
Children		
3–5 years	Systolic BP ≥ 116	Systolic BP ≥ 124
	Diastolic BP ≥ 76	Diastolic BP ≥ 84
6–9 years	Systolic BP ≥ 122	Systolic BP ≥ 130
	Diastolic BP ≥ 78	Diastolic BP ≥ 86
10–12 years	Systolic BP ≥ 126	Systolic BP ≥ 134
	Diastolic BP ≥ 82	Diastolic BP ≥ 90
Adolescents		
13–15 years	Systolic BP ≥ 136	Systolic BP ≥ 144
	Diastolic BP ≥ 86	Diastolic BP ≥ 92
16–18 years	Systolic BP ≥ 142	Systolic BP ≥ 150
	Diastolic BP ≥ 92	Diastolic BP ≥ 98

Source: Report of the Second Task Force on Blood Pressure Control In Children. Reprint of the Task Force Report by the National Heart, Lung, and Blood Institute, Dallas, American Heart Association, 1987.
BP = blood pressure.

TABLE 14–5. METHODS PHYSICIANS CAN USE TO PROMOTE PREVENTION OF HYPERTENSION IN CHILDREN

Objective	Target	Strategy
To reduce the risk of high blood pressure and obesity	Parents, children < 2 years old	Education of the parent about the use of salt as well as healthy eating patterns
To measure blood pressure in all children 3 years of age and older	Physicians, clinics, parents, children	To measure the blood pressure of all children during health visits

take over time increases blood pressure in individuals who are salt sensitive. The desire for salt may be an acquired taste, and it seems reasonable to initiate moderate salt use in childhood, which might preclude its subsequent overuse.

In Table 14–5 the objectives, target groups, and strategies to optimize blood pressure awareness in childhood and the preventive measures that may be helpful in reducing hypertension are identified. The goal of children's blood pressure assessment and follow-up is twofold: to identify children with secondary hypertension and those with severe primary hypertension who require evaluation and therapy, and to prevent in all children the acquisition of life style factors (obesity, excessive salt intake, and sedentary activity patterns) that contribute to excessive rise in blood pressure with aging.

LEVELS OF BLOOD CHOLESTEROL

Background

Major epidemiological studies in adults have established a strong positive association between total and low density lipoprotein (LDL) cholesterol levels and the incidence of coronary artery disease morbidity and mortality. Among adults dying of coronary artery disease, more than one third have a total cholesterol level higher than 240 mg/dl, a level at which the rate of coronary artery disease is twice that when total cholesterol is less than 200 mg/dl. Equally important, studies of adults carried out over time periods as short as 3 to 7 years have shown that lowering elevated cholesterol levels lowers the risk of coronary artery disease. Evidence linking higher blood cholesterol levels in children and adolescents with atherosclerotic lesions in coronary and other arteries is accumulating. Because the atherosclerotic process antedates clinical mani-

festations by years and even decades, it seems prudent to minimize or reduce known adult risk factors in younger as well as older groups. Such an approach is even more justified when reductions in risk are not associated with adverse side effects. Public, physician-based, and family-based education is likely to affect life styles in such a way that lower blood cholesterol levels will be seen in later years. An important aspect of addressing blood cholesterol levels in children should be positive emphasis on promotion of cardiovascular health and the avoidance of negative approaches like labeling children with higher cholesterol levels as being at risk.

Assessment and Intervention

Two strategies are recommended: the population strategy of maintaining lower blood cholesterol levels in all children, and the individual strategy of identifying children at higher risk for premature heart disease because of high blood cholesterol levels, so targeted intervention can lead to lower blood cholesterol levels in these children.

Population Strategy

This strategy is recommended for all children older than 2 years and has an overall goal of introducing nutritional patterns in childhood that when maintained in adulthood will lower blood cholesterol levels of the adult population as a whole. These recommendations are consistent with those of the AHA, the National Cholesterol Education Program (NCEP) report of the Expert Panel on Population Strategies for Blood Cholesterol Reduction, and the NCEP Expert Panel on Blood Cholesterol Levels in Children and Adolescents. The recommendations emphasize implementation of the AHA's Step 1 diet to lower blood cholesterol levels and promote cardiovascular health in all adults and children more than 2 years of age.

1. Adequate nutrition should be achieved by eating a wide variety of foods.

2. Total calories sufficient to support normal growth and development and maintain desirable body weight should be consumed.

3. Total fat should provide an average of no more than 30 per cent of total calories.

4. Saturated fatty acids should provide less than 10 per cent of total calories.

5. Polyunsaturated fatty acids should provide up to 10 per cent of total calories.

6. Less than 300 mg cholesterol should be consumed per day.

Dietary guidelines can be implemented by easily understood educational programs for the public; by marketing, industrial cooperation through the media, and emphasis on preparation of appropriate foods by the food service industry; and in physicians' offices. Government and communities can provide guidance to make school lunches more heart healthy. Instruction on preparation of school lunches, alternate low-fat food choices (e.g., 1 per cent or skim milk rather than whole milk), and substitutions and understanding of food labels are examples of programs that can be developed. Children should be encouraged to consume 1 per cent or skim milk and other low-fat dairy products, major sources of calcium, an important constituent of bone. Bone mass appears to be related to intake of calcium during the years of bone mineralization, that peaks at about age 20.

Individual Strategy

With increasing public awareness of the link between cholesterol and heart disease, cholesterol screening is an acceptable method for introducing children and families to heart-healthy life patterns. The AHA recommends monitoring the cholesterol levels of children in families or environments in which adverse cardiovascular health factors are present, including premature coronary artery disease (at or below age 55) in parents, grandparents, aunts, or uncles; family history of hypercholesterolemia (parents with blood cholesterol levels higher than 240 mg/dl), or children for whom family history is not available. The physician may elect to screen the child for high blood cholesterol levels if one or more of the following risk factors are observed: hypertension, smoking, sedentary life style, obesity, excessive alcohol intake, certain medications associated with hyperlipidemias (e.g., oral contraceptives or anticonvulsives), or disease states such as diabetes mellitus or nephrotic syndrome.

Total cholesterol levels can be measured at any time of day in nonfasting patients because levels of total cholesterol do not vary appreciably with eating. LDL cholesterol levels can be measured in either serum or plasma but are usually determined indirectly by using the Friedewald formula: LDL cholesterol = total cholesterol − [HDL cholesterol + (triglycerides/5)]. A 12 hour fasting blood sample is necessary for these measurements.

In population studies, childhood cholesterol level is a good predictor of cholesterol levels as a young adult, particularly at the high and low extremes of distribution. However, because the correlation is imperfect, it cannot be definitely stated that a child with high cholesterol levels will have high cholesterol levels as an adult. Multiple measurements through puberty are therefore recommended before labeling the child hypercholesterolemic.

The AHA endorses the guidelines of the NCEP Expert Panel on Blood Cholesterol in Children and Adolescents in setting the following definitions for acceptable, borderline, and high total and LDL cholesterol levels in children and adolescents between 2 and 19 years: Acceptable levels of total cholesterol and LDL cholesterol are less than 170 mg/dl and less than 110 mg/dl, respectively; borderline levels, 170 to 199 mg/dl and 110 to 129 mg/dl; and high levels, higher than 200 mg/dl and higher than or equal to 130 mg/dl.

The levels of 170 mg/dl and 200 mg/dl approximate the 75th and 95th percentiles, respectively, for total cholesterol levels in American children. A long-term goal is to identify children whose cholesterol levels put them at increased risk of coronary artery disease as adults. The screening protocol varies according to the reason for testing (Fig. 14–2). The initial test for young people with at least one parent with high blood cholesterol (higher than 240 mg/dl), should be a nonfasting measurement of total cholesterol level. The NCEP pediatric panel suggests that a fasting lipoprotein profile be obtained in two clinical situations: when the child's or adolescent's total cholesterol level is higher than 200 mg/dl, and when young people are tested because of a documented history of premature cardiovascular disease in a parent, grandparent, aunt, or uncle (in some instances cardiovascular disease occurs in individuals with low HDL cholesterol levels but normal total blood cholesterol levels).

If nonfasting total cholesterol level is borderline (170 to 199 mg/dl), a second measurement of total cholesterol should be taken; and if the average is borderline or high, a fasting lipoprotein analysis should be obtained (Fig. 14–2).

Two children with the same total cholesterol level but different levels of HDL cholesterol will also have different levels of LDL cholesterol. The child with the higher HDL cholesterol level will have a lower LDL cholesterol level, and the child with the lower HDL cholesterol level will have a higher LDL cholesterol level.

In the Framingham Study, low HDL cholesterol levels were correlated with a higher risk of coronary artery disease in adults. Members of some families with isolated decreases in plasma HDL cholesterol levels are at risk of developing premature coronary artery disease. The NCEP considers an HDL cholesterol level of less than 35 mg/dl a risk factor in children and adolescents. Other risk factors associated with low HDL cholesterol include smoking and obesity. Hypertriglyceridemia is often associated with lower HDL levels.

Because the correlation between HDL cholesterol levels in the prepubertal and the postpubertal years is not very good, and significant problems remain in the laboratory standardization of the measurements of HDL cholesterol, determining HDL choles-

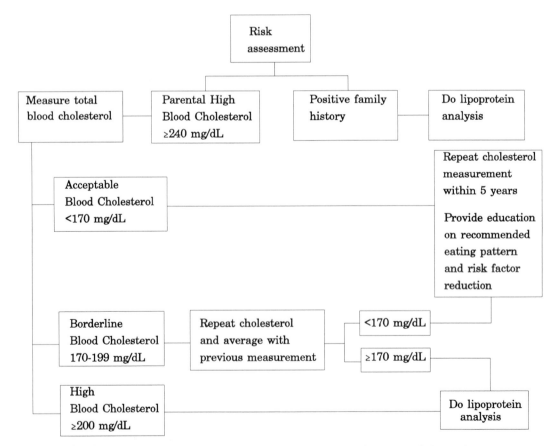

FIGURE 14–2. Flow chart of assessment of risk to determine need for second cholesterol measurement or lipoprotein analysis. Positive family history is defined as a history of premature (before age 55) cardiovascular disease in a parent or grandparent. (From Highlights of the Report of the Expert Panel on Blood Cholesterol Levels in Children and Adolescents. Reprint of the Pediatric Panel Report by the National Heart, Lung and Blood Institute. Dallas, American Heart Association, 1991. By permission.)

terol levels to assess risk is not recommended in children at present. However, HDL cholesterol levels much lower than 35 mg/dl or much higher than 70 mg/dl are, at least in part, genetically determined and may have some predictive significance.

The significance of elevated triglyceride levels measured in childhood for cardiovascular risk in adulthood is unknown. In general, triglyceride levels higher than 200 mg/dl are often related to obesity and will respond to weight reduction or decreasing fat content of the diet. Triglyceride levels higher than 500 mg/dl may suggest a genetic disorder of triglyceride metabolism.

What You Can Do

The above indications for determining cholesterol levels represent a minimum. As more is learned about the relation between elevated cholesterol and atherogenic lipo-

proteins, wider and more precise screening strategies may become apparent. Because elevated cholesterol level is in large part an inherited characteristic, it is of concern that a relatively small number of parents currently know their cholesterol level. Therefore, it seems reasonable for pediatric primary care providers to obtain parents' cholesterol measurements so a determination about the need for screening the child can be made.

All children with LDL cholesterol levels higher than 130 mg/dl should receive targeted intervention and follow-up (Fig. 14–3). As previously recommended by the AHA and, more recently, the NCEP pediatric panel an AHA Step 1 diet is the first approach to lowering elevated blood cholesterol levels.

Dietary education benefits the general population, but it is also the primary focus for intervention in children with hypercho-

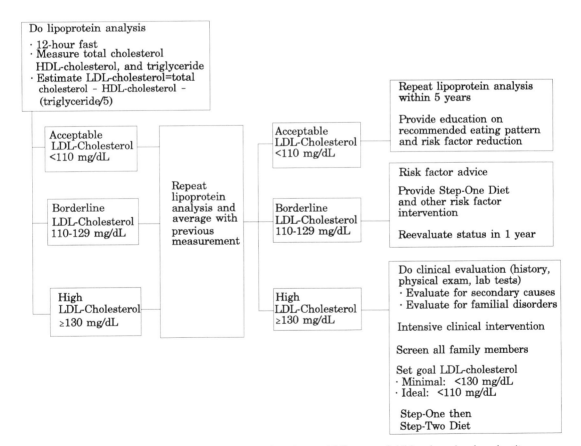

FIGURE 14–3. Flow chart of classification, education, and follow-up of children based on low density lipoprotein cholesterol levels. HDL = high density lipoprotein; LDL = low density lipoprotein. (From Highlights of the Report of the Expert Panel on Blood Cholesterol Levels in Children and Adolescents. Reprint of the Pediatric Panel Report by the National Heart, Lung, and Blood Institute. Dallas, American Heart Association, 1991. By permission.)

lesterolemia. Good aspects of a child's current diet should be used as the initial building block of a healthier nutritional intake.

If careful adherence to this diet for at least 3 months fails to achieve LDL cholesterol levels of less than 130 mg/dl, the Step 2 diet should be prescribed. This entails further reduction of the saturated fat intake to less than 7 per cent of calories and of the cholesterol intake to less than 200 mg/day. Adoption of the Step 2 diet requires careful planning to ensure adequacy of the nutrients, vitamins, and minerals. A registered dietitian or other qualified nutrition professional should be consulted at this stage, if this has not been done previously.

In general, as recommended by the NCEP pediatric panel, drug therapy to lower blood cholesterol levels is reserved for those 10 years of age or older who, while on a strict diet, either have LDL cholesterol levels higher than 190 mg/dl or have LDL cholesterol levels higher than or equal to 100 mg/dl and either a strong family history of premature coronary artery disease or two or more adult cardiovascular disease risk factors (i.e., low HDL cholesterol level, smoking, high blood pressure, obesity, or diabetes). The AHA endorses the recommendations of the NCEP pediatric panel report with respect to drug therapy. Children requiring drug therapy to lower blood cholesterol levels should be treated by physicians experienced in the management of lipid disorders in children.

Children with hypercholesterolemia will require nutritional intervention, long-term follow-up of cholesterol levels, nutritional guidance, and identification and avoidance of other risk factors. It is important to emphasize interactions among the different risk factors (e.g., the associations between obesity and increased LDL cholesterol levels and between smoking and decreased HDL cholesterol levels) as well as the ability of simple interventions to modify multiple risk factors simultaneously (e.g., exercise as a means of decreasing obesity, lowering blood pressure, and increasing HDL cholesterol levels). The physician's office or community clinic where cholesterol testing of patients and their families can reliably be performed is the perfect setting for the introduction of comprehensive risk factor assessment. An integrated approach involving the entire family will likely reduce the current high morbidity and public cost of coronary artery disease in the United States.

FAMILY HISTORY

Coronary artery disease (CAD) is familial; manifest CAD clusters in families. In some studies, a history of premature CAD in a first-degree relative has been found to be the single best predictor of risk even when patients with an inherited dyslipidemia are excluded. Therefore, a family history of CAD should be documented early in childhood. Because parents of infants and young children may be too young to have coronary artery disease themselves, a positive family history is defined as documented myocardial infarction, angiographic documentation of coronary artery disease, angina pectoris, or sudden cardiac death in parents, grandparents, aunts, or uncles at age 55 or younger.

If a positive family history is identified, information about cardiovascular risk and its modifiability should be introduced. The involved parent needs to be referred for evaluation if this has not been done previously. Because family history is still evolving in young families, it must be updated regularly; and if the family history becomes positive for coronary artery disease at any time, a review of cardiovascular risk and referral of the parents by the child's doctor are necessary. This process should be reciprocal; physicians making the diagnosis of heart disease in young adults should refer children and grandchildren for further evaluation.

INTERACTION OF RISK FACTORS

Identification of a child with multiple risk factors is important. The risk associated with any single identified factor is markedly affected by the intensity of any coexistent risk factors. Cross-sectional studies in adults have shown that patients with multiple risk factors have substantially increased cardiac risk compared with those with a single risk factor. In adults, it has also been shown that risk factors tend to cluster in an individual patient.

As an approach to identifying multiple risk factors, a cardiovascular health profile can be completed for each child (Fig. 14–4). Personal family history, smoking history (including passive smoking), blood pressure percentiles, weight-for-height chart, serum cholesterol level, and level of fitness can be used to develop a composite estimate of coronary artery disease risk and to direct man-

HEALTHY HEART TEST

Risk Factors

Family History (CAD <55 yrs)	☐ No	☐ Yes	
Family History (Hypercholesterolemia >240 mg/dl)	☐ No	☐ Yes	
Smoking	☐ No	☐ Parents	☐ Patient
Physical Activity	☐ Regular	☐ Occasional	☐ None
Weight	☐ Normal	☐ Overweight	☐ Obese
Blood Pressure	☐ Normal	☐ Borderline	☐ Hypertension
Cholesterol	☐ <170 mg/dl	☐ 170-199 mg/dl	☐ >200 mg/dl
LDL-Cholesterol	☐ <110 mg/dl	☐ 110-129 mg/dl	☐ >130 mg/dl
Reaction	OK	Concern	Action

FIGURE 14–4. Chart of cardiovascular risk factors. The more checks the patient has to the right, the more aggressive the primary physician should be in regard to intervention. CAD = coronary artery disease.

agement. This profile graphically demonstrates to children and their families their risk factors for future coronary artery disease.

CARDIOVASCULAR HEALTH SCHEDULE

The childhood years provide a unique opportunity for promotion of cardiovascular health. Parents actively seek advice and support from pediatric care providers, particularly when their children are in their infancy. Information provided at this vulnerable time can have an important impact on future life style. Plotting growth and blood pressure and following other health factors over time allows for early identification of life style elements that may contribute to the risk of cardiovascular disease later in life. Health promotion begins by focusing intervention at the child's developmental level. At the same time, educational intervention with the parents can be initiated so parents can serve as role models for their children while improving their own cardiovascular health. The cardiovascular health schedule described here (Table 14–6) calls

TABLE 14–6. CARDIOVASCULAR HEALTH SCHEDULE

Birth	• Family history for early coronary heart disease, hyperlipidemia → if positive, introduce risk factors: parental referral. • Start growth chart. • Parental smoking history—smoking cessation referral.
0–2 years	• Update family history, growth chart. • With introduction of solids, begin teaching about healthy diet (nutritionally adequate, low in salt, low in saturated fats). • Recommend healthy snacks as finger foods. • Change to whole milk from formula or breast feeding at approximately 1 year of age.
2–6 years	• Update family history, growth chart → review growth chart[a] with family (concept of weight for height). • Introduce prudent diet (< 30% of calories from fat). • Change to low-fat milk. • Start blood pressure chart at approximately 3 years of age[b]; review for concept of lower salt intake. • Encourage active parent-child play. • Lipid determination in children with positive family history or with parental cholesterol > 240 mg/dl (obtain parental lipid levels if necessary) → if abnormal, initiate nutrition counseling.
6–10 years	• Update family history, blood pressure, and growth charts. • Complete cardiovascular health profile with child; determine family history, smoking history, blood pressure percentile, weight for height, fingerstick cholesterol, and level of activity and fitness. • Reinforce prudent diet. • Begin active antismoking counseling. • Introduce fitness for health → life sport activities for child and family. • Discuss role of watching television in sedentary life style and obesity.
>10 years	• Update family history, blood pressure, and growth charts annually. • Review prudent diet, risks of smoking, fitness benefits whenever possible. • Consider lipid profile in all patients. • Final review of personal cardiovascular health status.

[a] If weight is > 120% of normal for height, diagnosis of obesity should be considered and the subject addressed with child and family.
[b] If three consecutive interval blood pressure measurements exceed the 90th percentile and blood pressure is not explained by height or weight, diagnosis of hypertension should be made and appropriate evaluation considered.

for identification of and education about known risk factors at a variety of times during routine pediatric care.

Birth

At either the prenatal or first neonatal visit, the primary care practitioner should obtain a careful family history for cardiovascular disease in the expanded first degree relative group. Family history is dynamic and therefore should be updated regularly. As noted previously, identification of a family history positive for cardiovascular disease should initiate a pattern of management for the parent and child.

At the initial pediatric visit, a parental smoking history should be obtained. Information about the negative impact of parental smoking on children and the risk associated with passive smoking should be communicated to parents, and smoking cessation should be strongly recommended. Information about smoking cessation should be available.

First Two Years

During the first 2 years of their child's life, parents have many questions about feeding. Issues like the introduction of solid foods provide openings for teaching parents about a healthy diet for children, one that is nutritionally adequate, low in salt, and low in saturated fats. When children begin eating independently, recommendations can be made about good snacks. At approximately 1 year of age, when the switch is usually made from breast milk or formula to cow's milk, the importance of whole milk as a source of calories at this age can be emphasized.

From Two to Six Years

At 2 years of age, the change can be made from whole milk to skim milk. This often promotes discussion of an appropriate diet. The prudent diet (AHA Step I) can be formally introduced at this time. Routine charting of weight and height allows early identification of children who are becoming overweight. The risk of obesity needs to be identified and the problem addressed early. Formal review of a child's growth chart is often revealing for a parent and can be very helpful in supporting recommendations for dietary change.

During the preschool years, when many physical skills are required, parents should be encouraged to participate in regular play with their children to enhance development of these skills. Family activities allow children to see their parents as models for an active life style and to learn activities they can enjoy throughout life; a link is established between fun and exercise. At approximately 3 years of age, formal recording of blood pressure should begin. Blood pressure needs to be interpreted in light of age, weight, and height; and charting is recommended to allow identification of those children with blood pressure at or higher than the 90th percentile. Recording blood pressures and reviewing the blood pressure course with patients and families leads naturally into discussion of avoidance of obesity and reduced salt intake, important for all patients. Three or more systolic and/or diastolic blood pressures higher than the 90th percentile for age uncorrected by weight and height should initiate a workup for hypertension as outlined by the Second Task Force on Blood Pressure.

Although the diagnosis of a dyslipidemia can be made in infancy, intervention is not usually recommended before age 2; a reasonable age for this assessment therefore appears to be 2 to 6 years. At this time, if the parents' lipid levels are unknown, parental lipid profiles should be obtained to identify those children who need lipid evaluation. Two determinations that show LDL cholesterol levels above the 95th percentile and/or HDL cholesterol levels below the 5th percentile strongly imply a genetic dyslipidemia.

From Six to Ten Years

In this age range, when children are still somewhat responsive to authority figures, the primary care physician can complete a cardiovascular health profile of the child. As stated previously, this composite estimate of CAD risk, based on family history, smoking history, blood pressure percentile, weight-for-height chart, fingerstick cholesterol, and level of fitness, is an effective teaching instrument. The profile can be used to emphasize all the important elements of cardiovas-

cular health, including the prudent diet that should be reinforced for this age group.

Because several studies indicate that exercise patterns established in childhood persist into adult life, reinforcing the need for regular exercise is important. To facilitate this, the subject of fitness can be formally introduced with the parent and child in this age range. Age-appropriate activities for the child can be recommended and increased family participation in regular activities of all kinds can be encouraged. The association of television watching with sedentary life style and obesity should be addressed.

Active antismoking counseling for the patient should also begin in this age group and be reinforced regularly.

More Than 10 Years

In this age range, when pediatric visits are generally limited to sports and camp physicals, the setting itself can be conducive to reviewing the benefits of fitness and smoking avoidance in preventing heart disease. A precollege or employment physical of a patient returning for a final pediatric visit is an ideal opportunity to review all the risk factors for heart disease. In epidemiological studies of children, the best correlation of adult cholesterol levels was with cholesterol levels obtained in the late teen years, so a lipid profile obtained at this age will be even more predictive than earlier ones of adult cholesterol levels. Because most of the turmoil of the teenage years has ended by the late teens, the patient may be better able to incorporate some of the information provided at this time. It is particularly important to review the significance of cardiovascular fitness because young adults often become much less active once they leave school. Because many young people seek no routine medical care over the next 10 to 20 years, strong recommendations for cardiovascular health promotion at this time can have an important effect.

CONCLUSION

The AHA's approach to cardiovascular health promotion in children, based on the identification of modifiable life style factors through routine pediatric care, is integrated with the child's developmental level. Smoking, hypertension, cholesterol, obesity, and physical activity have been reviewed in this chapter. The cardiovascular health schedule provides developmentally specific education to be implemented during routine pediatric visits. Cardiovascular health promotion linked to regular pediatric care has the potential to reduce the risk of atherosclerotic disease in both the individual child and the population at large.

SELECTED READINGS

1. The Health Consequences of Smoking: Cancer—A Report of the Surgeon General, US Department of Health and Human Services, Public Health Service. Office on Smoking and Health. Washington, DC, Government Printing Office, 1982.
2. Fielding JE: Smoking: Health effects and control (1). N Engl J Med 313:491–498, 1985.
3. Current Estimates from the National Health Interview Survey, United States. US Department of Health and Human Services Publ No. 86-1582. Washington, DC, Public Health Service, 1983, pp. 112–114.
4. The Health Consequences of Smoking: Chronic Obstructive Lung Disease—A Report of the Surgeon General. US Department of Health and Human Services, Publ. No. (PHS) 84-50205. Washington, DC, Government Printing Office, 1984, pp. 451–498.
5. Pacific Mutual Life Insurance Company: New Information. *In* Current Estimates From the National Health Interview Survey, United States. US Department of Health and Human Services Publ. No. (PHS) 86-1582. Washington, DC, Government Printing Office, 1983.
6. Working Group on Physician Behaviors to Reduce Smoking Among Hypertensive Patients: The Physician's Guide: How to Help Your Hypertensive Patients Stop Smoking. US Department of Health and Human Services Publ. No. 84-1271. Bethesda, National Institutes of Health, 1984.
7. Russell MAH, Wilson C, Taylor C, Baker CD: Effect of general practitioners' advice against smoking. BMJ 2:231–235, 1979.
8. Wilson D, Wood G, Johnston N, Sicurella J: Randomized clinical trial of supportive follow-up for cigarette smokers in a family practice. Can Med Assoc J 126:127–129, 1982.
9. Perry CL, Griffin G, Murray DM: Assessing needs for youth health promotion. Prev Med 14:379–393, 1985.
10. Kandel DB, Yamaguchi K: Developmental patterns of the use of legal, illegal, and medically prescribed psychotropic drugs from adolescence to young adulthood. NIDA Res Monogr 56:193–235, 1985.
11. Perry C, Killen J, Telch M, et al: Modifying smoking behavior of teenagers: a school-based intervention. Am J Publ Health 70:722–725, 1980.
12. Kwiterovich PO Jr: Diagnosis and management of familial dyslipoproteinemia in children and adolescents. Pediatr Clin North Am 37:1489–1523, 1990.
13. Lauer RM, Clarke WR: Use of cholesterol measurements in childhood for the prediction of adult hypercholesterolemia: the Muscatine Study. JAMA 264:3034–3038, 1990.
14. National Cholesterol Education Program Report of the Expert Panel on Blood Cholesterol Levels in Children and Adolescents, 1991. Bethesda, National Heart, Lung, and Blood Institute Information Center, 1991.
15. Castelli WP, Garrison RJ, Wilson PWF, et al: Incidence of coronary heart disease and lipoprotein cholesterol levels: the Framingham Study. JAMA 256:2835–2838, 1986.
16. Perry CL, Kleep KI, Sillers C: Communitywide strategies for cardiovascular health: the Minnesota Heart Health Program Youth Program. Health Educ Res 4(1):87–101, 1989.
17. Strong WB: Physical activity and children. Circulation 81:1697–1701, 1990.
18. Paffenbarger RS Jr, Hyde RT, Wing AL, Hsieh CC: Physical activity, all-cause mortality, and longevity of college alumni. N Engl J Med 314:605–613, 1986.
19. Wood PD, Stefanick ML, Dreon DM, et al: Changes in plasma lipids and lipoproteins in overweight men during weight loss through dieting as compared with exercise. N Engl J Med 319:1173–1179, 1988.
20. Dennison BA, Straus JH, Mellizs ED, Charney E: Childhood physical fitness tests: predictor of adult physical activity levels? Pediatrics 82:324–330, 1988.
21. Wilmore JH, Costill DL: Training for Sport and Activity: The Physiological Basis of the Conditioning Process. 3rd Ed. Boston, Allyn & Bacon, 1987.
22. Dietz WH Jr, Gortmaker SL: Do we fatten our children at the television set? Obesity and television viewing in children and adolescents. Pediatrics 75:807–812, 1985.
23. Taylor HJ, Jacobs DR Jr, Schucker B, et al: A questionnaire for the assessment of leisure time physical activities. J Chronic Dis 31:741–755, 1978.
24. Godin G, Shephard RJ: A simple method to assess exercise behavior in the community. Can J Appl Sport Sci 10:141–146, 1985.
25. Blair SN, Kohl HW III, Paffenbarger RS Jr, et al: Physical fitness and all-cause mortality: a prospective study of healthy men and women. JAMA 262:2395–2401, 1989.
26. Gortmaker SL, Dietz WH Jr, Sobol AM, Wehler CA: Increasing pediatric obesity in the United States. Am J Dis Child 141:535–540, 1987.
27. Van Itallie TB: Health implications of overweight and obesity in the United States. Ann Intern Med 103:983–988, 1985.
28. Wilmore JH: Ten tips to weight control. Sport Med Digest (in press).
29. Lohman TG, Roche AF, Martorell R (eds): Anthropometric Standardization Reference Manual. Champaign, IL, Human Kinetics Books, 1988.
30. Pollock ML, Wilmore J: Physical Activity in Health and Disease. 2nd Ed. Philadelphia, WB Saunders, 1990.
31. Report of the Second Task Force on Blood Pressure Control in Children—1987. Task Force on Blood Pressure Control in Children: National Heart, Lung, and Blood Institute, Bethesda, Maryland. Pediatrics 79:1–25, 1987.
32. Becque MD, Katch VL, Rocchini AP, et al: Coronary risk incidence of obese adolescents: reduction by exercise plus diet intervention. Pediatrics 81:605–612, 1988.

15

ENDOCARDITIS

Adnan S. Dajani

Infective endocarditis is a microbial infection of the endocardial (endothelial) surface of the heart. Heart valves, native or prosthetic, are the most frequently involved sites. Endocarditis can also involve ventricular septal defects, the mural endocardium, or intravascular foreign devices such as intracardiac patches and surgically constructed shunts. Infective endarteritis is a similar clinical illness involving arteries, including patent ductus arteriosus, the great vessels, aneurysms, or arteriovenous shunts. Although endocarditis is not common, it remains an important cause of morbidity and mortality in children with cardiovascular disease.

EPIDEMIOLOGY

The incidence of bacterial endocarditis in children ranges from 0.22 to 0.78 cases per 1000 hospital admissions and appears to be rising. The increase in incidence reflects increased survival of children with cardiovascular disease, an increase in the use of prosthetic intravascular devices, and more frequent insertion of long-term indwelling arterial and central venous catheters, particularly in the newborn in whom endocarditis therefore frequently involves the tricuspid valve. Endocarditis in neonates usually is not associated with congenital heart disease and in most patients has an atypical clinical course.

Beyond the neonatal period, the mean age of children with infective endocarditis is also increasing, perhaps owing to longer life expectancy resulting from improved overall therapy for children with heart disease.

PATHOPHYSIOLOGY

Several independent factors or events are required for the development of infective endocarditis. Preexisting structural heart disease is present in almost all patients who develop endocarditis (Table 15–1). Infection develops on injured endothelium or on damaged or abnormal heart valves on which blood-borne adherent organisms may lodge. Endothelial injury may result from persistently turbulent blood flow caused by a congenital cardiovascular defect, from chronic direct trauma as may be caused by indwelling intravascular catheters, or from cardiovascular surgical procedures. Despite the absence of preexisting cardiac disease, intravenous drug abuse is a high risk factor because it results in frequent bouts of bacteremia with invasive organisms. The tricuspid valve seems to be particularly at risk when this occurs. Congenital heart disease, with or without previous cardiac surgery, and indwelling intravascular catheters and devices are the most common underlying conditions in patients in developed countries. Rheumatic heart disease remains the major predisposing condition in many developing countries. Patients with surgically constructed systemic artery to pulmonary artery shunts, and those with prosthetic valves or other intracardiac prosthetic material are at particularly high risk for developing endocarditis. Previous bacterial endocarditis, even in the absence of heart disease, is considered by some authorities to be a risk factor for subsequent development of endocarditis.

Endothelial injury or damage results in collagen exposure and deposition of fibrin and platelets. If microorganisms adhere to

TABLE 15–1. CONDITIONS UNDERLYING INFECTIVE ENDOCARDITIS

Ventricular septal defect

Bicuspid aortic valve, with or without stenosis or regurgitation

Mitral valve prolapse with regurgitation

Rheumatic mitral or aortic regurgitation

Prosthetic heart valves and conduits

Indwelling vascular catheters, particularly central venous catheters

Intravenous drug abuse

Patent ductus arteriosus

Surgically constructed arterial shunts

Previous episode of infective endocarditis

---

these deposits, infective endocarditis ensues. Vegetations consisting of fibrin, platelets, and microorganisms may develop, and such vegetations become protected by a cover of fibrin and platelets. This protective sheath shelters the organisms from access by antimicrobial agents and host neutrophils. Most clinical manifestations and complications of endocarditis are directly related to either hemodynamic changes caused by the local infection or embolization from vegetations.

Bacteria are responsible for most cases of infective endocarditis, although fungi, chlamydia, rickettsiae, and viruses may also be a cause. Transient bacteremias occur frequently in humans, particularly during surgical or dental procedures and instrumentation involving mucosal surfaces or contaminated tissues. Transient bacteremias also may occur from chewing or tooth brushing. The ability of microorganisms to adhere to endocardial epithelial cells or to intravascular fibrin-platelet deposits is the critical first step in the development of endocarditis. Those bacteria that most frequently cause endocarditis can be shown experimentally to adhere more readily to normal aortic valve leaflets than do organisms that uncommonly cause endocarditis. What is more, specific products of these adherent bacteria enhance their ability to colonize the endocardium and fibrin-platelet deposits. Additionally, endocarditis-producing streptococci and staphylococci are potent stimulators of platelet aggregation, an action that enhances the formation of vegetations.

Certain immunologic factors also may play a role in the development of endocarditis. Gram-positive cocci cause endocarditis more often than gram-negative bacilli. Gram-positive bacteria resist the complement-mediated bactericidal activity of serum and phagocytosis that is required for their elimination. Only those few gram-negative bacteria that are serum-resistant are capable of producing endocarditis.

Humoral and cellular immune systems are stimulated as a result of endocarditis. This continuous antigenic challenge leads to increased production of specific antibodies and subsequent development of circulating immune complexes. Glomerulonephritis and the purpuric lesions sometimes seen in endocarditis are caused, at least in part, by immune complex deposits. Hypergammaglobulinemia and the development of rheumatoid factor in patients with long-standing disease are manifestations of the stimulation of the immune systems.

CLINICAL MANIFESTATIONS

Clinical presentation of patients with infective endocarditis is highly variable and may simulate many other diseases. Signs and symptoms are determined by the severity of the local cardiac disease and the extent of distant organ involvement secondary to embolization and circulating immune complexes. The spectrum of presentation varies from acute florid sepsis to indolent nonspecific subtle changes. *Infective endocarditis should be suspected in any child with an underlying cardiac condition who presents either with unexplained deterioration in cardiac function or with unexplained fever.*

Fever, the most common finding, often is low grade with no characteristic pattern, although high fever ($> 40°C$) and chills are not unusual. Fever is absent in about 10 per cent of cases, primarily neonates. Nonspecific symptoms are common and include malaise, fatigue, anorexia, and weight loss. Nausea, vomiting, and abdominal pain also may occur. *Arthralgia,* reported in about 25 percent of cases, is polyarticular and involves large joints.

Splenomegaly is the most common physical finding and is noted in about half of the patients. Appearance of a *new murmur* or change in a previous one is highly suggestive of infective endocarditis; it occurs, however, in only one fourth of the patients. *Petechiae* are seen in about one third of patients, especially those with long-standing disease. Splinter hemorrhages, Osler nodes, Roth spots, and Janeway lesions are characteristic of infective endocarditis but are rare, appearing in only 5 per cent of patients.

Neurologic findings, reported in about 20 percent of children with endocarditis, are manifestations of an infarct or an abscess. They may be the presenting feature of endocarditis or may occur long after the infection has been eradicated.

LABORATORY EVALUATIONS

Blood culture is the single most important procedure in the diagnosis of infective endocarditis. Some bacteria that cause endocarditis, such as coagulase-negative staphylococci and α-hemolytic streptococci are also frequent blood culture contaminants, particularly in infants and young children. It is essential therefore that meticulous aseptic techniques be observed when obtaining blood specimens for culture. At least three blood specimens should be drawn, preferably from different peripheral sites, and all samples should be obtained over a short period, no more than an hour or two. This method increases the yield of positive cultures and should differentiate a significant pathogen from a contaminant. A single positive blood culture is usually of little diagnostic significance. Bacteremia usually is continuous, so there is no need and no benefit from obtaining blood for culture during temperature spikes. Previous oral or parenteral antimicrobial therapy substantially reduces the yield from blood cultures. Blood obtained from patients who have received antimicrobics should be inoculated into special media to neutralize the antimicrobial effects. If not positive in a few days, blood cultures should be incubated for at least 3 weeks to allow for growth of fastidious organisms. Aerobic and anaerobic blood culture should be prepared routinely.

About 15 per cent of patients with clinically diagnosed endocarditis have negative routine blood cultures. Negative cultures may be due to previous antimicrobial administration or to fastidious or unusual organisms such as fungi, rickettsiae, *Chlamydia*, viruses, nutritionally deficient streptococci, *Brucella*, or anaerobes. Organisms are occasionally demonstrated by histologic examination or special staining of vegetations after surgical resection when blood cultures have been negative. Organisms also may be recovered from extracardiac embolic sites.

Echocardiography is the method of choice for the noninvasive assessment of valvar vegetations. Transesophageal echocardiography is more sensitive than transthoracic examination for left heart lesions, but the technique entails some risk and must be used with great care especially in small children. Vegetations may be present but not detected except at surgery or autopsy even with the most diligent echocardiographic examination.

A patient with infective endocarditis may have an elevated erythrocyte sedimentation rate, anemia, positive rheumatoid factor, and hematuria in varying frequencies.

MICROBIOLOGY

Many microorganisms can cause endocarditis in the pediatric population,[1] and the most common ones are listed in Table 15–2. Gram-positive cocci account for about 90 per cent of recoverable organisms. Oral α-hemolytic streptococci (*Streptococcus viridans*) and *Staphylococcus aureus* are the most frequent; jointly they account for 75 per cent of the gram-positive cocci. Pneumococci, enterococci, and β-hemolytic streptococci are less commonly encountered. The incidence of coagulase-negative staphylococcal endo-

TABLE 15–2. ETIOLOGIC AGENTS OF INFECTIVE ENDOCARDITIS IN INFANTS AND CHILDREN

Agent	Frequency
Streptococci	
α-Hemolytic	Most common
Enterococci	Rare
Pneumococci	Rare
β-Hemolytic	Uncommon
Others	Uncommon
Staphylococci	
S. aureus	Second most common
Coagulase-negative	Uncommon, but increasing
Gram-negatives	
Enterics	Rare
Pseudomonas spp.	Rare
HACEK[a]	Rare
Neisseria spp.	Rare
Fungi	
Candida spp.	Uncommon
Others	Rare

[a] *Hemophilus, Actinobacillus, Cardiobacterium, Eikenella,* and *Kingella.*

carditis is rising rapidly, particularly following cardiac surgery and in neonates.[2]

Gram-negative organisms seldom cause endocarditis in children, accounting for only about 5 per cent of positive cultures. Neonates, immunosuppressed patients, and intravenous drug abusers, however, are at an increased risk for gram-negative bacterial endocarditis. The HACEK group (*Hemophilus, Actinobacillus, Cardiobacterium, Eikenella, Kingella*) rarely cause endocarditis. Among this group *Hemophilus* is more common than the others in children. It can cause a subacute course of endocarditis and frequently results in emboli. *Neisseria gonorrhoeae*, another rare cause of endocarditis, may present as an acute illness, affecting previously normal valves and commonly resulting in valvar destruction.

Fungal endocarditis also is rare in children. Most cases occur following cardiovascular surgery, in neonates receiving hyperalimentation fluid or prolonged broadspectrum antimicrobial agents, and in other instances in which indwelling vascular catheters are used for extended periods.[3] *Candida albicans* is the most common fungal agent, although other *Candida* spp. have also been noted. *Aspergillus* spp. are the second most common fungi. *Histoplasma, Coccidioides, Cryptococcus*, and others may cause endocarditis, particularly in severely immunocompromised patients.

The clinical diagnostic microbiology laboratory can offer additional information that may be valuable for patient management. Measurement of the minimum inhibitory concentration (MIC) and minimum bactericidal concentration (MBC) of various antimicrobial agents against the isolated pathogen is helpful for determining if the organism is susceptible, tolerant, or resistant. MIC and MBC are almost always identical, and most laboratories report only the MIC. Antimicrobics should be used to attain serum concentrations well above the MIC (MBC). Within a day or two after starting antimicrobial therapy, it is desirable to determine a peak serum bactericidal titer (SBT), which is the highest dilution of the patient's serum that kills a standard inoculum of the isolated pathogen. Although it is not a standardized test, it is desirable to attain a peak SBT of at least 1:8. High SBTs are anticipated with most β-lactam antibiotics, and when these agents are used routine assays may not be necessary. If an aminoglycoside or vancomycin is used, it is imperative that serum peak and trough concentrations as well as peak SBTs be determined.

Repeat blood cultures should be performed to document the cessation of bacteremia. Blood should be cultured within a few days of starting antimicrobics to assess therapeutic efficacy. Blood cultures should be repeated once or twice within a few weeks of completion of antimicrobial therapy to detect possible relapse.

TREATMENT

Children in whom acute endocarditis is strongly suspected should be managed by a team that includes a pediatric cardiologist and a specialist in pediatric infectious disease. Dental evaluation is indicated as a precaution, regardless of whether a specific focus is identified.

Selection of the appropriate antimicrobial agent(s) is critical for the successful management of infective endocarditis.[4] Several general principles provide a basis for the current recommendations for treatment. Preferred regimens include (1) parenteral therapy, especially in infants and children; (2) prolonged course, usually 4 weeks or longer; (3) bactericidal agents; and (4) synergistic combinations, when applicable.

Table 15–3 summarizes recommended therapeutic choices for gram-positive cocci. Highly penicillin-susceptible streptococci (MIC < 0.1 µg/ml) include most α-hemolytic (viridans) streptococci, *S. bovis* (nonenterococcal group D streptococci), and group A streptococci. Aqueous crystalline penicillin G intravenously may be used alone for 4 weeks with excellent results. *Shorter courses with penicillin alone are not recommended.* Gentamicin may be used in conjunction with penicillin: gentamicin for the first 2 weeks and penicillin for either 2 or 4 weeks. Use of penicillin plus gentamicin for only 2 weeks has the obvious advantage of a shorter therapeutic course.[4]

Nutritionally deficient streptococci and α-hemolytic streptococci with an MIC between 0.1 and 0.5 µg/ml are preferably treated with a combination of penicillin for 4 weeks and gentamicin for 2 weeks.

Enterococci (*S. faecalis, S. faecium*, and *S. durans*) are rare causes of endocarditis in children. The usual penicillin MIC is above 2 µg/ml. Penicillin or ampicillin and an aminoglycoside act synergistically against these organisms. Enterococcal endocarditis is best

TABLE 15–3. TREATMENT REGIMENS FOR ENDOCARDITIS CAUSED BY GRAM-POSITIVE COCCI

Organism	Antimicrobial	Agent (/kg/24 hr)	Dose (/24 hr)	Max. Frequency of Dose	Duration of Administration (weeks)
Streptococci					
	For Patients Not Penicillin-Allergic				
Penicillin-susceptible (MIC < 0.1 µg/ml)	Penicillin G *or*	200,000 U	20 million U	q4h	4
	Penicillin G +	200,000 U	20 million U	q4h	2–4
	Gentamicin	7.5 mg	80 mg	q8h	2
Relatively-resistant to penicillin (MIC 0.1–0.5 µg/ml)	Penicillin G +	200,000 U	20 million U	q4h	4
	Gentamicin	7.5 mg	80 mg	q8h	2
Enterococci or other resistant streptococci (MIC > 0.5 µg/ml)	Ampicillin +	200 mg	12 gm	q4h	4–6
	Gentamicin	7.5 mg	80 mg	q8h	4–6
	For Penicillin-Allergic Patients				
MICs < 0.5 µg/ml	Vancomycin	40 mg	2 gm	q6h	4
MICs > 0.5 µg/ml	Vancomycin +	40 mg	2 gm	q6h	4–6
	Gentamicin	7.5 mg	80 mg	q8h	4–6
Staphylococci					
Methicillin-susceptible	Nafcillin *or*	200 mg	12 gm	q4h	4–6
	Oxacillin	200 mg	12 gm	q4h	4–6
Methicillin-resistant (including coagulase-negative staphylococci)	Vancomycin	40 mg	2 gm	q6h	4

See text for further details.

treated with ampicillin (or penicillin) plus gentamicin for 4 to 6 weeks.[5]

For penicillin-allergic individuals, vancomycin is recommended.[4] Eradication of susceptible streptococci (MICs < 0.5 µg/ml) can be accomplished with vancomycin alone for 4 weeks. Endocarditis due to enterococci or other resistant streptococci should be treated with a combination of vancomycin and gentamicin for 4 to 6 weeks.

For methicillin-susceptible staphylococcal endocarditis, methicillin may be substituted for nafcillin or oxacillin. The methicillin dose is 400 mg/kg/24 hr (maximum dose 12 gm) to be given every 4 hours for 4 to 6 weeks. Vancomycin should be used for methicillin-resistant staphylococci (both *S. aureus* and coagulase-negative staphylococci) and in patients allergic to penicillins. In patients who do not respond adequately to conventional therapy, rifampin may be used as a supplemental agent with a penicillinase-resistant penicillin or vancomycin.

Endocarditis caused by gram-negative bacteria requires individualized antimicrobial regimens. The identity of the specific organism and its susceptibility pattern are essential for selecting an appropriate regimen. In general, gram-negative endocarditis should be treated for at least 6 weeks with parenteral antimicrobics. An extended-spectrum penicillin (e.g., ticarcillin or piperacillin) or a third-generation cephalosporin (e.g., cefotaxime or ceftazidime), usually in combination with an aminoglycoside, are reasonable initial choices until the identity of the organism and its susceptibility pattern become available.

The prognosis for fungal endocarditis is poor, with high mortality and morbidity. Antifungal agents alone are usually inadequate; surgical intervention is often necessary. Several antifungal agents are in various stages of being assessed, but at this stage none has proved superior to amphotericin B. A "test" dose of amphotericin B of 0.1 mg/kg (maximum 1 mg) is administered initially. If it is well tolerated, it is followed by a dose of 0.5 mg/kg for 1 day and then 1 mg/kg/day for "maintenance." Minimum duration of therapy should be 6 to 8 weeks. Renal function and serum potassium concentrations should be carefully monitored. Surgery is probably best done after about 10 days of amphotericin B therapy and should consist in excision of the infected tissue with replacement of an infected valve (native or prosthetic).

Surgical intervention also may be necessary as part of the treatment of prosthetic valve endocarditis. Early replacement of an infected prosthetic valve may reduce the high mortality associated with such infections. The decision for surgical intervention and the timing of such intervention must be individualized. The usual indications for surgery include significant valvar obstruction, demonstration of a large vegetation, progressive heart failure secondary to valvar malfunction, persistent positive blood cultures after 10 to 14 days of appropriate antimicrobial therapy, and recurrent emboli or a single major embolus. Some suggest that all patients with staphylococcal endocarditis or all those who develop infection on a prosthetic valve soon after surgery should have a valve replacement. Occasionally, surgery is needed even in cases other than fungal or prosthetic valve endocarditis.

Antimicrobial therapy for patients with culture-negative endocarditis is directed at the most likely pathogens, but a careful and thorough workup must be completed before initiation of treatment. A combination of a penicillinase-resistant penicillin (nafcillin or oxacillin) plus gentamicin is a reasonable initial choice. For penicillin-allergic individuals, vancomycin plus gentamicin should be used. The duration of therapy must be individualized but is usually 4 to 6 weeks.

PREVENTION

Because of the high morbidity and mortality associated with infective endocarditis, any measure that can prevent the disease is advisable.[6] Endocarditis theoretically can be prevented by either repairing the underlying cardiac defect or reducing the likelihood of bacteremia in patients at risk. Ligation and division of a patent ductus arteriosus or patch closure of a ventricular septal defect with complete endothelialization of the patch leads to no increased risk for endocarditis.

Prophylactic antibiotics are recommended for children who are at risk to develop endocarditis when they undergo procedures that may induce bacteremia with organisms likely to cause endocarditis.[7] Recommended prophylaxis regimens are based primarily on in vitro studies, clinical experience, and experimental animal models. There are no adequate controlled clinical trials to validate the efficacy of such prophylaxis. Furthermore, it should be em-

phasized that endocarditis may occur despite appropriate antimicrobial prophylaxis.[8]

At-risk children include those with prosthetic heart valves, a history of endocarditis, congenital cardiac malformations (except isolated secundum atrial septal defect), rheumatic and other acquired valvar dysfunctions, hypertrophic cardiomyopathy, and mitral valve prolapse with regurgitation. Patients with rheumatic heart disease require bacterial endocarditis prophylaxis because antibiotics used to prevent streptococcal pharyngitis are not sufficient to provide protection against endocarditis (see Chapter 10). After cardiac surgery most patients still require endocarditis prophylaxis. Exceptions are patients who have had closure of either a patent ductus arteriosus or a ventricular septal defect in whom no residual shunt is present.

In general, dental or surgical procedures that induce bleeding from the gingiva or from the mucosal surfaces of the oral, respiratory, gastrointestinal, or genitourinary tracts require prophylaxis. Such procedures include tooth extraction, professional dental cleaning, gum surgery, tonsillectomy or adenoidectomy, bronchoscopy with rigid bronchoscope, esophageal dilatation, cytoscopy, and urethral catheterization or urinary tract surgery if urinary tract infection is present. Prophylaxis is most effective when given perioperatively and in doses to ensure adequate serum concentrations during and after a particular procedure.[6]

α-Hemolytic streptococci are the most common cause of endocarditis following dental, oral, or upper respiratory tract procedures. Prophylaxis for such procedures should be directed specifically against those organisms, which are generally susceptible to penicillin, ampicillin, or amoxicillin (Table 15–4). The standard general prophylaxis regimen is recommended even in patients who are at high risk to develop endocarditis (those with prosthetic valves, a previous history of endocarditis, or surgically constructed systemic-pulmonary shunts or conduits). Some medical authorities recommend a more stringent prophylactic regimen for these high-risk patients: ampicillin (50 mg/kg) plus gentamicin (2.0 mg/kg) to be given intramuscularly or intravenously 30 minutes before a procedure, to be repeated 6 to 8 hours after the initial dose. Penicillin-allergic patients who are at high risk may receive vancomycin (10 mg/kg IV

TABLE 15–4. RECOMMENDED PROPHYLAXIS FOR DENTAL, ORAL, OR UPPER RESPIRATORY TRACT PROCEDURES IN CHILDREN

Situation	Agent	Regimen
Standard general prophylaxis	Amoxicillin	50 mg/kg PO 1 hr before procedure (max. 3 gm), then half dose in 6 hr
Unable to take oral medications	Ampicillin	50 mg/kg IV or IM 0.5 hr before procedure (max. 2 gm), then half dose in 6 hr
Penicillin-allergic children	Erythromycin[a] *or* Clindamycin	20 mg/kg PO 2 hr before procedure (max. 1 gm), then half dose in 6 hr 10 mg/kg PO 1 hr before procedure (max. 300 mg), then half dose in 6 hr
Penicillin-allergic and unable to take oral medications	Clindamycin	10 mg/kg IV 0.5 hr before procedure (max. 300 mg), then half dose in 6 hr

Source: Modified from American Heart Association recommendations. JAMA *264*:2919–2922, 1990. Copyright 1990, American Medical Association.
[a] Ethylsuccinate or stearate.

over 1 hour starting 1 hour before the procedure).

Bacterial endocarditis following genitourinary or gastrointestinal tract surgery or instrumentation is primarily caused by enterococci.[6] Bacteremia due to gram-negative bacilli may follow such procedures, but endocarditis rarely is caused by these organisms. Prophylaxis is therefore directed primarily against enterococci (Table 15–5).

There are special situations in which the above recommendations may not apply. Surgical procedures through infected tissues require antimicrobial therapy directed against the most likely pathogen. Children who are receiving penicillin prophylaxis for prevention of rheumatic fever recurrence may have α-hemolytic streptococci in their oral cavities that are relatively resistant to penicillins. In such cases, an agent other than amoxicillin (e.g., erythromycin or clindamycin) should be selected for endocarditis prophylaxis. Finally, prophylaxis is recommended for patients who undergo open heart surgery, but such prophylaxis should be aimed primarily against staphylococci. A first-generation cephalosporin or vancomycin is a reasonable choice but should be used only perioperatively and for a short duration.

REFERENCES

1. Awadallah SM, Kavey R-EW, Byrum CJ, et al: The changing pattern of infective endocarditis in childhood. Am J Cardiol 68:90–94, 1991.

TABLE 15–5. RECOMMENDED PROPHYLAXIS FOR GENITOURINARY OR GASTROINTESTINAL TRACT PROCEDURES IN CHILDREN

Situation	Agent	Regimen
Standard general prophylaxis	Ampicillin *plus* Gentamicin	50 mg/kg IV or IM 0.5 hr before procedure (max. 2 gm), then same dose in 6 hr 2.0 mg/kg IV or IM 0.5 hr before procedure (max. 80 mg), then same dose in 8 hr
Penicillin-allergic children	Vancomycin *plus* Gentamicin	20 mg/kg IV over 1 hr starting 1 hr before procedure (max. 1 gm), then may repeat same dose in 8 hr 2.0 mg/kg IV or IM 1 hr before procedure (max. 80 mg), then may repeat same dose in 8 hr
Low-risk children	Amoxicillin	50 mg/kg PO 1 hr before procedure (max. 3 gm), then half dose in 6 hr

Source: Modified from American Heart Association recommendations. JAMA *264*:2919–2922, 1990. Copyright 1990, American Medical Association.

2. Etienne J, Eykyn SJ: Increase in native valve endocarditis caused by coagulase negative staphylococci: an Anglo-French clinical and microbiological study. Br Heart J *64*:381–384, 1990.

3. Dato VM, Dajani AS: Candidemia in children with central venous catheters: role of catheter removal and amphotericin B therapy. Pediatr Infect Dis J *9*: 309–314, 1990.

4. Bisno AL, Dismukes WE, Durack DT, et al: Antimicrobial treatment of infective endocarditis due to viridans streptococci, enterococci, and staphylococci. JAMA *261*:1471–1477, 1989.

5. Rice LB, Calderwood SB, Eliopoulos GM, et al: Enterococcal endocarditis: a comparison of prosthetic and native valve disease. Rev Infect Dis *13*: 1–7, 1991.

6. Dajani AS, Bisno AL, Chung KJ, et al: Prevention of bacterial endocarditis: recommendations by the American Heart Association. JAMA *264*: 2919–2922, 1990.

7. Imperiale TF, Horwitz RI: Does prophylaxis prevent postdental infective endocarditis? A controlled evaluation of protective efficacy. Am J Med *88*:131–136, 1990.

8. Van der Meer JTM, van Wijk W, Thompson J, et al: Efficacy of antibiotic prophylaxis for prevention of native-valve endocarditis. Lancet *339*:135–139, 1992.

16

DENTAL ISSUES FOR THE PRIMARY CARE PHYSICIAN

Carroll G. Bennett and Robert E. Primosch

Eruption of primary teeth proceeds along a predictable schedule as outlined in Table 16–1. Primary teeth provide all of the chewing functions until approximately age 6 to 7 years when the first permanent molars (6 year molars) erupt. They do not replace any primary (baby) teeth and are often overlooked and neglected. These permanent teeth have deep grooves and fissures on the chewing surface, a characteristic that unfortunately makes them susceptible to dental decay. Detailed information regarding tooth formation is available elsewhere for each of the primary and permanent teeth.[1]

SOFT TISSUE EVALUATION

The collar of tissue (gingiva) immediately adjacent to the teeth is tight, firm, and distinct, and about the same level throughout the mouth (Fig. 16–1). Areas of recession, swelling, bleeding, or changes in color, consistency, and contour of the gingiva indicate pathology. Healthy gingival tissue is critical in heart patients, as diseased periodontium under mastication can produce bacteremias capable of creating infective endocarditis.

The maxillary arch is ovoid in shape with some space between the anterior teeth (Fig. 16–2). This space is necessary, as the permanent incisors are larger. The anterior portion of the palate contains soft tissue ridges (rugae) that extend laterally from the midline and give this region a heavily textured surface. Spacing should also be present in the mandibular arch (Fig. 16–3).

EXAMINATION OF THE TEETH

The easiest way to determine the level of oral hygiene is to use a disclosing material, either a solution or a chewable tablet (Fig. 16–4). Teeth should also be examined for stains and calculus. Most preschool children do not have calculus, but older patients, especially adolescents, develop calculus on the lingual surfaces of the mandibular anterior teeth. Calculus is usually supragingival but cannot be removed by home care techniques and causes irritation to the gingival tissue. It appears as a chalky, hard buildup at the junction of the tooth crown and gingival collar. Poor hygiene and calculus accumulations are major causative factors of periodontal disease in children.[2]

Significant dental caries creates large, discolored defects on the involved teeth (Fig. 16–5). The lesions are usually yellowish brown and occur most often on the chewing surfaces of the molars. More subtle lesions appear as discolored pits and fissures on these same surfaces (Fig. 16–6) or as white, chalky spots on the smooth surfaces of teeth near the gingival junction. Once the enamel is penetrated and the underlying dentin is exposed to oral fluids, the carious lesion is nonreversible and must be treated by dental intervention. Accurate diagnosis of interproximal decay (between the teeth) requires intraoral dental radiographs. Figure 16–7 is a radiograph of the molars seen in Figure 16–6. The large, dark shadow on the first primary molar is a deep cavity.

Dental caries in the very young child may be caused by night feeding with a baby bot-

TABLE 16–1. CHRONOLOGY OF PRIMARY TEETH

Tooth	Eruption (month) Mean	Eruption (month) Range	Exfoliation (years, range)
Maxillary			
Central incisor	10	8–12	7–8
Lateral incisor	11	9–12	8–9
Cuspid	20	16–23	11–12
First molar	16	14–18	10–11
Second molar	29	25–33	11–12
Mandibular			
Central incisor	8	6–10	6–7
Lateral incisor	13	10–16	7–8
Cuspid	20	16–23	9–10
First molar	16	14–18	10–11
Second molar	27	23–31	11–12

tle. Nutrient materials placed in a nursing bottle, such as milk, soft drinks, and sweetened fruit juice, can cause extensive damage to the teeth if the child is permitted to feed at night when the flow rate of saliva decreases and the oral cavity becomes dry. Heavy plaque buildup occurs along the gingival margins, especially on the maxillary anterior teeth, causing a characteristic pattern of decay (Figs. 16–5 and 16–8). A more complete discussion of this important problem is available in a number of sources.[3,4]

Evaluation of teeth should include inspection for chipped, fractured, and worn areas. Children are accident prone, and anterior teeth are frequently injured. Damaged teeth turn dark (usually gray) several months after the accident if there has been pulpal

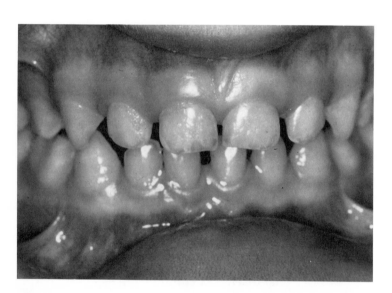

FIGURE 16–1. Normal healthy mouth of a 3-year-old. Gingival tissue is light pink and firm around the teeth, changing to red where it joins oral mucosa.

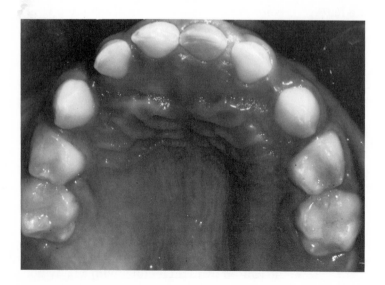

FIGURE 16–2. Healthy, well formed maxillary arch of a 4-year-old, with spacing throughout the anterior segment and typical ovoid shape.

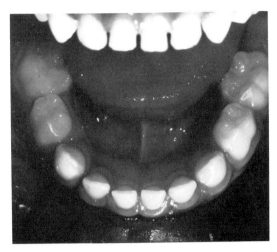

FIGURE 16–3. Healthy, well formed mandibular arch of a 4-year-old, with good anterior spacing and contact between the posterior molars.

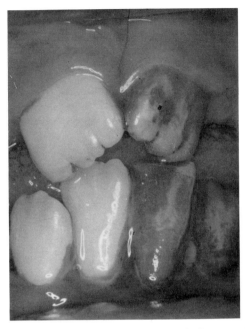

FIGURE 16–4. Disclosing solution applied to anterior teeth. Clean teeth on the left do not retain the stain. Plaque pattern is seen on the right side.

involvement. Extraction of these teeth may be required in children with heart disease because failure of endodontic therapy can increase the risk of infective endocarditis or a brain abscess. Children active in organized sports should be fitted by their dentist with an athletic mouth guard to prevent dentofacial trauma.

PREVENTIVE MEASURES

Home Care Techniques

Prevention of dental disease is particularly important for children with systemic health problems. The foundation of an effective preventive dental program is daily oral hygiene. Parents must be taught the proper techniques and must be responsible for brushing the child's teeth for the first 6 to 7 years.

Up to age 18 months, a soft cloth wrapped around the parent's index finger can be used to remove debris from the teeth, gum pads, and tongue. After carefully cleaning the teeth, a small amount of toothpaste can be placed on a small, soft bristle, toothbrush and the child allowed to brush over the bath-

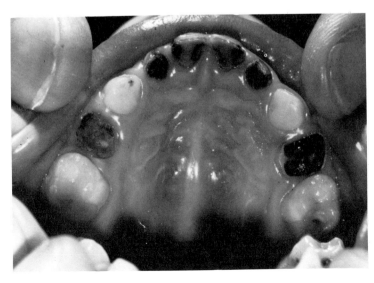

FIGURE 16–5. Extensive dental caries involving the maxillary anterior teeth and the first primary molars. Dental crown of first molars has decayed nearly even with the soft tissue.

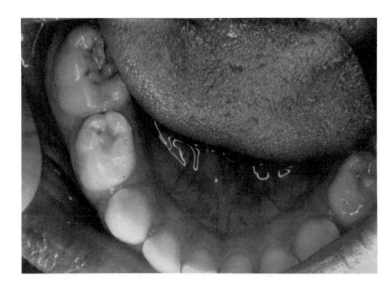

FIGURE 16–6. Stained pits and fissures on the first and second primary molars in the mouth of a 4-year-old.

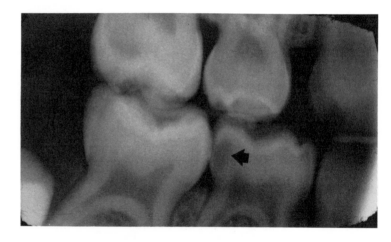

FIGURE 16–7. Dental roentgenogram showing a large interproximal carious lesion (arrow) on the distal surface.

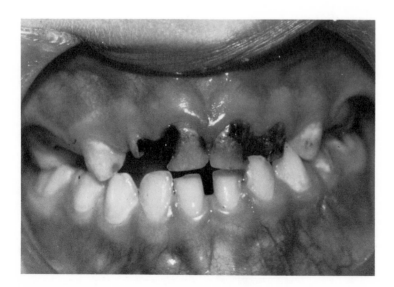

FIGURE 16–8. Classic nursing bottle decay involving the maxillary anterior teeth. Mandibular incisors are protected by the tongue during feeding and are usually caries-free.

room sink. This practice reinforces the importance of oral hygiene. As the child erupts more teeth, at around age 2 years, the soft cloth should be replaced by a small, soft-bristle toothbrush. The parent must still perform the brushing, although the child should be encouraged to participate after the teeth are cleaned by the parent.

As the child grows older, tooth brushing can be done at the bathroom sink with the parent standing behind the child. An American Dental Association (ADA)-approved fluoride toothpaste is strongly recommended. Usually by age 4 years the spaces between the posterior teeth have closed, and these surfaces can be cleaned only with dental floss. The parent should floss the child's teeth three or four times each week. Special floss holders are available that make it easier. A thin, waxed dental floss is recommended. High-quality toothbrushes with polished, rounded-end, soft bristles are available in a number of head sizes.

The child who develops new dental caries over a short period can benefit from daily home fluoride treatment. An ADA-approved over-the-counter fluoride mouth rinse should be used at night in the older school-age child after thorough brushing. Low concentration fluoride solutions have an effect on plaque pH and help remineralize early enamel changes. Illustrated brochures on brushing and flossing are available for purchase from the ADA. A brochure, "Dental Care for Children with Heart Disease," is available from the American Heart Association.

Systemic Measures

The most effective agent available for the prevention of dental decay is fluoride. Children between the ages of 6 months and 9 years receive major systemic benefit from fluoride because it alters the hydroxyapatite crystal in enamel, making the tooth more decay-resistant. Fluoride functions both topically, when applied to erupted teeth, and systemically, if ingested while enamel is being formed. Major segments of the population benefit from fluoride added to the drinking water supply. There are many families, however, who drink water from private wells or small systems that contains no fluoride.

Children not receiving the benefit of optimally fluoridated drinking water should receive a fluoride supplement. The dose (Table 16–2) depends on the age of the child and the amount of fluoride present in the drinking water. Most state water system laboratories have the ability to analyze water samples for fluoride content. This analysis should be done before prescribing supplemental systemic fluoride. Other sources of fluoride (e.g., schools) should also be evaluated. Excessive fluoride ingestion can result in dental fluorosis, an alteration in the enamel surface appearance that ranges from white opaque spots in its mildest form to brown-yellow defects in its most severe form. For infants and very young children, daily fluoride drops are recommended. For older children, a daily chewable tablet provides a topical benefit to the erupted teeth and a systemic benefit to the developing teeth.

Office Procedures

An important component of any preventive dentistry program is a routine dental office evaluation at either 6- or 12-month intervals. It is especially important for patients with heart disease, especially those with cyanotic heart disease, because such patients seem particularly prone to dental disease. Dental office visits for these children should begin by age 2 years. During these visits the teeth are cleaned, the calculus removed if present, and necessary dental roentgenograms obtained. Topical fluoride is applied, as this periodic office treatment is much more concentrated than the home fluoride daily rinse.

Regular visits also allow the dentist to use pit and fissure sealants soon after eruption of the permanent posterior teeth. This material is a special liquid composite solution that penetrates the narrow pits and fissures on the chewing surfaces, preventing bacte-

TABLE 16–2. DAILY FLUORIDE SUPPLEMENT DOSAGE

Age	Supplement (mg fluoride/day) According to Fluoride Content of Drinking Water		
	<0.3 ppm	*0.3–0.7 ppm*	*>0.7 ppm*
Birth to 2 years	0.25	0	0
2–3 Years	0.50	0.25	0
3–14 Years	1.00	0.50	0

Source: Accepted Dental Therapeutics, American Dental Association. 40th Ed. Chicago, 1984.

rial penetration into these areas that cannot be kept clean. The enamel is pretreated with a mild acid solution that leaves the surface with microporosities that bind the sealant to the enamel surface.

ORAL MANIFESTATIONS AND HEART DISEASE

There are few oral manifestations whose etiology is specific to cardiovascular disease in children. One can note abnormalities in the mouth that are associated with a patient's cardiac status, including the type and severity of heart disease and the intake of certain medications. Cyanosis may be more apparent in the mucous membranes of the mouth than it is elsewhere, particularly in black infants. Delayed tooth formation and eruption occurs in 20 per cent of patients with cyanotic heart disease.[5] Chronic hypoxemia predisposes an individual to an increased number of defects, which in turn result in increased dental caries. Increased frequency of dental caries also is a consequence of poor oral hygiene, a cariogenic diet as might be given by overindulgent or compensating parents, and use of cariogenic medications. Digoxin elixir, for example, contains 30 per cent sucrose and can have a significant cariogenic effect for selected individuals.[6] Some patients, particularly those with cyanotic heart disease, require iron supplementation, which can lead to staining of the teeth. Gingival bleeding is more common with patients with high hematocrits, particularly those over 60 per cent. Gingival bleeding also may be a consequence of anticoagulant medication.

SPECIFIC ISSUES

Bacterial Endocarditis Prophylaxis

Antibiotic prophylaxis against bacterial endocarditis should be given to most children with heart disease who undergo dental procedures that may result in a transient bacteremia. Table 16–3 gives the most commonly used antibiotic schedule for dental procedures. For complete information see Chapter 15.

TABLE 16–3. BACTERIAL ENDOCARDITIS PROPHYLAXIS FOR DENTAL PROCEDURES: STANDARD REGIMEN IN PATIENTS AT RISK

Initial amoxicillin[a] dose: PO, 1 hour before procedure

< 15 kg (33 lb)	750 mg
15–30 kg (33–66 lb)	1500 mg
> 30 kg (66 lb)	3000 mg (maximum adult dose)

Second amoxicillin[a] dose: PO, one-half initial dose, 6 hours after initial dose

[a] For amoxicillin/penicillin-allergic patients, see details in Chapter 15.

The risk of bacteremia is related to the health of the teeth and gums, as it may result from even simple mastication in a neglected mouth. Most dental manipulations create a risk for endocarditis, although it is generally agreed that simple adjustment of orthodontic appliances and the shedding of primary teeth do not require antibiotic prophylaxis.

Dental procedures are not necessarily identifiable as the predisposing event in patients who develop bacterial endocarditis. Guntheroth[7] reported that none of 18 pediatric patients with infective endocarditis received recent dental treatment. Other reports reveal a similarly low prevalence of dental extractions preceding infective endocarditis. Scrupulous oral hygiene clearly is superior for reducing the risk of infective endocarditis than is any recommended chemoprophylaxis regimen.

Physicians treating a patient with infective endocarditis should remember to perform a careful examination of the patient's teeth. Dental consultation is then obtained if there is disease or if there is uncertainty regarding dental status.

Anticoagulated Patients

Vigorous local hemostatic measures can be effective in preventing excessive blood loss if appropriate warfarin therapy (prothrombin time between 1.5 to 2.0 times the control) is maintained for minor surgical procedures. Patients receiving warfarin should be switched to heparin therapy at least 2 days before a planned surgical procedure in which there may be a risk of significant bleeding. Heparin effect can be rapidly reversed for a short period should it be necessary in order to accomplish the procedure safely. Need for this alternative therapy regimen should be compelling enough to justify its use, particularly for dental procedures.

Precardiac Surgery Evaluation

Prior to an elective surgical procedure, the dentist must be given an opportunity to perform a thorough dental evaluation of the pediatric cardiac patient. Ideally, this evaluation should occur 1 to 2 months prior to the scheduled surgery in order to allow adequate time for consultation, counseling, treatment, and healing without undue stress to the patient and parents. Preoperative dental evaluation and treatment should reduce the risk of intraoperative and postoperative infection.

Transplant Patients

Whenever possible, patients should receive needed dental treatment prior to heart transplantation.[8] After heart transplantation the patient is immunocompromised and therefore at high risk for infection. Prophylactic antibiotics are recommended following invasive dental procedures, although there is not uniform agreement on this point. See Chapter 18 for further discussion. Medical consultation may be required to assess the need for supplemental corticosteroid therapy preceding stressful dental procedures. Patients taking large doses of steroids in the equivalent of 20 mg hydrocortisone (5 mg prednisone) daily or more for longer than 1 month require supplemental therapy for dental procedures that are determined to be stressful or painful. Some patients receiving immunosuppressive therapy may already be taking large doses of steroids and may be adequately covered without supplementation.

Cyclosporin A is known to cause gingival hyperplasia, which is confined to the keratinized tissue and usually is limited to the interdental papillae (Fig. 16–9). The hyperplastic response is not related to drug dosage but, rather, to individual patient susceptibility (sensitivity of human gingival fibroblasts) and the amount of local irritants present.[9] Gingival hyperplasia can be treated by gingivectomy, but recurrence is common if regular, strict oral hygiene measures are not practiced by the patient. Oral infection (herpes, candidiasis) and ulceration of the mouth are additional complications observed in patients undergoing immunosuppression.

Qualified dentists should be available to the transplant team to ensure consultation and necessary dental care prior to and after transplantation. Postoperative susceptibility to oral infection suggests that an aggressive treatment plan should be used, all possible sources of infection eliminated, and proper oral hygiene measures emphasized. A complete dental protocol for transplant patients would include a complete clinical and radiographic examination, complete oral prophylaxis, plaque control, oral hygiene instructions, restoration or removal of infected teeth, and daily oral topical fluoride and chlorhexidine rinses.

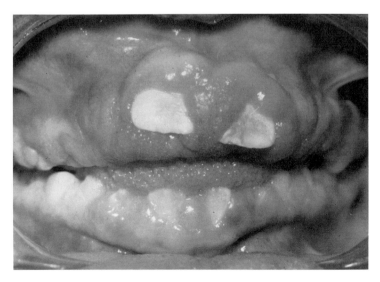

FIGURE 16–9. Cyclosporin A hyperplasia of the gingival tissue. Crowns of the posterior teeth have been covered completely.

Cooperation and Interaction with Dentists

Cooperation between the dentist and the physician minimizes the risk of dental problems. Parents must be informed as to the need for prophylactic antibiotic coverage required for dental procedures. The physician and dentist should discuss the regimen for antibiotic coverage, drug therapy, and other considerations such as anticoagulation status and supplemental steroid usage prior to initiation of any dental procedure. The physician should be informed as to the nature of the procedure and a mutual agreement reached as to the best approach for the specific child.

The physician should stress the importance of receiving optimal oral health care. Regular oral health evaluation with emphasis on oral disease prevention is essential to reduce the potential for endocarditis.

REFERENCES

1. Mathewson RJ, Primosch RE, Robertson D: Fundamentals of Pediatric Dentistry. 2nd Ed. Chicago, Quinteissence Publishing, 1987, pp. 15–19.
2. Wei SHY: Pediatric Dentistry—Total Patient Care. Philadelphia, Lea & Febiger, 1988, pp. 542–554.
3. Pinkham JR: Pediatric Dentistry. Philadelphia, WB Saunders, 1988, p. 165.
4. American Academy of Pediatric Dentistry: Pediatric Dental Care: An Update for the 90's. Chicago, AAPD, 1991, pp. 21–22.
5. Hakala PE, Haavikko K: Permanent tooth formation of children with congenital cyanotic heart disease. Proc Finn Dent Soc 70:63–66, 1976.
6. Feigal RJ, Gleeson MC, Beckman TM, et al: Dental caries related to liquid medication intake in young cardiac patients. J Dent Child 51:360–362, 1984.
7. Guntheroth WG: How important are dental procedures as a cause of infective endocarditis? Am J Cardiol 54:797–801, 1984.
8. Harms KA, Bronny AT: Cardiac transplantation: dental considerations. J Am Dent Assoc 112:677–681, 1986.
9. Ross PJ, Nazif MM, Zullo T, et al: Effects of cyclosporin A on gingival status following liver transplantation. J Dent Child 56:56–59, 1989.

17

GENETIC ISSUES OF CONGENITAL HEART DEFECTS

Jaime L. Frías

Congenital heart defects (CHD), with an estimated prevalence of 8 to 10 per 1000 live births,[1-3] constitute a heterogeneous group of malformations with various etiologies. We have generally considered and taught that in approximately 10 per cent of the cases CHD is genetically determined. Another 3 per cent are the result of environmental causes, and the remaining 87 per cent can be attributed to multifactorial mechanisms (Table 17–1).[2,4,5] Genetic etiology includes chromosomal and monogenic (mendelian) abnormalities. Among the chromosomal disorders, trisomy 21 is by far the most common, with reported incidences varying between 4 and 10 per cent of all children with CHD.[5-7] Other trisomies are rare as causes of CHD, although cardiac malformations in patients with some of them, such as trisomy 13 and trisomy 18, are of common occurrence.[8] Turner syndrome, caused by complete or partial monosomy of the X chromosome, has an incidence of less than 1 per cent among children with CHD.[7] Because of its recognized association with coarctation of the aorta, however, it should be suspected in any girl with this malformation and short stature.

Monogenic (mendelian) mechanisms have been considered to account for about 3 per cent of all cases of CHD.[9] Most of the cases are multiple congenital anomaly syndromes, such as the Noonan, Holt-Oram, or Carpenter syndrome, among others. Single-gene-determined isolated CHD has been considered to be rare, but autosomal dominant inheritance has been demonstrated in

at least one type of atrial septal defect and in some families with idiopathic hypertrophic subaortic stenosis.[9] Gene localization for these two defects has been provisionally assigned to chromosome 6. Others have suggested, however, that the gene for idiopathic hypertrophic subaortic stenosis is on chromosome 14.[9a] Continued advances in molecular genetics will most probably provide identification of increasing numbers of single-gene-determined CHD. (For a description of mendelian disorders with CHD the reader is referred to McKusick's catalog of mendelian inheritance.[10])

A few environmental factors, including exposure to certain drugs and chemicals, infectious agents during pregnancy, and maternal metabolic disturbances, are known to produce patterns of anomalies that include CHD in a significant proportion of affected patients.[2,5,9,11] These syndromes are outlined in Table 17–2, together with the observed incidence of CHD and the most frequent type of cardiac lesions found in each of them.

Multifactorial inheritance has been proposed to account for most patients with isolated CHD. In simple terms, multifactorial inheritance presupposes that a genetic predisposition caused by several genes makes an individual susceptible to the effect of an environmental factor. Mathematic models and animal experimentation support this hypothesis, but proof of its existence in humans is empiric. As we see later in the chapter, there is now reason to consider that single gene defects account for a much

TABLE 17–1. ETIOLOGY OF CONGENITAL HEART DEFECTS

Etiology	%
Genetic	10
Chromosomal	7
Monogenic	3
Environmental (drugs and chemicals, viruses, maternal diseases)	3
Multifactorial	87

larger proportion of CHD. The concept of multifactorial inheritance, then, may become less attractive.

GENETIC APPROACH TO THE CHILD WITH CHD

The physician caring for a child with CHD should be aware of the genetic implication of the malformation in order to provide the family with initial information and to consider whether to refer the patient for genetic evaluation and counseling. To assess the nature of the disorder and its risk of

TABLE 17–2. ENVIRONMENTALLY INDUCED DISORDERS WITH CHD

Disorder	Pts. with CHD (%)	Predominant Heart Defect(s)[a]
Rubella syndrome	50	PDA, peripheral PS
Diabetic embryopathy	3–5	TGV, VSD, CoA
Maternal phenylketonuria	30	TOF, VSD, ASD
Thalidomide embryopathy	15	TOF, TGV, DORV
Isotretinoin embryopathy	25	TOF, TGV, IAA-B
Fetal alcohol syndrome	35	VSD, ASD, TOF
Fetal hydantoin syndrome	10	PS, AS, PDA
Fetal trimethadione syndrome	50	VSD, TOF

Source: Modified from Noonan[5] and Nora and Nora.[9]
[a] AS = aortic stenosis; ASD = atrial septal defect; CoA = coarctation of the aorta; DORV = double outlet right ventricle; IAA-B = interrupted aortic arch, type B; PDA = patent ductus arteriosus; PS = pulmonic stenosis; TGV = transposition of the great vessels; TOF = tetralogy of Fallot; VSD = ventricular septal defect.

recurrence in future offspring, the clinical geneticist must obtain from the pediatric cardiologist a precise definition of the type of CHD present in the patient, not only from an anatomic point of view but, more importantly, in terms of its pathogenesis. Genetic evaluation should include (1) a complete review of the family history to ascertain other affected family members and establish a pattern of inheritance; (2) a detailed analysis of the pregnancy, including the presence of specific maternal diseases and exposure to potentially teratogenic agents; and (3) a careful evaluation of the patient, looking for the presence of associated anomalies in an effort to identify recognized associations, known syndromes, or unidentified patterns of malformation. Laboratory studies, such as chromosome or molecular analysis, are indicated in specific instances.

CARDIAC APPROACH TO THE CHILD WITH A DYSMORPHIC SYNDROME, GENETIC OR NONGENETIC

It is useful for the primary care practitioner to be aware of specific cardiac defects that are associated frequently with dysmorphic syndromes. For example, 50 per cent of patients with Down syndrome have a cardiac abnormality, the most common of which is an endocardial cushion defect, particularly a complete atrioventricular canal. An endocardial cushion defect causes a characteristic electrocardiographic pattern in almost all cases (see Chapter 3). It seems reasonable therefore to obtain an electrocardiogram on all patients with Down syndrome, many of whom are now identified soon after birth, regardless of whether ab-

TABLE 17–3. SYNDROMES WITH CHD

Syndrome	Pts. with CHD (%)	Predominant Heart Defect(s)
Down	50	ECD, VSD, TOF
Turner	20	CoA
Noonan	65	PS, ASD, ASH
Marfan	60	MVP, AoAn, AR
Trisomy 18	90	VSD, PDA
Trisomy 13	80	VSD, PDA
DiGeorge	80	IAA-B, TA
Williams	75	SVAS, peripheral PS

Abbreviations as in Table 17–2 plus: AoAn = aortic aneurysm; AR = aortic regurgitation; ASH = asymmetric septal hypertrophy; ECD = endocardial cushion defect; MVP = mitral valve prolapse; SVAS = supravalvular aortic stenosis; TA = truncus arteriosus.

normal cardiac findings are noted. Similarly, identification of a child with Turner syndrome should alert the practitioner to be diligent when examining the patient for possible coarctation of the aorta; the presence of Noonan syndrome suggests the possibility of pulmonic stenosis; and Marfan syndrome raises concern regarding the ascending aorta and aortic valve as well as mitral valve prolapse. Table 17–3 summarizes information in these and other syndromes. Tables 17–2 and 17–3 indicate that some cardiac defects, such as ventricular septal defect and tetralogy of Fallot, occur in many syndromes and embryopathies, whereas others are less common.

PATHOGENIC DEFINITION OF THE CARDIOVASCULAR MALFORMATION

Knowledge of developmental mechanisms involved in the production of CHD[12–15] has improved our understanding of relations between specific cardiac malformations and extracardiac anomalies. Five pathogenic mechanisms may operate during early embryogenesis to produce CHD: (1) abnormal proliferation and migration of cells from the branchial arch mesenchyme and the neural crest; (2) changes in the proportion of right and left heart blood flow; (3) abnormalities in the process of programmed cell death; (4) abnormalities in extracellular matrix formation; and (5) abnormalities in targeted growth. Table 17–4 depicts cardiac malformations that may result from each proposed mechanism.[12,15] Note that although morphologically dissimilar malformations may have a common pathogenetic mechanism, morphologically similar defects may result from markedly different developmental processes. This situation pertains, for example, for the various types of ventricular septal defect, each of which may be produced by a different pathogenic mechanism. Recognition of this hypothesis is of major importance for genetic counseling and may also shed light on the pathogenesis of the malformations associated with these defects. For instance, observation of a correlation between DiGeorge sequence and interrupted aortic arch type B (interrupted aortic arch types A and B are discussed in Chapter 6), persistent truncus arteriosus, and tetralogy of Fallot[13,16] supports the hypothesis that the DiGeorge sequence, same as all

TABLE 17–4. CLASSIFICATION OF CHD BY PATHOGENETIC MECHANISMS

Abnormalities of Mesenchymeal Tissue Migration (conotruncal defects)
Subarterial ventricular septal defect
Aorticopulmonary window
Double-outlet right ventricle
Tetralogy of Fallot
D-Transposition of the great vessels
Truncus arteriosus communis
Interrupted aortic arch, type B
Pulmonary atresia with ventricular septal defect

Altered Cardiac Hemodynamics
Coarctation of the aorta with intact ventricular septum
Hypoplastic left heart syndrome
Aortic valvular stenosis
Interrupted aortic arch, type A
Atrial septal defect, secundum type
Pulmonary atresia without ventricular septal defect
Perimembranous ventricular septal defect

Abnormalities in Programmed Cell Death
Muscular ventricular septal defect
Ebstein anomaly

Abnormalities of Extracellular Matrix
Endocardial cushion defects

Targeted Growth Defects
Total anomalous pulmonary venous return
Partial anomalous pulmonary venous return
Single atrium

conotruncal defects, is the result of an abnormality in the development and migration of neural crest cells. Three other syndromes in which the most commonly observed congenital cardiac malformations are also conotruncal defects are the CHARGE association, hemifacial microsomia, and the Shprintzen syndrome.[17–19] It is logical to assume that the noncardiac malformations in these syndromes also are the consequence of abnormal mesenchymal tissue proliferation and migration.[20]

Analogous correlations have been observed in two teratogen-induced patterns of congenital anomalies: the thalidomide and isotretinoin embryopathies. With both disorders the characteristic cardiac malformations are conotruncal: tetralogy of Fallot, transposition of the great vessels, and double-outlet right ventricle in the thalidomide embryopathy[21,22]; and tetralogy of Fallot, transposition of the great vessels, and interrupted aortic arch type B in the isotretinoin embryopathy.[23] These observations are consistent with the hypothesis that abnormalities in the development and migration of neural crest cells play a significant role in the pathogenesis of multiple anomaly syndromes.[12,24]

FAMILY HISTORY

A careful family history spanning at least three generations should be obtained during the evaluation of any child with CHD in an effort to identify affected relatives. The possibility of consanguinity should be investigated, as it is a clue for autosomal recessive inheritance and a recognized factor for increased risk of recurrence. As we discuss later in the chapter, the risk of recurrence increases if close relatives are also affected. Concordance of a malformation present in a patient with a defect(s) found in relatives should be analyzed in light of pathogenic mechanisms discussed above, rather than on the basis of purely anatomic definition.[15]

It would be best if family history data are documented with medical records. Relatives suspected of having a cardiac abnormality or known to be affected ought to be examined by a cardiologist to define the diagnosis. The value of this approach has been well demonstrated. For example, prospective clinical and echocardiographic studies in first-degree relatives of patients with complete atrioventricular canal or with hypoplastic left-heart syndrome, disclosed unsuspected heart malformations that, although of less clinical significance than those observed in the probands, were part of the same pathogenetic spectrum.[25,26]

Relatives of patients with syndromic CHD should be carefully evaluated for minor manifestations of the disorder. It is especially important in those with mendelian syndromes that are known to have a high degree of variability of expression (e.g., Noonan syndrome, Kartagener syndrome, hypertelorism-hypospadias syndrome, and Waardenburg syndrome).

ASSOCIATED EXTRACARDIAC ANOMALIES

In most patients CHD occurs as an isolated malformation, but approximately one third have associated anomalies and 10 to 15 per cent have specific dysmorphic syndromes. The reported incidence of associated extracardiac anomalies ranges from 7.7 to 45.0 per cent.[5,6,27] This wide variation is the result of different methodologies used

in the various studies, such as the type of patients with CHD included in the analysis, the definition of an associated anomaly, the retrospective or prospective nature of the study, and the inclusion of autopsy reports. Early reports[27,28] were limited to simple enumeration of identified anomalies; but more recent studies, by careful analysis of the data, have attempted to identify known patterns of malformation and to correlate the nature of the extracardiac anomalies with the type of CHD found in the patients. This method has shed light, as mentioned before, on the pathogenesis of CHD and revealed some of the patterns of malformation associated with them.[6,19,23]

A prospective study of 1016 children with congenital heart defects[6] identified 135 (13.3 per cent) who had recognized syndromes, embryopathies, or associations (Table 17–5). This percentage is higher than

TABLE 17–5. RECOGNIZABLE PATTERNS OF MALFORMATION IN 135 CHILDREN WITH CHD

Disorder	No. of Cases
Chromosomal Syndromes	
Down syndrome	43
Trisomy 18	2
Turner syndrome	3
Duplications/deletions	5
Other	3
Total	56 (41.5%)
Nonchromosomal Patterns of Malformation	
Noonan syndrome	14
Cardiofacial association	7
Williams syndrome	5
Ivemark complex (asplenia)	3
Ellis-van Creveld syndrome	2
Holt-Oram syndrome	2
Neurofibromatosis	2
VATER association	2
Shprintzen syndrome	1
Marfan syndrome	1
Marden-Walker syndrome	1
Dubowitz syndrome	1
Opitz syndrome	1
Frontonasal dysplasia	1
CHARGE association	1
Prune belly sequence	1
Multiple anomalies/mental retardation	7
Total	52 (38.5%)
Teratogen-induced Patterns	
Rubella embryopathy	13
Fetal alcohol syndrome/effects	10
Suspected viral embryopathy	3
Hydantoin-barbiturate syndrome	1
Total	27 (20.0%)

Source: Adapted from Kramer et al.[6] Copyright 1987, American Medical Association.

those observed in other studies[27–29] probably owing to the prospective nature of this study and the special emphasis placed on detection of both major and minor extracardiac anomalies, as well as on syndrome recognition.

Previous reports[5,29] have cited incidences of chromosomal abnormalities ranging between 5 and 7 per cent of children with CHD. A higher prevalence was reported in the Baltimore-Washington Infant Study,[7] a population-based case-control study that sought to identify risk factors for cardiovascular malformations. Of 2102 infants with CHD, they found 271 (12.9 per cent) who also had a chromosome abnormality, in contrast to only two cases among 2328 randomly selected control subjects. In their study, Down syndrome occurred in 10.4 per cent of infants with CHD. The predominant lesion, as expected (60 per cent), was an endocardial cushion defect.

Some studies have demonstrated a correlation between the type of CHD and the incidence of associated extracardiac anomalies.[28] In the New England Regional Infant Cardiac program,[30] a cooperative group of 11 New England hospitals reporting all infants with significant CHD diagnosed during the first year of life, 25 per cent had extracardiac anomalies. The incidence was more than 33 per cent in those with endocardial cushion defect, patent ductus arteriosus, or cardiac malposition defects. Lower prevalences, between 20 and 32 per cent, were found in infants with ventricular septal defects, tetralogy of Fallot, coarctation of the aorta, or single ventricle, and less than 10 per cent in those with transposition of the great vessels or pulmonary atresia with intact ventricular septum. In another study of 881 patients without specific patterns of malformation,[6] 68 (7.7 per cent) had major extracardiac anomalies and 369 (41.9 per cent) minor extracardiac anomalies. Among the children with major anomalies, those with tetralogy of Fallot had a higher incidence (15.7 per cent) than did the rest of the group (6.8 per cent). Similar figures have been reported by others.[28,30]

Specific major malformations have been found to have a higher prevalence than expected in children with CHD, including tracheoesophageal fistula, anal atresia, vertebral abnormalities, omphalocele, and diaphragmatic hernia.[5,28,31] Some authors have found urinary tract anomalies in up to 15 per cent of children with CHD,[32] whereas others have noted no difference between cardiac patients and normal controls.[6,33–35] Many pediatric cardiologists examine the urinary tract after angiography at cardiac catheterization in an effort to identify asymptomatic malformations.

Few studies have included evaluation of minor congenital extracardiac anomalies in patients with CHD. This lack is unfortunate, as such anomalies may serve not only as indicators of abnormal morphogenesis but also as clues in the diagnosis of specific patterns of malformation.[36,37] Kramer et al.[6] observed that the frequency of minor anomalies in patients with CHD whom they studied was significantly higher than in healthy children. They did not find, however, a correlation between the type of CHD and the frequency of minor extracardiac anomalies, as they did with major extracardiac anomalies.

RECURRENCE RISKS

The incidence of CHD in the siblings of an affected child is, on average, 1 to 3 per cent.[4,9] These empiric figures vary depending on the type of lesion present in the patient and, in accordance with the multifactorial model, with the number of affected relatives and the presence of consanguinity. Suggested risks of recurrence for any type of CHD in siblings are listed on Table 17–6.

TABLE 17–6.   RISK IN SIBLINGS FOR THE RECURRENCE OF ANY CONGENITAL HEART DEFECT

	Suggested Risk (%)	
Defect	*One Sibling Affected*	*Two Siblings Affected*
Ventricular septal defect	3.0	10
Patent ductus	3.0	10
Atrial septal defect	2.5	8
Tetralogy of Fallot	2.5	8
Pulmonary stenosis	2.0	6
Coarctation of the aorta	2.0	6
Aortic stenosis	2.0	6
Transposition	1.5	5
Endocardial cushion	3.0	10
Fibroelastosis	4.0	12
Hypoplastic left heart	2.0	6
Tricuspid atresia	1.0	3
Ebstein anomaly	1.0	3
Truncus	1.0	3
Pulmonary atresia	1.0	3

Source: Data from Nora and Nora.

These risks range from 1 to 4 per cent if one sibling is affected and three times that if two siblings are affected.[38]

Individuals with CHD are surviving to adulthood in increasing numbers, creating interest in defining the risks of recurrence in their offspring. The assumption that, as first-degree relatives, these risks ought to be similar to those observed among siblings has been challenged. Rose et al.[39] studied the incidence of CHD in the children of 219 probands (100 male and 119 female), each having one of four selected defects: atrial septal defect, coarctation of the aorta, aortic valve stenosis, or complex dextrocardia. Of the 385 live infants born to both male and female probands, 40 (10.4 per cent) had a CHD. Excluding minor defects (e.g., Wolff-Parkinson-White syndrome and mitral valve prolapse) the recurrence risk was 8.8 per cent. This figure is considerably higher than the 1 to 3 per cent risk of recurrence in siblings reported by Nora and Nora.[4] Rose et al. also observed that the risk of recurrence was higher in children of affected mothers (27/207 = 13 per cent) than in children of affected fathers (13/178 = 7.3 per cent) ($p < 0.001$). Whittemore,[40] in a prospective study of 252 women with different types of CHD, found that 65 (15.7 per cent) of their 413 offspring had a cardiac malformation. After excluding probands with genetic syndromes or positive family history, the observed risk was 13 per cent. A higher risk of recurrence in offspring of affected mothers than in children of affected fathers also has been reported by Nora and Nora.[41] The risks identified in children of affected fathers were of the same magnitude as those observed in siblings. A population-based epidemiologic study[15] estimated the risk of recurrence in siblings, grouping the specific defects according to their pathogenetic mechanism.[12] These data are difficult to interpret owing to the relatively small size of the data subsets, but they suggest that there is a familial predisposition to pathogenetically related malformations (e.g., bicuspid aortic valve, coarctation of the aorta, and hypoplastic left heart syndrome within the flow lesions) rather than to specific anatomic defects. Much more data are needed before it is possible to provide a sound basis for the assessment of risk figures in CHD.

Rein et al.[42] described a consanguineous kindred that demonstrated various conotruncal malformations whose presence suggested monogenic inheritance. These findings suggest that at least some nonsyndromic cases of CHD may be the result of single gene defects rather than of multifactorial mechanisms. Progress in genetic science may in fact identify a much larger population of single gene defects as etiologic factors in CHD. Some cardiologists and geneticists even now believe that the multifactorial inheritance hypothesis will become obsolete.

REFERENCES

1. Ferencz C, Rubin JD, McCarter RJ, et al: Congenital heart disease: prevalence at live birth. Am J Epidemiol 121:31–36, 1985.
2. Pierpont ME, Moller JH: Congenital cardiac malformations. In Pierpont ME, Moller JH (eds): Genetics of Cardiovascular Disease. Amsterdam, Martinus Nijhoff, 1986, pp. 13–24.
3. Calgren LE, Ericson A, Källen B: Monitoring of congenital cardiac defects. Pediatr Cardiol 8:247–256, 1987.
4. Nora JJ, Nora AH: The evolution of specific genetic and environmental counseling in congenital heart diseases. Circulation 57:205–213, 1978.
5. Noonan JA: Association of congenital heart disease with syndromes or other defects. Pediatr Clin North Am 25:797–816, 1978.
6. Kramer H, Majewski F, Trampisch HJ, et al: Malformation patterns in children with congenital heart disease. Am J Dis Child 141:789–795, 1987.
7. Ferencz C, Neill CA, Boughman JA, et al: Congenital cardiovascular malformations associated with chromosome abnormalities: an epidemiologic study. J Pediatr 114:79–86, 1989.
8. Schinzel AA: Cardiovascular defects associated with chromosomal aberrations and malformation syndromes. In Steinberg AG, et al (eds): Progress in Medical Genetics, New Series. Vol. 5. Philadelphia, WB Saunders, 1983, pp. 303–379.
9. Nora JJ, Nora AH: Genetic epidemiology of congenital heart diseases. In Steinberg AG, et al (eds): Progress in Medical Genetics, New Series. Vol. 5. Philadelphia, WB Saunders, 1983, pp. 91–137.
9a. Geisterfer-Lowrance AAT, Kass S, Tanigawa G, et al: A molecular basis for familial hypertrophic cardiomyopathy: a beta cardiac myosin heavy chain missence mutation. Cell 62:999–1006, 1990.
10. McKusick VA: Mendelian Inheritance in Man. Catalogs of Autosomal Dominant, Autosomal Recessive, and X-linked Phenotypes. 9th Ed. Baltimore, The Johns Hopkins University Press, 1990.
11. Tikkanen J, Heinonen OP: Maternal exposure to chemical and physical factors during pregnancy and cardiovascular malformations in the offspring. Teratology 43:591–600, 1991.
12. Clark EB: Mechanisms in the pathogenesis of congenital cardiac malformations. In Pierpont ME, Moller JH (eds): Genetics of Cardiovascular Disease. Amsterdam, Martinus Nijhoff, 1986, pp. 3–11.
13. Van Mierop LHS, Kutsche LM: Cardiovascular anomalies in DiGeorge syndrome and importance

of neural crest as a possible pathogenetic factor. Am J Cardiol 58:133–137, 1986.

14. Kirby ML: Cardiac morphogenesis–recent research advances. Pediatr Res 21:219–224, 1987.

15. Boughman JA, Berg KA, Astemborski JA, et al: Familial risks of congenital heart defect assesses in a population-based epidemiologic study. Am J Med Genet 26:839–849, 1987.

16. Van Mierop LHS, Kutsche LM: Interruption of the aortic arch and coarctation of the aorta: pathogenetic relations. Am J Cardiol 54:829–834, 1984.

17. Young D, Shprintzen RJ, Goldberg RB: Cardiac malformations in the velocardiofacial syndrome. Am J Cardiol 46:643–648, 1980.

18. Ardinger HH, Clark EB, Hanson JW: Cardiovascular anomalies in craniofacial disorders: pathogenetic and epidemiologic implications. Proc Greenwood Genet Center 4:81–82, 1984.

19. Graham JM, Meill E, Pagon RA, et al: Cardiovascular conotruncal defects in CHARGE association: evidence for neural crest involvement. Pediatr Res 19:235A, 1985.

20. Thomas IT, Frías JL: The heart in selected congenital malformations: a lesson in pathogenetic relationships. Ann Clin Lab Sci 17:207–210, 1987.

21. Lenz W, Knapp: Die thalidomid-embryopathie. Deutsch Med Wochenscher 24:1232–1242, 1962.

22. Frías JL, Leonardo VS: Talidomida: Antecedentes bibliograficos. *In* Martínez ML (ed): Mediacamentos y Teratogenia: Revisión Bibliográfica y Situación en España. Madrid, Ministerio de Sanidad y Consumo, 1989, pp. 35–40.

23. Lammer EJ, Chen DT, Hoar R, et al: Retinoic acid embryopathy: a new human teratogen. N Engl J Med 313:837–841, 1985.

24. McCredie J: Neural crest defect: a neuralanatomic basis for classification of multiple malformations related to phocomelia. J Neurol Sci 28:373–387, 1976.

25. Disegni E, Pierpont ME, Bass JL, et al: Two-dimensional echocardiographic identification of endocardial cushion defect in families. Am J Cardiol 55:1649–1652, 1985.

26. Berg KA, Astemborski JA, Boughman JA, et al: Heart defects in first degree relatives of infants with hypoplastic heart syndrome (HLHS). Am J Hum Genet 41:A47, 1987.

27. Boesen I, Melchoir JC, Terslev E, et al: Extracardiac congenital malformations in children with congenital heart disease. Acta Paediatr Scand 146: 28–33, 1963.

28. Greenwood RD, Rosenthal A, Parisi L, et al: Extracardiac abnormalities in infants with congenital heart disease. Pediatrics 55:485–492, 1975.

29. Lamy M, de Grouchy J, Schweisguth O: Genetic and non-genetic factors in the etiology of congenital heart disease: a study of 1188 cases. Am J Hum Genet 9:17–41, 1957.

30. Fyler DC: Report of the New England Regional Infant Cardiac Program. Pediatrics 65(Suppl): 376–459, 1980.

31. Richards MR, Merritt KK, Samuels MH, et al: Congenital malformations of the cardiovascular system in a series of 6,053 infants. Pediatrics 15: 12–32, 1955.

32. Engle MA: Associated urologic anomalies in infants and children with congenital heart disease. *In* El Shafie M, Klippel CH (eds): Associated Congenital Anomalies. Baltimore, Williams & Wilkins, 1981, pp. 137–142.

33. Humphry A, Munn JD: Abnormalities of the urinary tract in association with congenital cardiovascular disease. Can Med Assoc J 95:143–145, 1966.

34. Hoeffel JC, Mery J, Worms AM, et al: Frequence de l'association des malformations cardiaques et urinaires. Sem Hop Paris 54:9–12, 1978.

35. Boioli F, Damascelli B, Musumeci R, et al: Contributo clinico-estatistico allo studio delle malformazioni reno-ureterali asintomatiche (204 casi in 2120 pazienti). Radiol Med 54:888–903, 1968.

36. Marden PM, Smith DW, McDonald MJ: Congenital anomalies in the newborn infant, including minor variations: a study of 4412 babies by surface examination for anomalies and buccal smear for sex chromatin. J Pediatr 64:357–371, 1964.

37. Leppig KA, Werler MM, Cann CL, et al: Predictive value of minor anomalies: I. Association with major malformations. J Pediatr 110:530–537, 1987.

38. Nora JJ, Nora AH: Update on counseling the family with a first-degree relative with a congenital heart defect. Am J Med Genet 29:137–142, 1988.

39. Rose V, Reynold JMG, Lindsay G, et al: A possible increase in the incidence of congenital heart defects among offspring of affected parents. J Am Coll Cardiol 6:376–382, 1985.

40. Whittemore R: Genetic counseling for young adults who have a congenital heart defect. Pediatrician 13:220–227, 1986.

41. Nora JJ, Nora AH: Maternal transmission of congenital heart disease: new recurrence risk figures and the question of cytoplasmic inheritance and vulnerability to teratogens. Am J Cardiol 59: 459–463, 1987.

42. Rein AJJT, Dollberg S, Gale R: Genetics of conotruncal malformations: review of the literature and report of a consanguineous kindred with various conotruncal malformations. Am J Med Genet 36:353–355, 1990.

18

HEART AND LUNG TRANSPLANTATION IN CHILDREN

David Baum and Daniel Bernstein

Heart transplantation in children, initially attempted in 1968,[1] was first performed successfully in 1974 at Stanford,[2] and a small number of teenagers received heart transplants over the next 6 years.[3] Introduction of the immunosuppressant cyclosporine in 1980 markedly improved survival in adult recipients, resulting in a rapid increase in the number of cardiac transplant centers and stimulation of new interest for the pediatric age group. Encouraged by increasing success, pediatric transplant centers extended their recipient selection to include younger children and infants. At present, the number of pediatric heart transplant centers is sufficiently large to accommodate the needs of most areas in the United States, Canada, and western Europe. In recent years, survival rates and the quality of life after transplantation have improved to such an extent that heart transplantation is now considered an accepted therapeutic modality for children with end-stage heart disease and no other therapeutic alternative.

Successful cardiac transplantation requires a team approach involving physicians, nurses, social workers, and a responsible recipient family. Among the physicians involved, the local physician has a key role, as this individual must provide general pediatric care while collaborating in the management of special medical and psychosocial needs of recipients and their families. The primary care physician must be attentive to subtle, nonspecific clinical signs that can occur after transplant. Illnesses that affect these children following transplantation are often related to immunosuppression or

graft rejection. A high level of suspicion and prompt use of diagnostic studies can reduce morbidity and mortality.

SURVIVAL AND QUALITY OF LIFE

Children severely ill with serious heart disease usually derive great benefit from heart transplantation. Because most are not expected to live more than 6 to 12 months without transplant, their life expectancy on average with transplant is usually markedly prolonged. Cumulative survival in Stanford pediatric recipients (Fig. 18–1) suggests that an additional 5 years of life can be anticipated in 65 per cent of cases and 10 years in 55 per cent; even 15 additional years is a reasonable possibility for some.

Not only is life prolonged, but the quality of life is dramatically improved. Children recover quickly and are discharged from the hospital within a few weeks of transplantation. Young patients gain strength with remarkable rapidity and become capable of activities commensurate with normal individuals of comparable age.

Physical rehabilitation is begun; and, when applicable, school work is resumed before leaving the hospital. Ordinarily, recipients remain normally active and participate in usual activities so long as they remain free of significant complications.

Once a feeling of well-being is regained, appetite increases and nutritional status is improved. Caloric restriction and salt limitation are stressed, particularly for those receiving corticosteroids. General improve-

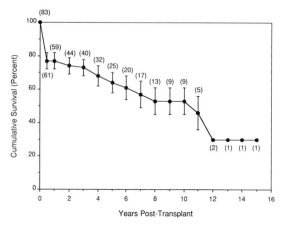

FIGURE 18–1. Cumulative survival determined by the Cutler-Ederer calculation for 83 patients, ages 0.07 to 17.9 years, who received heart transplants between August 1, 1974 and May 29, 1992 at the Stanford University Medical Center. Numbers of living recipients are in parentheses. Mean ± 1 standard error is shown. There are no standard errors beyond 11 years because of the small numbers of recipients.

ment is demonstrated in other ways. Illness requiring hospitalization has been found to be relatively infrequent and, in fact, progressively less with time. In a Stanford study involving pediatric recipients, rehospitalization for illness averaged 7 days per year per patient during the initial posttransplant year.[2] By the fifth year, rehospitalization averaged less than 1 day per year per patient. A small group of recipients had long hospitalizations, but the posttransplant course in one fourth of the patient group studied was sufficiently benign that rehospitalization for illness did not occur at all. Considering the options, heart transplantation offers a reasonable alternative to an incapacitated child with short life expectancy.

INDICATION FOR TRANSPLANTATION

Cardiomyopathy has been the most common indication for heart transplantation during childhood, accounting for two thirds of children accepted as candidates. Most of the patients accepted for transplant have had either idiopathic or viral cardiomyopathies. Several have had endocardial fibroelastosis, and a small number had anthracycline (doxorubicin, daunorubicin) cardiomyopathy resulting from chemotherapy used for treating malignancy. Congenital heart disease has been the underlying disorder in the remaining one third of patients. Some have had in-

operable cardiac anomalies, but an increasing number have undergone surgery for congenital heart disease with subsequent development of severe myocardial dysfunction unresponsive to medication.

RECIPIENT SELECTION

Candidates for acceptance into a cardiac transplantation program must be carefully selected, predominantly on the basis of lack of a suitable therapeutic alternative. Potential transplant recipients must be evaluated in the cardiac catheterization laboratory to rule out significant pulmonary vascular disease. Potential recipients with mildly elevated pulmonary vascular resistance can receive transplants provided the resistance is less than 6 Wood units and preferably is responsive to oxygen or vasodilators. Patients with more severe pulmonary vascular disease have a much higher risk of postoperative right ventricular failure and considerably poorer postoperative prognosis. In turn, such patients may be considered for heart–lung transplantation. Systemic infection, liver or renal dysfunction, severe undernutrition, or any illness that would be aggravated by immunosuppression can be expected to increase mortality and may be a contraindication to cardiac transplantation.

In the selection process, patients and their families meet with a social worker who is a member of the transplant team. The family support system is evaluated, and the likelihood of compliance with the complicated posttransplant medical regimen is assessed. Such preacceptance evaluation also helps the team prepare for language and cultural differences. Important economic considerations involving third-party payment and nonmedical costs such as transportation, the cost of living away from home, and lost wages are discussed and assistance provided when possible. This point is of immediate importance because, once accepted to the transplant program, families are usually required to move to an area close to the transplant center.

Informed consent is a key element of the selection process. Whenever possible patients who are minors should be permitted to be involved in the transplant decision to the extent of their abilities. When presenting the possibility of transplantation, both the potential risks and benefits must be carefully explained. We strongly encourage families who are weighing the possibility of transplant to meet with families who already have experienced the procedure and its consequences. Such interaction provides an invaluable perspective, a better informed consent, and often the beginning of a much needed support system.

TRANSPLANTATION

Donor availability is a serious problem in the pediatric age group. Under most circumstances, 1 to 2 months may be required to obtain a suitable donor heart. The wait may be considerably longer, however, if the child's requirements are complicated by patient size, immunologic matching, or an unusually large group of competing recipients waiting at centers within the region. It is essential therefore for the candidate's family to understand that the transplant candidate may not survive the wait for a donor. Potential recipients are listed on one of two computerized registries (Unified Network for Organ Sharing or North American Coordinating Organization). Donor hearts are selected by ABO blood group, body weight, and heart size. Because graft ischemic time of more than 4 hours is associated with high surgical mortality, long distance procurement is avoided whenever possible. Cardiac grafts are not taken from donors with preexisting severe cardiac disease, systemic illness, active infection, or demonstrable cardiac dysfunction.

Immunosuppression is initiated preoperatively to diminish the risk of rejection, and heart transplantation is performed utilizing hypothermic cardiopulmonary bypass by the method originally described by Lower and Shumway.[4] The transplant procedure is highly organized, minimizing the time between graft procurement and completing of transplant.

Maintenance immunosuppression is usually accomplished with three drugs: cyclosporine, azathioprine, and corticosteroids. Some centers utilize two of the drugs (e.g., cyclosporine and azathioprine), and in a few only cyclosporine is given. A high level of immunosuppression is maintained early after transplantation, as the risk of acute rejection is greater during that period. Later, as the risk of rejection decreases, the degree of immunosuppression is gradually dimin-

ished. While tapering immunosuppression, the pediatric recipient is monitored clinically. Echocardiography plays a key role in this surveillance, but most centers depend on endomyocardial biopsy using a flexible pediatric bioptome for definitive diagnosis of acute rejection. While in the hospital, reverse isolation is practiced to reduce the risk of infection.

Cyclosporine blood levels also are monitored because the pharmacokinetics of this drug are so variable and because blood concentration usually correlates with both drug effectiveness and toxicity. The serum level of cyclosporine is measured by enzyme immunoassay.

In the absence of serious complications, hospitalization for heart transplantation ranges from 2 to 4 weeks. After discharge, close follow-up in the outpatient department is required for an additional 2 to 6 weeks for purposes of added surveillance, adjustment of medications, and parental guidance.

GRAFT REJECTION

Graft rejection is a major risk in pediatric heart transplant recipients. The risk of acute rejection is greatest during the first 3 to 6 months after receiving a cardiac allograft. Despite immunosuppression, most patients develop at least one episode of rejection within the first year of transplantation. Although transplant recipients remain at risk for the remainder of their lives, rejection is much less common after the early postoperative period. Rejection is certainly a threat to well-being, and it is crucial for the family to realize that most rejection episodes respond to therapy.

Clinical symptoms of acute graft rejection may include unusual fatigue, shortness of breath, diaphoresis, dizziness, loss of appetite, and abdominal discomfort. Clinical signs include persistent increase in heart rate, fever, abnormal diastolic heart sounds (S_3, S_4, or both), distant and indistinct heart sounds, hepatomegaly, fluid retention, poor peripheral perfusion, electrocardiographic reduction in voltage, arrhythmia and heart block, and radiographic evidence of cardiac enlargement and increased pulmonary vascular congestion. Use of cyclosporine has had the unintended result of diminishing sensitivity of noninvasive indices suggestive of allograft rejection. As a result, most episodes occur in the absence of detectable symptoms. Making matters worse, most symptoms associated with rejection are non-specific and may be the result of other causes (e.g., infection). It is necessary, therefore, to maintain graft surveillance throughout posttransplant life and to remain alert to the possibility of rejection when transplant recipients present with unexplained symptoms. It is also necessary to remember that recipients are prone to develop other complications that must be considered once rejection is ruled out and symptoms remain unexplained.

Echocardiography performed by an experienced pediatric cardiologist is a valuable noninvasive diagnostic modality for cardiac graft surveillance and diagnosis. Demonstration of reduced ventricular function or development of significant pericardial effusion generally warrants endomyocardial biopsy.

Because echocardiography is neither completely reliable nor highly sensitive for detection of acute rejection, most transplant centers depend on endomyocardial biopsy for periodic rejection surveillance as well as for definitive diagnosis. When performing a biopsy, several pieces of right ventricular tissue are obtained in large infants and young children with the assistance of a flexible pediatric bioptome. These specially designed pediatric bioptomes permit myocardial biopsy with low risk. Interpretation of myocardial biopsy specimens has been standardized with specific criteria developed by the International Society for Heart and Lung Transplantation.[5] Mild cardiac rejection is diagnosed when a sparse cellular infiltrate is present without myocyte necrosis. Moderate and severe rejection are associated with myocyte necrosis as well as cellular infiltrate. The degree of involvement further determines the severity of rejection.

Management is guided by clinical and biopsy observations. When mild rejection is found, immunosuppression is not significantly altered, but a repeat biopsy specimen is taken within 10 to 14 days. Mild rejection progresses to moderate rejection in approximately one third of recipients; the remainder of cases resolve spontaneously. When moderate or severe rejection is detected, a supplementary course of corticosteroids is administered. During the first posttransplant year and in patients with severe or symptomatic rejection, a 3-day course of intravenous methylprednisolone (15 mg/kg/day) is administered, and the biopsy is repeated 10 to 14 days later to assess response to therapy. Children with few previous episodes of rejection who develop asymptomatic, moderate rejection after the initial posttransplant year are given a brief course of oral prednisone (1 mg/kg bid for 3 days, tapering to twice the prerejection maintenance dose over the next 2 weeks). Persistent rejection is usually managed with a second course of corticosteroids and subsequent rebiopsy. When rejection remains despite treatment with corticosteroids, a course of murine antihuman T-lymphocyte antibody (OKT3) may be given over a 2-week period. Total lymphoid irradiation is a valuable therapeutic modality in cases of medically unresponsive rejection. Aside from treating refractory rejection, it may also produce long-term graft tolerance. The ultimate treatment for graft rejection is retransplantation, which is performed only when all forms of medical therapy fail. Although retransplantation is potentially life-saving, the outcome is less successful than after the initial transplant procedure.

INFECTION

Infection is the most serious complication of chronic immunosuppression representing a major cause of both morbidity and mortality in cardiac transplant patients. It accounts for almost one third of all deaths in pediatric recipients. The incidence of infection is greatest during the first 3 to 6 months after transplant, roughly paralleling that of acute rejection.

Serious infection is frequently the result of opportunistic microorganisms, and viruses are common etiologic agents. Although the usual minor viral illnesses of childhood are well handled by transplant recipients, viral infections caused by cytomegalovirus, herpes simplex with visceral involvement, or varicella-zoster are serious and require careful attention. Prophylaxis with varicella-zoster immune globulin (VZIG) should be given, when possible, within 96 hours of varicella exposure. Acyclovir is frequently useful for treatment of herpes simplex and varicella-zoster infections.

Cytomegalovirus (CMV) infection,

whether a primary infection, reactivation, or superinfection, is of particular importance to the heart transplant recipient. Primary infection is the most severe and is often the consequence of a CMV-negative recipient receiving a heart from a CMV-positive donor. The infection is usually disseminated, with pulmonary involvement, and difficult to manage. Of the available antiviral agents, ganciclovir appears to be the most effective. Reactivation implies development of viral replication following transplantation in a CMV-positive recipient who receives a heart from a CMV-negative donor. Reactivation can occur also after transplantation from a CMV-positive donor, but in this case CMV activation may be a superinfection, that is, due to the CMV strain transplanted along with the donor heart. Distinguishing between reactivation and superinfection usually is not possible, nor is it clinically useful. CMV is of additional consequence in that it is associated with a high incidence of graft rejection, graft coronary artery disease, and graft loss. CMV antibody status should be determined in the recipient and donor prior to transplantation. The fatality rate with CMV status mismatch at transplant is greatest in instances in which the transplant recipient is antibody-negative and the graft donor CMV-positive. One would like to ensure a match in CMV status in the recipient and the donor, but the shortage of pediatric heart donors restricts the practicality of this approach.

Bacterial infections similarly are frequent. The most common sites of infection are lung, blood, urinary tract, and less commonly the sternotomy site and central nervous system, in that order. Organisms most commonly isolated include Enterobacteriaceae, *Pseudomonas*, *Serratia*, *Staphylococcus*, *Hemophilus*, *Streptococcus*, and to a lesser extent *Legionella* and *nocardia*. Polymicrobial infections occur, and many sites may be involved.

A significant number of posttransplant infections are due to fungi and protozoa. Fungal infections are often associated with bacterial and viral infections. With visceral involvement, fungal infection must be treated vigorously, because it is associated with disproportionately high morbidity and mortality.

Indwelling catheters require meticulous care, as they are particularly vulnerable to infection in immunosuppressed individuals.

When the suspected site of infection is a catheter, replacement must be considered.

CORONARY ARTERY DISEASE

As length of survival has increased, graft coronary artery disease has become an increasingly common disorder. It develops in approximately 15 per cent of pediatric recipients. Graft coronary disease differs from the natural atherosclerotic process in several respects. The natural disorder is found primarily in older people, although it may occur at a younger age in patients with certain diseases such as diabetes. Atherosclerosis in nontransplant patients generally develops slowly and has a predilection for male individuals; it involves the two main coronary arteries located on the epicardial surface. Stenoses are focal and are caused by asymmetric plaques. In contrast, graft coronary artery disease is a combination of the usual atheromatous lesions and an unusual diffuse obliterative process. The latter abnormality involves secondary and tertiary branches of the main epicardial arteries. Angiographically, distal obliterative changes are characterized by diffuse, concentric narrowing. Narrowed vessels frequently end abruptly or by rapid tapering in lumen diameter. In the cardiac graft, distal obliterative obstruction is the predominant abnormality.

This graft disorder has been found during late infancy and at any time thereafter. Graft coronary disease may develop shortly after transplant and progress rapidly. Because neural regeneration does not take place after transplant, cardiac allografts do not become reinnervated, making it difficult for transplant recipients to experience angina pectoris with coronary ischemia. The earliest sign of serious coronary artery disease may be myocardial infarction, development of congestive heart failure, ventricular arrhythmia, or even sudden death. Because of the insidious nature and potentially rapid progression of this disease, coronary arteriography is advised on an annual basis and more often when necessary.

In contrast to natural coronary atherosclerosis, graft coronary disease is not amenable to coronary angioplasty or coronary bypass surgery because of its diffuse nature and involvement of small vessels. At present there is no persuasive evidence that dietary modification is an effective preventive measure.

Elective retransplantation is the only currently available therapy for severe allograft coronary artery disease. Only patients at high risk of death from the disorder are considered for retransplantation.

MALIGNANCY

Advances in immunosuppressive therapy have led to improved survival and quality of life, but the accomplishment has been made at the cost of an increased incidence of tumors among cardiac recipients. The frequency of cancers common in the general population is not increased, but certain uncommon malignancies occur more often in graft recipients: lymphoma, squamous cell carcinoma of the lip and skin, and carcinoma of the kidney and liver (see Chapter 16).

In both adult and pediatric transplant recipients a form of lymphoma referred to as lymphoproliferative disease is the most common of all tumors and has been observed in 10 per cent of pediatric heart recipients. When it occurs, evidence of the disorder appears between 3 and 6 months after transplant. If detected during the first year after transplantation, it is usually unifocal and responsive to therapy. Later presentation often is associated with disseminated tumor, and mortality is high. Persistent unexplained fever, anemia, recurrent unresponsive gastroenteritis, or persistent unexplained pneumonia or atelectasis is cause for suspicion of this disease. Presentation may be in the form of isolated lymphadenopathy or lesions in the liver, spleen, gastrointestinal tract, lung, or kidney. The importance of careful physical examination for early detection of this disease cannot be overemphasized.

Vulnerability to malignancy is associated with immunosuppression. There is considerable evidence supporting a relation between Ebstein-Barr viral infection and the development of lymphoproliferative disease. It has been proposed that lymphoproliferative disease in immunosuppressed recipients occurs as a result of impaired T cell control over Ebstein-Barr virus-actuated T cell proliferation.[6]

When lymphoproliferative disease is suspected in transplant recipients the possibility must be pursued. Valuable diagnostic aids include excisional biopsy of enlarged lymph nodes, magnetic resonance imaging or computed tomography for suspected tumor in the head, chest, and abdomen, and endoscopy with biopsy for examination of the gastrointestinal tract. Immediate reduction in immunosuppression is advised when the diagnosis is confirmed. A course of acyclovir of at least 6 months' duration is recommended because of the relation between the Ebstein-Barr virus and lymphoproliferative disease. Upon reducing immunosuppression, particular attention must be given to the potential for the development of an acute graft rejection.

SIDE EFFECTS OF MEDICATION

Undesired effects may occur as a result of immunosuppressive agents. Renal dysfunction and blood pressure elevation are common in pediatric recipients given cyclosporine.

Impaired renal function demonstrated by elevated serum urea nitrogen and creatinine levels may be found within weeks of beginning cyclosporine. Most pediatric recipients develop a gradual increase in serum creatinine levels during the initial year following transplantation. Thereafter, creatinine values tend to stabilize. When creatinine levels exceed 1.5 mg/dl, reduction of the cyclosporine dose is considered. Improvement in renal function is obtained in most patients by decreasing the cyclosporine dose. Development of renal failure requiring dialysis or renal transplantation fortunately is rare.

Hypertension is common among recipients given cyclosporine. The incidence of blood pressure elevation is increased when corticosteroids are given in conjunction with cyclosporine. Because blood pressure elevation is frequent during the early posttransplant period, sodium limitation and administration of a diuretic are routine in many centers. In addition, vasodilators may be required early until the risk of rejection falls and the corticosteroid dosage can be safely reduced.

Growth may be impaired in young pediatric heart transplant recipients given corticosteroids. Return to normal growth can be expected upon tapering the dose to an alternate-day regimen or by eliminating the drug entirely.

Neurologic complications occur infrequently. During the immediate postoperative period they are usually related to perioperative ischemic events. Late neurologic difficulties are more often secondary to cyclosporine toxicity. Headache, tremor, and seizures may appear but generally resolve with dose reduction.

Some side effects are largely cosmetic but require attention, particularly in teenagers. Corticosteroids, taken over a long period, may result in a cushingoid appearance, increased appetite and obesity, and acne. Hypertrichosis may develop in young patients receiving cyclosporine. A depilatory agent is often useful in adolescent girls for whom excessive hair is troubling. Gingival hyperplasia develops in many children receiving cyclosporine. When pronounced, it may become painful and even interfere with eating. If sufficiently severe, periodontal surgery frequently is helpful.

Rarely, chronic corticosteroid administration produces orthopedic difficulties, such as osteoporosis and vertebral collapse. Aseptic necrosis of the major weight-bearing joints has been seen in a few adolescent recipients.

Azathioprine may cause bone marrow depression. This complication may be produced or made more severe by certain viral infections such as that caused by cytomegalovirus. When marrow function becomes depressed, azathioprine is temporarily discontinued as a precautionary measure, and the drug is not restarted until the white blood cell count exceeds 5000/cu mm. With renewed marrow function, the drug may be restarted at a small dose and progressively increased, using the peripheral white blood cell count as a guide.

EMOTIONAL CONSIDERATIONS

Heart transplantation is stressful for cardiac graft recipients and their families. It is particularly difficult for teenagers. Changes in physical appearance induced by immunosuppressive medication are especially troublesome for adolescents to whom body image is of considerable importance. Teenagers seeking independence and those who have gained a sense of invulnerability may decide to disregard their complex medical regimen. The potential for graft rejection is particularly threatening for the young person fearful of death and may be cause for great anxiety or depression. Patience, understanding, and emotional support from family and health care providers are essential for young graft recipients. Depression, rebelliousness, and thoughts of suicide are serious. These potentially life-threatening reactions are reason for immediate counseling. They cannot be disregarded.

TRANSPLANTATION IN THE NEONATE

Heart transplantation has become an option for neonates with serious, unrepairable congenital heart disease. Introduced by Bailey et al.,[7] neonatal cardiac transplantation has become a successful surgical alternative. Survival and quality of life are good for neonatal recipients. Donor availability, however, is a major problem. Monitoring of rejection in these patients also is a challenge.

HEART–LUNG AND LUNG TRANSPLANTATION

Heart–lung transplantation is a resource for pediatric patients with congenital heart disease and serious pulmonary vascular disorders.[8] The vascular abnormality may be (1) of a nature that produces pulmonary hypertension (e.g., the Eisenmenger complex); or (2) a type with vascular anomalies that preclude surgical palliation or repair (e.g., severe, diffuse hypoplasia of the entire pulmonary arterial tree). Experience with childhood heart–lung transplantation is relatively small. Results are not as good as those for pediatric heart transplantation, but it does represent a reasonable alternative for those with no remaining option. Acute rejection can occur in the heart, the lung, or both; but detection of pulmonary rejection is more difficult. In addition to the usual complications of heart transplantation, there is the additional possibility of pulmonary obliterative bronchiolitis, a process thought to be related to rejection.

Single-lung or double-lung transplantation is a newer procedure. These operations have been performed successfully in children with lung disease but without heart disease. Lung transplants are performed in patients with disorders such cystic fibrosis and advanced lung disease, primary pulmonary hypertension with no associated cardiac anomaly, and anomalies involving the lung (e.g., diaphragmatic hernia). In addition, unilateral lung transplantation has been used in patients with pulmonary atresia and hypoplastic pulmonary arteries. In this situation, a graft conduit is inserted between the right ventricle and the transplanted pulmonary artery. The number of pediatric recipients of isolated lung transplants is even smaller than those with heart–lung transplants, but short-term results are encouraging.

REFERENCES

1. Kantrowitz A, Haller JD, Joos H, et al: Transplantation of the heart in an infant and an adult. Am J Cardiol 22:782–790, 1968.
2. Baum D, Bernstein D, Starnes VA, et al: Pediatric heart transplantation at Stanford: results of a 15-year experience. Pediatrics 88:203–204, 1991.
3. Bernstein D, Starnes VA, Baum D: Pediatric heart transplantation. Adv Pediatr 37:413–439, 1990.
4. Lower R, Shumway NE: Studies on orthotopic homotransplantation of the canine heart. Surg Forum 11:18–19, 1960.
5. Billingham M, Cary N, Hammond M, et al: A working formulation for the standardization of nomenclature in the diagnosis of heart and lung rejection; heart rejection study group. J Heart Transplant 9:587–593, 1990.
6. Nalesnik MA, Makowa L, Starzl TE: The diagnosis and treatment of post-transplant lymphoproliferative disorders. Curr Probl Surg 25:371–472, 1988.
7. Bailey LL, Nehlsen-Cannarella SL, Doroshow RW, et al: Cardiac allotransplantation in newborns as therapy for hypoplastic left heart syndrome. N Engl J Med 315:949–951, 1983.
8. Starnes VA, Marshall SE, Lewiston NJ, et al: Heart-lung transplantation in infants, children, and adolescents. J Pediatr Surg 26:1–4, 1991.

19

CARDIOVASCULAR SURGERY

Daniel G. Knauf, Daniel J. O'Brien, and James A. Alexander

Since the first report in 1939 of a surgical procedure to close a patent ductus arteriosus[1] and the first report in 1945 of a palliative procedure for a cardiac abnormality,[2] the science and practice of cardiovascular surgery have made continuous advances in the scope, safety, and success of surgical procedures for congenital heart defects. This progress has come about as a result of more accurate clinical diagnosis, improved surgical techniques, and diligent postoperative care. Lower risk and improvement of benefits associated with repair of even devastating congenital heart deformities is a credit to all of the practitioners and scientists engaged in this work. This chapter reviews some of the more common cardiovascular surgical procedures by presenting a brief description of the technique, expected short-term results, and long-term outcome emphasizing the role of the pediatric physician in monitoring patient progress.

PREOPERATIVE EVALUATION

Preoperative surgical planning for a child with congenital heart disease includes detailed anatomic and hemodynamic diagnosis as may be provided by echocardiography and cardiac catheterization. The surgeon's interest also is directed toward evaluation and management of those processes that might increase the risk of an otherwise elective, straightforward procedure.

Prior to surgery it is important that the patient be free of acute infection and of bacterial overselection caused by current (or recent) antibiotic administration. General medical problems that could complicate the patient's clinical course must be investigated. This evaluation includes serum electrolytes, renal and hepatic function tests, and clotting studies including platelet count, prothrombin time, and partial thromboplastin time.

A specific concern for patients who undergo extracorporeal circulation is the presence of cold agglutinins in the serum. Cold agglutinin disease may follow a viral infection or an episode of *Mycoplasma* pneumonia and is hazardous under the circumstance of significantly lowering body temperature, as occurs during cardiopulmonary bypass. The presence of cold agglutinins usually is temporary; therefore elective open heart surgery should be delayed for a few months to allow their natural removal from the bloodstream.

Patients at risk for the presence of hemoglobinopathies, particularly sickle cell (SS) disease, should be evaluated appropriately. The concern is the reaction of the red blood cell to hypothermic extracorporeal circulation. Patients with SS disease can safely undergo open heart surgery,[3] but their management requires careful planning and coordinated effort by staff from cardiovascular surgery, anesthesiology, pediatric cardiology, and pediatric hematology.

Concern about the use of blood and blood components during and after cardiac surgery has led to frequent requests that only directed donation of blood be utilized. This procedure usually can be worked out with the blood bank so all components (e.g., fresh frozen plasma and platelets) from a directed donor unit of blood are kept together, reducing the risk that would occur with exposure to multiple donors. Autologous donation of blood is not applicable to infants and young children but is an option for some older children and adolescents.

Patients scheduled for elective cardiovascular surgery should undergo a thorough examination of the teeth and gums. Appropriate treatment can eliminate a common potential source of bacteremia with its attendant risks during the perioperative period. Dental caries are of less concern than inflammatory periodontal disease (see Chapter 16).

CLOSED HEART SURGICAL PROCEDURES

Coarctation of the Aorta

Coarctation of the thoracic aorta during the neonatal period often is manifested by severe congestive heart failure. Physical examination plus appropriate noninvasive studies, particularly echocardiography, should lead to a nearly complete clinical diagnosis. Prostaglandin E_1 may be of benefit by opening the ductus arteriosus, thereby allowing improved systemic arterial perfusion, especially to the lower body. Other pharmacologic intervention, such as diuretics and inotropic agents, particularly dobutamine, help stabilize the patient, following which surgical correction should be accomplished without delay.

In the neonate and young infant use of the subclavian artery as an on-lay, in-continuity patch (Fig. 19–1B) for correction of coarctation has proved safe and reliable for immediate and long-term correction.[4,5] The left arm loses its major blood supply, but collaterals are abundant in the shoulder area and often a pulse returns in the left brachial or radial artery by 2 to 3 years of age. The procedure may result in decreased growth of the left arm to a slight degree. Some surgeons may try to preserve subclavian flow while correcting the coarctation by relocating the subclavian orifice.[6] Some centers are also using this technique effectively in the older infant and child.

Clinical presentation of coarctation in the older infant and child commonly occurs during a routine physical examination when the patient is found to have weak or absent arterial pulses in the lower extremities together with mild upper extremity hypertension. These patients are asymptomatic, and therefore appropriate clinical evaluation and surgical intervention can be arranged electively. There are several surgical techniques currently in use to correct coarctation in the child. Our group has had significant short- and long-term (up to 10 years) success using a Dacron patch to enlarge the aorta (Fig. 19–1A). This technique is not widely used, however, because of concern regarding aneurysm formation at the surgical site. We have not seen this complication in 37 patients who have undergone angiographic and magnetic resonance imaging 3 to 9 years after operation. Our success may result because our technique does not include resection of the coarctation shelf, which we believe can weaken the aortic wall. However, the potential for the occurrence of aneurysms (both true and false) in the surgical area warrants continued postoperative evaluation at regular intervals.[7]

Resection of the coarcted segment with an

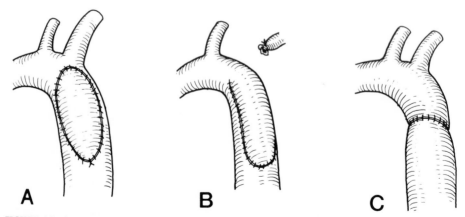

FIGURE 19–1. Repair of coarctation. (*A*) Dacron patch aortoplasty. (*B*) Subclavian flap aortoplasty. (*C*) Resection with end-to-end anastomosis. (Artwork by D. J. O'Brien.)

end-to-end anastomosis (Fig. 19–1C) is preferred by some surgical groups because this technique removes the entire area of coarctation, thereby eliminating the possibility of aneurysm formation in the area of abnormal aortic tissue. Interrupted sutures are placed on half the aortic circumference to allow unrestricted growth. Recurrence of obstruction at the anastomosis is still a recognized complication. Long-term results are good, particularly when surgery is accomplished early in childhood.[8]

Postoperative management also reflects the different age groups in which coarctation of the aorta presents. The newborn typically is in heart failure preoperatively. Surgical correction of coarctation provides immediate relief of the obstruction, but pharmacologic therapy with diuretics and other agents may be required for some time postoperatively, particularly if left ventricular dysfunction or associated intracardiac abnormalities remain. During the immediate postoperative period close attention is also paid to respiratory and metabolic status, feeding, and clinical status of the surgical repair. Infants who have had successful relief of their aortic obstruction should be symptomatically improved to a significant degree.

Surgical repair of coarctation of the aorta in the older infant and child may be followed during the immediate postoperative period by the occurrence of paroxysmal, sometimes severe, systemic hypertension, regardless of the surgical technique utilized. If such hypertension occurs it must be aggressively treated in the intensive care unit. Mesenteric arteritis that can lead to an acute abdomen is a known complication following coarctation repair. For this reason complete gastrointestinal rest generally is recommended during the first few postoperative days.

Long-term management of the patient who has had surgical repair of coarctation of the aorta is concerned primarily with monitoring blood pressure for the purpose of identifying residual or recurrent obstruction as well as the patient who may develop systemic hypertension despite excellent anatomic relief of the obstruction. Attention must be paid to proper techniques of measuring blood pressure, particularly in the infant or small child in whom there is a propensity to use blood pressure cuffs that are too small, thereby causing an erroneously high reading to be obtained. Blood pressure should be measured in both arms and in one leg (avoiding measurement in a leg whose femoral artery may have been compromised by catheterization or surgery) using a mercury manometer. Automated methods are satisfactory for screening purposes but should not be relied on for accuracy in this patient population. Auscultatory blood pressure in the right arm is obtained to document systolic and diastolic pressures. Pressure in the left arm is measured as well because the technique of coarctation repair or the abnormality itself may compromise flow to the left arm and it should be documented. Blood pressure in the leg is measured by the Doppler technique and is most easily accomplished by placing the cuff on the calf and monitoring the Doppler signal over either the posterior tibial artery or the dorsalis pedis artery. Doppler systolic pressure should also be obtained from the brachial artery so equivalent methods are being compared. In the normal individual the systolic blood pressure is higher in the foot than in the arm because of the artifact of distal pulse wave amplification described in Chapter 1. After successful coarctation repair, systolic pressure in the foot may still be 5 to 10 mm Hg less than that in the right brachial artery, despite the absence of anatomic obstruction, because the pulse wave may be damped slightly as it travels through the surgical site.

The older child may require substantial antihypertensive therapy during the first week or two after surgery, as suggested earlier. This therapy often can be reduced within a relatively short period and most commonly can be discontinued entirely after a month or two. Some patients, particularly older children, may require long-term antihypertensive therapy because of their tendency to develop essential hypertension. Patients who have had surgical repair of coarctation of the aorta probably will never be free of the need for regular medical evaluation to monitor their blood pressure. If other congenital cardiac abnormalities are present, they should be treated accordingly. Keep in mind that most patients with coarctation of the aorta have a bicuspid aortic valve and therefore require prophylaxis against bacterial endocarditis. Long-term follow-up of patients after coarctation of the aorta repair also includes monitoring left ventricular size and function by appropriate techniques. Periodic chest roentgenograms are recommended to monitor the surgical site for possible aneurysm formation.

Systemic Artery to Pulmonary Artery Shunts

A systemic artery to pulmonary artery shunt is performed to palliate those congenital cardiac abnormalities characterized by severe hypoxemia due to inadequate pulmonary blood flow. The most common shunt is the classic Blalock-Taussig procedure, or subclavian artery to pulmonary artery end-to-side anastomosis[2] (Fig. 19–2A). This procedure is named after surgeon Alfred Blalock and pediatric cardiologist Helen Taussig, who devised this operation, the first surgical therapy applied to a congenital heart abnormality. Most commonly the subclavian artery originating from the innominate artery is used to construct this anastomosis. In the patient with a left aortic arch, therefore, the shunt would be accomplished on the right; and in the patient with a right aortic arch, the shunt would be accomplished on the left. Prior to undertaking this surgery it is the cardiologist's responsibility to determine if there is an aberrant subclavian artery, as this abnormality precludes a standard Blalock-Taussig procedure. The surgeon ordinarily ligates the vertebral artery to prevent a steal syndrome from developing. The Blalock-Taussig shunt can be done at any age and in almost any size infant. In those individuals in whom the surgeon believes that a Blalock-Taussig shunt is not appropriate, a similar shunt can be constructed using a polytetrafluoroethylene (PTFE) graft (Gore-Tex) (Fig. 19–2B). This graft is placed from the side of the subclavian artery to the side of the pulmonary artery and can be accomplished on either side of the body.[9] It also can be constructed using an aberrant subclavian artery; this so-called modified Blalock-Taussig shunt generally preserves flow to the arm because the subclavian artery is not obstructed. The shunt often does not function as well or as long, however, as a native Blalock-Taussig shunt.

There has been some surgical enthusiasm for placing PTFE grafts centrally between the ascending aorta and pulmonary trunk (Fig. 19–2C) to obtain a better distribution of pulmonary blood flow and in an attempt to promote better bilateral growth of pulmonary arteries, particularly when they are hypoplastic.[10] It remains to be seen if this theoretical benefit will be realized.

We recommend low-dose aspirin therapy for patients with PTFE grafts to minimize platelet aggregation on the endothelial lining of the graft. This hazard is created because the endothelial lining that develops is patchy.

Postoperative follow-up of patients who have systemic artery to pulmonary artery shunts includes monitoring the continuous murmur that should develop, measuring hematocrit, percutaneously (noninvasively) assessing oxygen saturation, and, if necessary, measuring arterial blood gas. Hematocrit should be evaluated, preferably by automated measurement of a sample drawn from a large vein, with the frequency of measurement depending on the age of the patient and the clinical estimation of shunt size. Measurements every 6 months are probably the minimum required. A significant rise in hematocrit, an obvious decrease in the intensity of the continuous murmur, increased cyanosis, and decreased exercise tolerance suggest decreasing pulmonary blood flow and therefore the need for reevaluation and possibly further therapy. Blood pressure should not be measured in an arm whose arterial blood supply has been used to construct a shunt because the reading is not accurate.

Venous Shunts

It is possible to divert systemic venous return directly into the lungs by connecting the venae cavae to the pulmonary arteries. The first operation of this type, in which the superior vena cava and right pulmonary artery are connected end to end, was developed by William Glenn.[11] A modification of

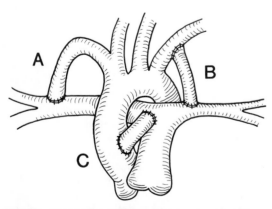

FIGURE 19–2. Systemic artery to pulmonary artery shunts. (*A*) Blalock-Taussig shunt. (*B*) Modified Blalock-Taussig shunt. (*C*) Central shunt. (Artwork by D. J. O'Brien.)

the Glenn procedure, allowing superior vena cava flow into both pulmonary arteries (Fig. 19–3), is used as precursor to the Fontan procedure and is known as the hemi-Fontan or bidirectional Glenn.[12] In 1971 Francis Fontan[13] developed an operation for tricuspid valve atresia in which the right atrium is anastomosed to the pulmonary arterial system by means of a conduit. The Fontan procedure now has been modified for use not only in patients with tricuspid atresia but also in those with almost all forms of single ventricle, or univentricular, anatomy.

Staging the Fontan procedure by initially creating a venous shunt to direct superior vena cava flow into the right (Glenn) or both (hemi-Fontan or bidirectional Glenn) pulmonary arteries seems to allow adaptation of the patient to the moderately low-output state that results. Children palliated with these types of venous shunt continue to be clinically cyanotic. The optimal age for subsequent total correction by completing the modified Fontan procedure is becoming younger as experience with these procedures increases. There is some evidence, however, that surgery in children under 4 years old is less successful.[14]

Follow-up of children with venous shunts includes clinical assessment of hypoxemia, hematocrit, facial plethora, and assessment of other signs of diminished flow through the superior vena caval drainage system. Technical problems at the anastomotic site or development of increasing pulmonary vascular resistance may cause upper body and cerebral venous hypertension. This problem can be serious and may require urgent reassessment and treatment if a correctable cause indeed exists.

OPEN HEART SURGICAL PROCEDURES

Cardiac surgery with extracorporeal circulation (open heart surgery) is available for patients of all ages and for all defects. There are no cardiovascular malformations that inherently are beyond the scope of current surgical techniques if one accepts the possibility of heart and heart–lung transplantation. There may be patients who for one of several reasons are not suitable candidates for a surgical procedure, but it is not the defect itself that creates this circumstance. Heart and heart–lung transplantation are discussed in Chapter 18. Some postoperative rhythm disturbances are reviewed in Chapter 11. The specific defects are described in the chapters on clinical findings.

Some aspects of patient care following open heart surgery are common to most defects, including those under consideration in this section. At the time of discharge from the hospital many patients are taking one or more medications, for example, digoxin, diuretics, systemic arterial vasodilators, anticoagulants, potassium, and iron. Most of these medications are planned for administration over a short period, often just until the first postoperative reevaluation. Restriction of a child's activity after open heart surgery is recommended primarily to protect the patient from trauma to the surgical incisions and the underlying sternotomy rather

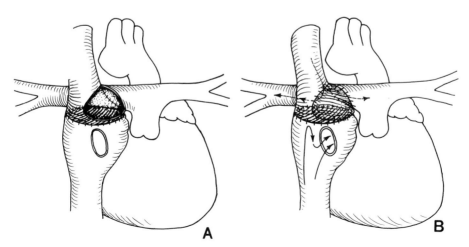

FIGURE 19–3. Venous shunt (bidirectional Glenn). (*A*) Cavo-atrio-pulmonary artery anastomosis with occlusive dam. (*B*) Augmentation of anastomosis with a homograft or pericardial patch. (Artwork by D. J. O'Brien.)

than out of concern for the physical exertion itself.

There are specific medical concerns during the first few weeks after surgery and discharge from the hospital. Any episode of fever should be reported and evaluated, particularly in regard to the possibility of bacterial infection. Respiratory symptoms should be investigated for the possibility of infection, pleural fluid accumulation, or paralysis of a diaphragm due to phrenic nerve injury. Wound concerns range from simple problems such as protrusion of a suture to more serious possibilities such as infection. Postpericardiotomy syndrome is an inflammatory process whose etiology may be related to cytomegalovirus exposure.[15] The syndrome is characterized by fever, chest pain that may radiate into the shoulder, pericardial friction rub, and pericardial effusion. The syndrome may begin during the first week after operation but often is not recognized until after discharge from hospital. Treatment with aspirin generally is successful, although some patients require a short course of steroid therapy.

Patients are scheduled to return for their initial postoperative evaluation approximately 1 month after surgery. This visit may be with the cardiovascular surgeon or the pediatric cardiologist. The complexity of this evaluation depends on the type of surgery that was accomplished, if residual abnormalities persist, and suspicion of a complication. The evaluation may include an electrocardiogram to evaluate cardiac rhythm and chamber enlargement; a chest roentgenogram to evaluate size and shape of the mediastinal shadow (heart size, pericardial effusion), pleural fluid, pulmonary parenchymal changes, and position of the diaphragms; and hematocrit, hemoglobin, or both for patients who had cyanotic heart disease, anemia at discharge, or other hematologic concerns. Echocardiography is accomplished if there are specific indications for doing so. Other laboratory tests, such as electrolytes or prothrombin time, may be indicated by specific patient concerns.

Determination that postoperative status is satisfactory with no evidence of complication likely results in a reduction of medication usage and removal of restrictions in regard to exercise. The next return for cardiology evaluation may be scheduled for 6 to 12 months, and during this time the primary care physician has the responsibility of monitoring the patient and evaluating concerns that exist or develop. Unexplained fever should be treated with respect, particularly in a patient who remains at risk for bacterial endocarditis (see Chapter 15). If suspicion of endocarditis occurs, three blood specimens for culture should be obtained before considering use of antibiotics. These samples can be drawn in rapid succession (from different sites), as success in recovery of an organism relates only to number of samples. Onset of heart failure is a major concern but fortunately is rare. Its occurrence should prompt referral to the pediatric cardiologist. Chest pain is common after operation and is sometimes as difficult to evaluate in this group as it is in those without heart disease or surgery. Most chest pain is related to muscular discomfort secondary to the operation. A careful history and physical examination should allow the physician to reassure the patient and the patient's family that the problem is not serious. The presence of a friction rub, abnormal chest sounds, or a change in cardiac auscultation all suggest that a more significant problem exists and that consultation with the cardiologist is indicated. Development of a significant cardiac rhythm disturbance, respiratory distress, or onset (or worsening) of cyanosis should alert the primary physician that a significant complication may be present.

Fortunately, most complications of surgery appear within the first few months after operation. Infection remains a threat at any time. The natural history of whatever residual hemodynamic abnormality persists also may affect long-term status.

Atrial Septal Defect

An ostium secundum atrial septal defect should be surgically closed. The risk of complications is minimal, certainly less than 2 per cent; and the risk of mortality is also at an absolute minimum, well under 1 per cent. The repair is either by direct suture closure of the defect or by placing a patch that can be fashioned from the patient's pericardium. The surgeon has the responsibility of identifying pulmonary venous return, as these patients ordinarily do not undergo preoperative cardiac catheterization, and echocardiography might not identify a single anomalous pulmonary vein. The coronary sinus is identified, particularly if it is large because of the presence of a left superior vena cava; and prominent venous valves are noted. These structures are important only because they can cause confusion for an inexperienced surgeon, creating a risk of misidentification of the defect.

A sinus venosus atrial septal defect is closed in a similar fashion. This type of defect usually is accompanied by partial anomalous venous return of some of the right lung to the superior vena cava. A type of baffle procedure is required to direct the anomalous pulmonary vein return into the left atrium. Preoperative evaluation by the pediatric cardiologist should have identified the presence of this associated abnormality. The surgeon must be careful to avoid injury to the sinoatrial node or to its arterial blood supply.

An ostium primum atrial septal defect, a form of endocardial cushion defect, is almost always associated with a cleft in the anterior leaflet of the mitral valve that can cause mitral regurgitation. The surgeon's challenge, in addition to proper closure of the atrial septal defect, is proper management of the mitral valve so as to reduce the degree of regurgitation without creating mitral stenosis.

Short-term results of atrial septal defect repair should be excellent, with few complications and near-zero mortality. Long-term results similarly are excellent. The onset of an atrial or atrioventricular conduction abnormality as a complication of the surgical procedure ordinarily is confined to the first few months after operation. It is unusual for cardiac rhythm disturbances to appear many years after an atrial septal defect repair, but this complication can occur.[16] As a result, it would be wise for the primary physician to obtain an electrocardiogram every 2 to 3 years. Bacterial endocarditis prophylaxis is required indefinitely for patients who had an ostium primum defect but not beyond 6 months after operation for other atrial septal defect repairs. There should be no restrictions of patient activity.

Clinical findings following atrial septal defect repair should be nearly normal after closure of a secundum or sinus venosus defect. A grade I-II/VI pulmonary flow murmur may persist, but S_2 is normal (unless widened slightly by some degree of right ventricular conduction delay), and there is no diastolic murmur. The electrocardiogram may continue to show a pattern of right ventricular conduction delay, but there should be no direct evidence of right ventricular hypertrophy. Some patients with a secundum atrial septal defect have associated mitral

valve prolapse; if so, the characteristic auscultatory findings should have been present preoperatively. These patients require endocarditis prophylaxis if there is evidence of mitral regurgitation. Closure of the defect may result in resolution of the mitral valve prolapse.

After repair of an ostium primum atrial septal defect function of the mitral valve must be followed. A grade I/VI murmur of mitral regurgitation is common and should not increase in intensity. The electrocardiogram continues to demonstrate a left and superior axis, but evidence of right ventricular hypertrophy should disappear. More significant mitral regurgitation may cause left atrial or left ventricular enlargement (or both). Complete heart block, a significant risk in years past, rarely occurs and is not a risk beyond the short term after operation. Bacterial endocarditis precautions are required indefinitely.

Patients who have had repair of a secundum or sinus venosus atrial septal defect can be discharged from care by the cardiologist a year or two after surgery if no hemodynamic abnormality remains. As mentioned, the primary physician should monitor the electrocardiogram during succeeding years. After repair of an ostium primum atrial septal defect, evaluation every year or two by the cardiologist is appropriate in order to monitor the status of the mitral valve.

Ventricular Septal Defects

Most operations to close a ventricular septal defect are accomplished in infants who have a left-to-right shunt of sufficient magnitude to cause significant symptoms, such as congestive heart failure and growth retardation.[17] A ventricular septal defect is considered large if right and left ventricular systolic pressures are equal (i.e., an unrestrictive defect) and pulmonary blood flow is at least twice systemic blood flow. Such defects likely will be 10 mm or more in diameter and are unlikely to close spontaneously.

Elevated pulmonary vascular resistance can occur in patients who have an unrestrictive ventricular septal defect. The cardiologist must identify such patients early in infancy so development or progression of this potentially devastating complication can be prevented. The defect must be closed usually before 1 year of age to treat these patients successfully.[18]

A large muscular ventricular septal defect can be difficult to manage, particularly if it is located close to the left ventricular apex. That position precludes closure from the right ventricular side of the septum, and most surgeons prefer not to incise the left ventricle. Large midmuscular defects can be closed from the right ventricle, although some residual shunt often remains; these defects also are amenable to transcatheter device closure, a technique currently under development. Large muscular defects that cannot be managed by direct closure techniques (e.g., the large apical defect) may be palliated by pulmonary artery banding. Some of these defects spontaneously decrease in size sufficiently that subsequent surgical closure is not necessary, although a second operation to remove the pulmonary artery band is required.

Surgical technique to close a large ventricular septal defect requires placement of a patch, usually of Dacron. If possible, the defect is closed through the tricuspid valve, avoiding a right ventricular incision. Care is taken to avoid injury to either the tricuspid valve or the aortic valve, both of which are in proximity to the defect.[19] Permanent complete heart block due to suture injury of the atrioventricular node or bundle of His is a threat, but current surgical technique and experience has reduced this risk to 1 to 2 per cent. Patients who develop permanent complete heart block require an internal electronic pacemaker. Transient atrioventricular block is seen during the first few days after operation in approximately 10 per cent of patients. Once it resolves, recurrence is unlikely.

Short-term outcome of ventricular septal defect closure is excellent. Significant morbidity risks should be under 5 per cent and mortality risk under 2 per cent. The presence of a significant heart murmur after operation should be apparent before the patient leaves the hospital and identified as to possible cause, such as tricuspid regurgitation, aortic regurgitation, or a residual ventricular septal defect. Differentiating the murmurs of tricuspid regurgitation and residual ventricular septal defect may require echocardiography. The electrocardiogram demonstrates right bundle branch block in all patients who have had a right ventriculotomy and even in some of those whose defect was closed through the tricuspid valve. An occasional patient also has a left anterior hemiblock pattern, suggesting injury to the left anterior division of the left bundle branch.

Long-term outcome after ventricular septal defect closure also is excellent. Tricuspid regurgitation and aortic regurgitation rarely appear if not detected within the first month after operation. The same is true for a residual ventricular septal defect. Later onset does occur, however, and the primary care physician may be the first to have an opportunity to recognize that one of these complications is present. Therefore careful auscultation at each clinical visit is important. If a residual ventricular septal defect occurs, it is almost always small; and its management is not different from a naturally occurring small ventricular septal defect. No restrictions on physical activity are necessary except in the patient who has aortic regurgitation. Such patients should be examined frequently during the first 6 to 12 months after operation to establish stability, and as they progress into later childhood they should be advised away from activities that involve significant weight lifting. Patients who had transient atrioventricular block also should be followed closely, although development of complete heart block fortunately is rare.

Patients who have no residual hemodynamic abnormality may be discharged from care by the cardiologist several years after surgery, although there is a tendency to follow these patients long term. Those with residual abnormalities are followed at appropriate intervals, usually annually if their status is stable. Precautions against bacterial endocarditis are discontinued if no hemodynamic abnormality remains.

Endocardial Cushion Defect (Atrioventricular Canal Defects)

An endocardial cushion defect presents a more complex problem to the surgeon. Success in closure of the left-to-right shunt has been excellent, but correction of atrioventricular valvar insufficiency has been less rewarding. The ostium primum complex (ostium primum atrial septal defect with cleft mitral valve) should be correctable with minimal residual abnormality as discussed above. Partial atrioventricular canal includes both atrial and ventricular level shunts together with mitral regurgitation, but the ventricular septal defect is small. Shunt closure usually is complete, but management of atrioventricular valve regurgitation is challenging. In fact, avoiding residual significant mitral regurgitation can be more difficult with a partial canal than with a complete canal. A complete atrioventricular canal, the defect commonly seen in Down syndrome, includes large atrial and ventricular septal defects together with a common atrioventricular valve. Repair should be done during infancy, as this group is at most risk for development of obstructive pulmonary vascular disease.[20] Surgical correction of partial and complete atrioventricular canal is accomplished by placing a patch, which may need to be large, on the atrial and ventricular septal defects. Repair of the atrioventricular valve abnormality can require substantial reconstruction.

Short-term result of repair of atrioventricular canal defects is excellent.[21] Mortality risk should be less than 5 per cent. These patients commonly have residual mild atrioventricular valvar insufficiency, which ordinarily can be controlled pharmacologically. The systolic murmur of mitral regurgitation is heard, although it may be located more over the midprecordium than over the apex. Unfortunately, in a few patients progression of valvar insufficiency may be rapid, leading to signs and symptoms of congestive heart failure during the early postoperative period. Most patients who subsequently require reoperation, some of whom need atrioventricular valve replacement, become markedly symptomatic within the first 6 months after their initial surgical procedure. During these first few months the primary care physician, in addition to the pediatric cardiologist, must watch carefully for tachypnea, poor feeding, fluid retention, or other signs of congestive heart failure. Pharmacologic control of severe mitral insufficiency seldom is successful, and reoperation is likely. Residual left-to-right shunts are uncommon. A ventricular shunt causes a characteristic systolic murmur that may, however, be difficult to distinguish from the murmur of mitral regurgitation. An atrial shunt requires echocardiography for detection, as characteristic physical findings are not present.

Long-term results depend on function of the mitral valve.[21] If mitral regurgitation is mild, these patients do well. Endocarditis may be the only significant risk. With more severe mitral regurgitation, however, progression may occur, leading to congestive heart failure and the need for further surgery as just described. Patients in whom some degree of elevated pulmonary vascular resistance has been documented preoperatively must be monitored carefully for increasing resistance after surgery, as this complication can occur despite the absence of either residual left-to-right shunt or significant mitral regurgitation. Clinical signs include a noticeable increase in the intensity of the pulmonic component of the second sound; onset of a medium- to high-frequency early diastolic murmur of pulmonic regurgitation; increasing right ventricular hypertrophy on electrocardiogram (although the presence of right bundle branch block after operation can make it difficult to identify). Uncertainty from clinical and echocardiographic data suggests the need for cardiac catheterization to clarify patient status.

All of these patients require bacterial endocarditis prophylaxis indefinitely. Physical activity is not restricted unless the patient has significant residual hemodynamic abnormalities. Annual evaluation by a cardiologist is continued indefinitely.

Tetralogy of Fallot

Repair of tetralogy of Fallot includes closure of the ventricular septal defect by a Dacron patch, relief of right ventricular outflow obstruction by excision of obstructing muscle, and pulmonic valvotomy if indicated (Fig. 19–4A); surgery also includes closure of a shunt if one was placed previously. Patients with severe infundibular stenosis and a hypoplastic pulmonic valve annulus may need to have a patch placed from the right ventricle across the annulus onto the pulmonic trunk (Fig. 19–4B). This technique necessarily destroys the function of the pulmonic valve, creating pulmonic regurgitation; but such regurgitation generally is well tolerated. More complex forms of tetralogy, such as those with pulmonic valve atresia, may require use of an extracardiac conduit (Fig. 19–4C). Most commonly it is a cryopreserved homograft obtained from fresh cadavers.[22] The conduit is placed from the right ventricular outflow tract to the pulmonary arteries. The presence of a valve within the homograft provides improved hemodynamics, and pliability of the homograft tissue affords easier technical placement than that required with Dacron valved conduits.

Short-term results of repair of uncomplicated tetralogy of Fallot are good at all ages, including the infant.[23] Mortality should be less than 5 per cent and significant morbid-

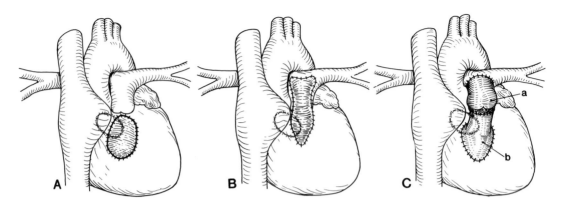

FIGURE 19–4. Repair of tetralogy of Fallot. (*A*) Right ventricular infundibulectomy with patch closure. (*B*) Transannular infundibulectomy patch. (*C*) Extracardiac valved conduit. a = pulmonary homograft; b = PTFE tubular extension of homograft. (Artwork by D. J. O'Brien.)

ity less than 10 per cent. All patients have a residual murmur of right ventricular outflow tract obstruction, although stenosis may be mild. Pulmonic valve regurgitation is common and causes a low-frequency diastolic murmur that may replace the pulmonic component of S_2. Almost all patients have right bundle branch block on electrocardiogram. A residual ventricular septal defect occurs in fewer than 10 per cent of patients and usually is small, requiring no specific therapy. Complete heart block due to trauma to the conduction system now is a rare complication. Its occurrence and management are as described previously for repair of an isolated ventricular septal defect.

Long-term results after repair of uncomplicated tetralogy of Fallot remain excellent.[24,25] A residual ventricular septal defect is rarely large enough to be a significant problem; pulmonic valve regurgitation is well tolerated although less so if residual right ventricular outflow tract obstruction is present. Ventricular premature beats are seen frequently on routine electrocardiogram. Exercise stress testing may reveal more significant ventricular ectopy, including short runs of ventricular tachycardia. There is evidence to suggest that ventricular ectopy in the presence of residual right ventricular hypertension is a significant risk factor for sudden death. The primary care physician should be alert to the occurrence of symptomatic ectopy. Initially such symptoms should be carefully investigated by means of 24-hour electrocardiographic monitoring. Electrophysiologic catheterization techniques may then be necessary for proper diagnosis and therapeutic decisions.

Homograft conduits provide excellent short-term results for repair of complex tetralogy of Fallot, but their long-term durability remains a matter of concern. Serial echocardiography reliably assesses both stenosis and regurgitation of the homograft valve. Immediately after operation patients receive digitalis, diuretics, and an afterload reducing agent. They require these medications for longer periods than do patients with simple forms of tetralogy of Fallot. Typically, the diuretics and afterload reduction may be discontinued within the first few months after operation, but inotropic support with digitalis is continued for approximately 6 to 12 months. Close follow-up by the pediatric cardiologist is required to monitor function of the right ventricle and homograft conduit.

Bacterial endocarditis prophylaxis is required indefinitely in all patients following surgical repair of tetralogy of Fallot. Physical activity is not significantly restricted unless there is a specific reason for doing so based on residual hemodynamic abnormality. Patients should be evaluated annually by a cardiologist. At longer intervals this evaluation likely must include some specific investigation of right ventricular function, usually by echocardiography, and evaluation of the conduction system by 24-hour electrocardiographic monitoring and exercise stress testing.

Transposition of the Great Vessels

Two surgical techniques have been used to manage transposition of the great vessels. First, redirection of venous inflow by an atrial baffle procedure was reported by Senning in 1959.[26] A similar, apparently less complicated, method was described in 1964 by Mustard.[27] Second, Jatene et al. in 1976 described a technique for exchanging the pulmonic trunk and aorta, thereby anatomically correcting the defect[28] (Fig. 19–5A,B). It is necessary to move the coronary arteries so they remain with the aorta (Fig. 19–5C,D). The Jatene (or arterial switch) operation and its modifications has now become the most popular procedure for surgical management of transposition of the great vessels.[29] In patients with simple transposition, the arterial switch must be accomplished during the neonatal period, as the left ventricle must be at near-systemic pressure levels in order to assume function as the systemic arterial ventricle. Patients with transposition who have a significant ventricular septal defect may maintain high left ventricular pressure, thereby allowing arterial switch later during infancy.

The short-term results of both procedures are good. The mortality risk with the Senning (or Mustard) procedure should be below 5 per cent and may be less than 2 per cent.[30] The mortality risk of the Jatene procedure is higher, approaching 10 per cent for newborns in some reports. This risk should decrease and become comparable to (or better than) the Senning method as experience is gained. Short-term morbidity associated with the Senning and Mustard procedures includes right ventricular dysfunction, tricuspid regurgitation, cardiac rhythm disturbance, systemic venous obstruction, especially of the superior vena cava (much more common after the Mustard technique), pulmonary venous obstruction, and left ventricular outflow tract obstruction, which may be progressive. All of these problems explain the popularity of the Jatene procedure, which for the most part avoids each of them. Morbidity does occur with the Jatene procedure, however; obstruction of the aorta or, more often, the pulmonic trunk can develop within months after operation. Modifica-

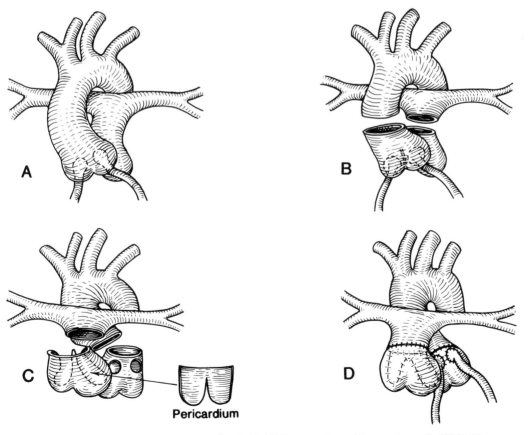

FIGURE 19–5. Jatene procedure (arterial switch). (*A*) Transposition of the great vessels. (*B*) Division of great vessels and creation of aortocoronary buttons. (*C*) LeCompte maneuver to place the aorta posteriorly. Pericardial patch to replace aortocoronary buttons. (*D*) Completed arterial and coronary switch. (Artwork by D. J. O'Brien.)

tions of the operation have made both of these complications less frequent. Coronary artery injury or myocardial ischemia may also occur, although use of continuous nitroglycerine infusion starting in the operating room and continuing for several days after operation can apparently decrease the incidence of coronary artery spasm and myocardial ischemic damage.

Long-term results for the Senning and Mustard procedures are variable. Patients with no right ventricular dysfunction and no left ventricular outflow obstruction continue to do well without evidence of deterioration. Whether it will be true for a lifetime remains to be seen. Disturbances of cardiac rhythm remain a concern particularly after the Mustard operation.[31,32] Holter monitoring is indicated at regular intervals, especially in patients with junctional rhythm. There are no long-term data available following the Jatene procedure, as it is a relatively recent development, particularly in terms of its application to the newborn. Concerns regarding coronary artery growth exist on theoretic grounds.

All of these patients must be evaluated by a cardiologist at intervals of 6 to 12 months. Bacterial endocarditis prophylaxis is indicated indefinitely. Restriction on physical activity depends on ventricular function and cardiac rhythm.

Complex Cardiac Anomalies With a Single Functioning Ventricle

Surgical treatment of tricuspid atresia, pulmonary atresia with intact septum, single ventricle, and other complex lesions for which a two-ventricle repair is not feasible has expanded remarkably since the 1970s. The Fontan procedure, in which the right atrium and its systemic venous return is isolated from the rest of the heart and attached to the pulmonary arterial tree either directly or by means of a conduit, has been expanded to include many more lesions than its first use for tricuspid atresia.[13] Interestingly, the surgical outcome remains best for the patients with tricuspid atresia.[33]

Direct anastomotic connection between the right atrial appendage and the right pulmonary artery or main pulmonary artery has led to decreased use of conduits and valves. The surgical objective is to create as large an anastomotic area as possible, thereby permitting unobstructed flow into the pulmonary arteries. Initial management of the infant with inadequate pulmonary blood flow includes construction of a shunt as described earlier in the chapter. Patients treated initially with a systemic artery to pulmonary artery shunt can be better prepared for a Fontan procedure by replacing the arterial shunt with a venous shunt, such as the bidirectional Glenn (hemi-Fontan).[12] This repair appears to allow technically easier reconstructive procedures on the pulmonary arteries as well as physiologic adaptation to the lower pressure venous shunts. Unfortunately, venous shunts seem less predictable in terms of their performance than do arterial shunts. Subsequent completion of the Fontan procedure to include inferior vena caval flow (Fig. 19–6) may lead to fewer early and late complications.[34]

Short-term results of Fontan-type operations are satisfactory and seem to be improving as larger surgical series report decreasing mortality, reaching below 10 per cent in recent years.[33] Many centers report that patients with tricuspid atresia are the best surgical candidates. Some groups believe that operation in children under 4 years of age increases mortality,[14] whereas others report no difference based on age.[35] Morbidity includes fluid retention, low cardiac output, pleural effusion, hepatic dysfunction, ascites, and protein-losing enteropathy. Postoperative patients may no longer be hypoxemic, but exercise tolerance initially may be decreased. Fortunately, most such patients improve during the first postoperative year. Medical therapy with digoxin, diuretics, and vasodilators often is continued for many months. Many groups routinely anticoagulate postoperative Fontan procedure patients for 3 to 6 months because of the increased risk of thrombus formation due to slow blood flow, especially in the atria. The patients are followed closely by the cardiologist. The primary physician should be alert to the development of complications, which may manifest as increasing signs of congestive heart failure, sudden weight gain suggesting fluid retention, and respiratory distress; a neurologic event due to a left-sided embolism is rare but can occur.

Long-term results are becoming available.[36] Patients with the fewest risk factors at the time of surgery (i.e., those who are clinically the best candidates) have a 4-year survival rate of approximately 80 per cent, including those patients who were operated on when they were under 4 years of age.[14] Concern regarding function of the single

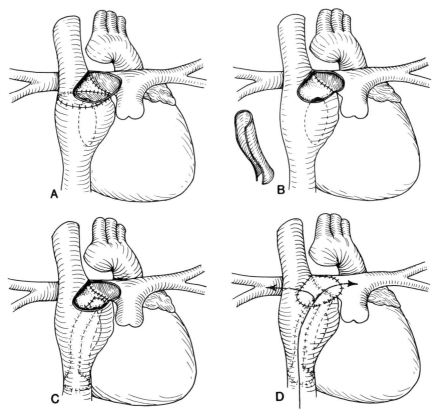

FIGURE 19–6. Modified Fontan procedure. (A) Previous bidirectional Glenn shunt with occlusive dam. (B) Removal of dam and preparation of intercaval conduit (PTFE). (C) Intercaval conduit in place with open ASD. (D) Augmentation of atrial-pulmonary anastomosis with a homograft or pericardial patch. (Artwork by D. J. O'Brien.)

ventricle over many years has led to speculation that many of these patients eventually will become candidates for heart transplantation. Patients are followed closely by the cardiologist, usually at 6-month intervals. Evidence of increased ventricular dysfunction (e.g., signs of congestive heart failure, onset of a murmur of atrioventricular valve regurgitation) should prompt an earlier return visit. Bacterial endocarditis prophylaxis is required. Medical therapy may be continued indefinitely. Patients can be allowed reasonable physical activity, although it must be recognized that their ability to increase cardiac output is limited.

SPECIAL CONSIDERATIONS

Valve Replacement

Reparative techniques for management of valvar insufficiency and stenosis have progressed remarkably, but valve replacement

still occurs in the pediatric population. In addition to lack of growth of the valve annulus, long-term problems of valve dysfunction as well as thrombotic or embolic complications are increased in the pediatric population because of younger age and because it is more difficult to manage anticoagulation. Need for dental interventions, childhood accidents and trauma, teenage behavior and life style, and pregnancy are a few of the variables that make anticoagulation management in the pediatric population more difficult than it is for adult patients. Unfortunately, no safe substitute for warfarin has been found. Some groups do not routinely use warfarin for some types of mechanical aortic valves, using aspirin, dipyridamole, or both as a milder form of anticoagulation.[37] Antibiotic prophylaxis for dental or surgical interventions is mandatory.

Porcine valves avoid the complications of anticoagulation; but, particularly in the pediatric population, they are subject to relatively early calcification and degeneration, which in turn leads to reoperation and replacement. Use of aortic homografts may allow longer, complication-free, reoperation-free intervals,[22] but this possibility has yet to be explored.

Anticoagulation

Aspirin is given to patients with Gore-Tex conduits to minimize endothelial buildup within the graft. The once-daily dose required is small, ranging from 37.5 mg in an infant to 300.0 mg in an adult. Aspirin should be discontinued temporarily with the occurrence of a febrile illness to minimize the possibility of Reye syndrome.

Attention to detail and strict management is necessary for patients receiving warfarin. The prothrombin time should be checked every 3 to 4 weeks and more frequently if it is not stable with a given warfarin dosage. It should be maintained at approximately 1.5 times control. Other medications, both prescription and over-the-counter, interfere with administration of warfarin, and prolongation or shortening of the prothrombin time may result. This information should be conveyed to both patients and parents as well as to other health care providers in order to minimize the administration of such drugs. Occasionally, it is necessary to discontinue warfarin temporarily. For example, warfarin is teratogenic and must be stopped during pregnancy. Elective surgical and dental procedures also may require discontinuing warfarin. In these situations anticoagulation is maintained with heparin. Discontinuation of anticoagulation should never be undertaken without first creating a coordinated management plan involving all of the physicians involved in the patient's care.

REFERENCES

1. Gross RE, Hubbard JP: Surgical ligation of a patent ductus arteriosus: report of first successful case. JAMA *112*:729–731, 1939.
2. Blalock A, Taussig HB: The surgical treatment of malformations of the heart in which there is pulmonary stenosis or pulmonary atresia. JAMA *128*:189–202, 1945.
3. Esseltine DW, Baxter MRN, Bevan JC: Sickle cell states and the anaesthetist. Can J Anaesth *35*:385–403, 1988.
4. Moulton AL, Brenner JI, Roberts G, et al: Subclavian flap repair of coarctation of the aorta in neonates. J Thorac Cardiovasc Surg *83*:220–235, 1984.
5. Goldman S, Hernandez J, Pappas G: Results of surgical treatment of coarctation of the aorta in the critically ill neonate: including the influence of pulmonary artery banding. J Thorac Cardiovasc Surg *91*:732–737, 1986.
6. Meier MA, Lucchese FA, Jazbik W, et al: A new technique for repair of aortic coarctation: subclavian flap aortoplasty with preservation of arterial blood flow to the left arm. J Thorac Cardiovasc Surg *92*:1005–1012, 1986.
7. Mendelsohn AM, Crowley DC, Lindauer A, et al: Rapid progression of aortic aneurysms after patch aortoplasty repair of coarctation of the aorta. J Am Coll Cardiol *20*:381–385, 1992.
8. Cohen M, Fuster V, Steele PM, et al: Coarctation of the aorta: long-term follow-up and prediction of outcome after surgical correction. Circulation *80*:840–845, 1989.
9. Donahoo JS, Gardner TJ, Zahka K, et al: Systemic-pulmonary shunts in neonates and infants using microporous expanded polytetrafluoroethylene: immediate and late results. Ann Thorac Surg *30*:146–150, 1980.
10. Ullom RL, Sade RM, Crawford FA Jr: The Blalock-Taussig shunt in infants: standard v. modified. Ann Thorac Surg *44*:539–543, 1987.
11. Glenn WWL: Circulatory bypass of the right side of the heart: IV. Shunt between superior vena cava and distal right pulmonary artery: report of clinical application. N Engl J Med *259*:117–120, 1958.
12. Hopkins RA, Armstrong BE, Serwer GA, et al: Physiological rationale for a bidirectional cavopulmonary shunt. J Thorac Cardiovasc Surg *90*:391–398, 1985.
13. Fontan F, Baudet E: Surgical repair of tricuspid atresia. Thorax *26*:240–248, 1971.
14. Bartmus DA, Driscoll DJ, Offord KP, et al: The modified Fontan operation for children less than 4 years old. J Am Coll Cardiol *15*:429–435, 1990.
15. Paloheimo JA, von Essen R, Klemola E, et al: Subclinical cytomegalovirus infections and cytomegalovirus mononucleosis after open heart surgery. Am J Cardiol *22*:624–630, 1968.
16. Bricker JT, Gillette PC, Cooley DA, et al: Dysrhythmias after repair of atrial septal defect. Tex Heart Inst J *13*:203–208, 1986.
17. Van Hare GF, Soffer LJ, Sivakoff MC, et al: Twenty-five year experience with ventricular septal defect in infants and children. Am Heart J *114*:606–614, 1987.
18. Yeager SB, Freed MD, Keane JF, et al: Primary surgical closure of ventricular septal defect in the first year of life: results in 128 infants. J Am Coll Cardiol *3*:1269–1276, 1984.
19. Richardson JV, Schieken RM, Lauer RM, et al: Repair of large ventricular septal defects in infants and small children. Ann Surg *195*:318–322, 1982.
20. Chin AJ, Keane JF, Norwood WI, Castaneda AR: Repair of complete common atrioventricular canal in infancy. J Thorac Cardiovasc Surg *84*:437–445, 1982.
21. Studer M, Blackstone EH, Kirklin JW, et al: Determinants of early and late results of repair of atrioventricular (canal) defects. J Thorac Cardiovasc Surg *84*:523–542, 1982.
22. Kay PH, Ross DN: Fifteen years experience with the aortic homograft: the conduit of choice for right ventricular outflow tract reconstruction. Ann Thorac Surg *40*:360–364, 1985.
23. Groh MA, Meliones JN, Bove EL, et al: Repair of

tetralogy of Fallot in infancy: effect of pulmonary artery size on outcome. Circulation *84*(Suppl III): 206–212, 1991.

24. Kirklin JW, Blackstone EH, Kirklin JK, et al: Surgical results and protocols in the spectrum of tetralogy of Fallot. Ann Surg *198*:251–265, 1983.

25. Katz NM, Blackstone EH, Kirklin JW, et al: Late survival and symptoms after repair of tetralogy of Fallot. Circulation 65:403–410, 1982.

26. Senning A: Surgical correction of transposition of the great vessels. Surgery 45:966–980, 1959.

27. Mustard WT: Successful two-stage correction of transposition of the great vessels. Surgery 55: 469–472, 1964.

28. Jatene AD, Fontes VF, Paulista PP, et al: Anatomic correction of transposition of the great vessels. J Thorac Cardiovasc Surg 72:364–370, 1976.

29. Wernovsky G, Hougen TJ, Walsh EP, et al: Midterm results after the arterial switch operation for transposition of the great arteries with intact ventricular septum: clinical, hemodynamic, echocardiographic, and electrophysiologic data. Circulation 77:1333–1344, 1988.

30. Trusler GA, Williams WG, Izukawa T, et al: Current results with the Mustard operation in isolated transposition of the great arteries. J Thorac Cardiovasc Surg 80:381–389, 1980.

31. Vetter VA, Tanner CS, Horowitz LN: Electrophys-

iologic consequences of the Mustard repair of d-transposition of the great arteries. J Am Coll Cardiol *10*:1265–1273, 1987.

32. Gewillig M, Cullen S, Mertens B, et al: Risk factors for arrhythmia and death after Mustard operation for simple transposition of the great arteries. Circulation *84*(Suppl III):183–192, 1991.

33. Mair DD, Hagler DJ, Puga FJ, et al: Fontan operation in 176 patients with tricuspid atresia: results and a proposed new index for patient selection. Circulation 82(Suppl IV):164–169, 1990.

34. Balaji S, Gewillig M, Bull C, et al: Arrhythmias after the Fontan procedure: comparison of total cavopulmonary connection and atriopulmonary connection. Circulation 84(Suppl III):162–167, 1991.

35. Kirklin JK, Blackstone EH, Kirklin JW, et al: The Fontan operation: ventricular hypertrophy, age, and date of operation as risk factors. J Thorac Cardiovasc Surg 92:1049–1064, 1986.

36. Driscoll DJ, Offord KP, Feldt RH, et al: Five- to fifteen-year follow-up after Fontan operation. Circulation 85:469–496, 1992.

37. Verrier ED, Tranbaugh RF, Soifer SJ, et al: Aspirin anticoagulation in children with mechanical aortic valves. J Thorac Cardiovasc Surg 92: 1013–1020, 1986.

20

LIFE STYLE ISSUES

Hugh D. Allen and Wayne H. Franklin

In addition to specific concerns regarding one's medical status, individuals who have cardiovascular disease face other matters that are part of their present and future life styles and life choices. These issues include schooling, employability, insurability, exercise and sports, sexuality, developmentally related problems, and choice of health care provider. These subjects are of particular concern to the adolescent and young adult, so our emphasis in this chapter is directed accordingly. Comment regarding a particular cardiac abnormality is included only when needed to elucidate specific life style issues.

SCHOOLING

Most young people who have congenital heart disease are inherently neither physically nor socially different from their peers. Patients who may be predicted to have permanently impaired ability to perform manual work should prepare for careers not requiring excessive physical exertion. School experiences and choices should be directed to accommodate such limitations.

Most young people who have heart disease limiting their educational choices seem to acquire the insight to anticipate this reality and develop their own educational directions. The long-term Natural History Study (NHS II) of patients with certain congenital heart defects (ventricular septal defect, aortic valvar stenosis, pulmonary valvar stenosis) who were followed over several decades[1] demonstrated that these patients achieved higher educational levels than did their peers. Most finished high school, and 50 per cent graduated from college. College attendance was not hampered by the type or

severity of these particular defects; and, as a matter of fact, patients who had Eisenmeger syndrome had the highest college graduation rate of any group in the Natural History Study. These data suggest that many young people recognize, or at least adapt to, possible future limitations related to their cardiac status. Not all patients are this realistic, however. Some of these young people therefore may be helped by supportive questioning and (gentle) direction.

The physical environment in high school and college can be difficult for students with certain cardiac malformations. For example, those with exercise-limiting conditions, such as cyanosis, can have difficulty climbing stairs during the brief period between classes. Many schools now are well equipped for the physically challenged, but most of these youths do not wish to consider themselves different from their peers. Most are ambulatory and do not want to draw attention to their condition by riding an elevator or being late for class. Indeed, such a patient may compensate by overexerting physically or may act out emotionally in response to demands that are reasonable for a healthy person but excessive for the patient.

The practitioner cannot know about any of these problems unless appropriate questions are asked. Young people usually do not volunteer this information; and when they are asked, they minimize it. More information is forthcoming one-on-one than in the presence of parents. During office visits, therefore, in addition to meeting with a parent and the patient, some time should be allocated to talking with the young person alone. If a problem is uncovered, the practitioner should then work with the patient, the family, school nurses, and others who can help so the school experience is as normal as possible.

EMPLOYABILITY

The Natural History Study[1] showed that young adults with congenital cardiac malformations usually find employment on a par with their peers. In addition to ordinary problems related to finding employment, however, the type of job may be limited by the young person's condition, employer attitudes, and availability of benefits.

Certain cardiac conditions prevent employment in environments that may pose risk or hazard to the patient or others. Patients who have pacemakers should not work in the presence of magnetic fields. Those with physically restricting conditions should not do manual labor, and patients at significant risk for sudden death should not be in control of the safety of others, as would an airline pilot.

Some of these concepts often are misunderstood by employers, who equate congenital cardiac malformations, repaired or not, with coronary artery disease; they do not hire such candidates, no matter how well qualified for the position. The cardiologist and primary care physician must be advocates for the patient by educating employers specifically and the public in general.

Many employed patients are unable to progress in their professions because of "job lock," a phenomenon created by the availability of guaranteed benefits for them (or their dependents) in one company or field that may not be available in another area of opportunity because of a preexisting condition exclusion in the new company's benefit package (see insurability section below). An individual's advancement may not be possible despite the person being the best and most logical candidate for a given position. This limitation leads to job dissatisfaction and frustration. The best advice at present for such a person, nevertheless, is to stay where benefits are assured rather than run the risk that significant medical expenses will be incurred because surgery or further diagnostic procedures become necessary before insurance coverage is again available.

INSURABILITY

Many young people who have congenital cardiac malformations cannot obtain appropriate health insurance regardless of the severity of their abnormality. At a 1991 symposium on health insurability of the adolescent and young adult with heart disease,[2] a study was reported demonstrating that more than 50 per cent of this population was uninsured or underinsured.[3] This population is growing in size as a result of improving medical care and surgical techniques. Medical care is inconsistent, however. The Natural History Study showed that even though they had been followed annually before age 21, the average patient was seen only every 10 years thereafter—despite the fact that health care costs were decidedly lower after the age of 21 than before.[4]

Small businesses in particular may experience difficulty obtaining group health insurance if the industry uses claims experience instead of community rating. Community rating averages premium costs and places everyone into an insurance pool. Claims experience, on the other hand, can be less expensive because it is based on individual experience. For example, if a company (group) hires only healthy people who have no anticipated health care costs, premiums are lower. Individuals with a preexisting condition who are brought into a small group may noticeably increase the premium cost for that group, resulting in a negative incentive to hire people who have any cardiac history. Preexisting condition exclusions may allow such an individual to be hired, albeit without health insurance, an unfortunate circumstance for these young people to say the least. Young adults with congenital heart disease usually are healthy, with the exception of having to deal with their congenital heart malformation, and should not be burdened with concerns about whether to seek medical aid that they may not be able to afford individually. Our health care, insurance, and legislative systems should be able to develop a program that permits this expanding population to obtain appropriate health insurance at an affordable cost.

Obtaining life insurance also may be difficult for individuals with congenital heart defects, even those with minor defects. Some information does exist on this subject based on deliberations that took place between pediatric cardiology representatives of the American Heart Association and the insurance industry.[5] In this document, for example, individuals with a small ventricular septal defect characterized as having a typical murmur, normal chest roentgenogram, and normal electrocardiogram were recommended for insurability at standard risk.

Other common congenital cardiac defects are reviewed according to severity with recommendations regarding insurability. Insurance companies do not necessarily follow these recommendations, but there are companies that do. Parents who insist on purchasing life insurance for their children should be counseled to seek those companies that have endorsed these recommendations so they can avoid paying excessive premiums.

EXERCISE AND SPORTS

The topics of exercise and sports can be related to specific cardiac abnormalities. Much of the information in this section is a review of how the authors manage patients. For the major literature on the topic, the reader is referred specifically to the report of Mitchell et al. on the 16th Bethesda conference on cardiovascular abnormalities in the athlete and their recommendations regarding eligibility for competition.[6] This conference made specific recommendations regarding patients with congenital and acquired heart disease by reviewing the available literature and, when there was no literature on the subject, by consensus. General recommendations regarding exercise in normal children are contained in Chapter 14.

The topic of exercise and sports usually is not discussed by either the primary physician or the pediatric cardiologist when the patient is an infant because it does not seem germane. Many parents, however, faced with their infant having a congenital heart lesion, develop the notion that their child will become a "cardiac cripple." Their concerns are expressed by such questions as: "Will I be able to play ball with her?" "Will he be able to go to a regular school, or will he need home tutors?" These concerns occur to parents of a child with a hemodynamically insignificant ventricular septal defect as well as to parents of a child with tetralogy of Fallot. Guidance and reassurance from the primary care physician, beginning during early childhood (and even infancy), go far toward making modifications in exercise behavior during adolescence easier.

Discussion of exercise and sports with a patient who had a congenital cardiac malformation should be as positive as possible. The physician should direct the patient toward activities that maintain physical fitness while having fun and yet avoid significant risk. This method is more productive than simply listing the activities that should be limited. This is not to say that the patient should not be warned about activities that entail significant risk. The thrust of the discussion, however, should be on what *can* be done rather than what *cannot*.

Sports and other physical activities can be grouped based on their physical and emotional requirements. Some sports have a high degree of isometric activity, that is, an activity in which a muscle develops a large force with minimal muscular or joint movement (weight lifting). Other sports have a large amount of isotonic activity, that is, sports in which large muscular and joint movements occur with little change in force (tennis). Other sports have large isotonic and isometric exercise occurring together (ice hockey). Furthermore, some sports have a higher risk of injury (gymnastics).

Thorough understanding of the patient's cardiac defect must be known prior to recommending activities. Most patients with acyanotic forms of congenital heart disease have either valvar abnormalities (e.g., pulmonic or aortic) or a left-to-right shunt (e.g., atrial septal defect, ventricular septal defect). Valvar defects are usually graded trivial, mild, moderate, or severe; and left-to-right shunt lesions are graded trivial, small, medium, and large. These patients may have had previous surgery, or they may not have required surgery.

Cyanotic forms of congenital heart disease can be considered mild, moderate, or severe in relation to the intensity of hypoxemia expressed (e.g., by the degree of hematocrit elevation). Patients with these conditions usually have had one or more operations. Surgery may be palliative (e.g., a Blalock-Taussig shunt for tetralogy of Fallot) or reparative (arterial switch procedure for transposition of the great arteries). Patients who have had only palliative surgery for a cyanotic form of congenital heart disease remain hypoxemic to some degree and may have significantly limited exercise tolerance. Exercise recommendations therefore must take this condition into account. Those who have had a reparative procedure may not have any degree of hypoxemia and may not require any exercise limitations.

Primary myocardial disease, such as hypertrophic obstructive cardiomyopathy or chronic dilated cardiomyopathy, may be congenital or acquired. Myocardial diseases may be static or progressive. In the latter case, exercise recommendations probably change over time for a specific patient.

Patients who participate at the organized, competitive level usually experience external pressure to perform in addition to internal motivation. This pressure can come from coaches, teammates, and parents and may force the patient to perform beyond that which feels comfortable.

Patients with acyanotic forms of congenital heart disease, such as valvar aortic stenosis, are often asymptomatic. Aortic stenosis deserves particular attention because it is a frequent abnormality, especially in boys, and because when severe there is a risk, albeit small, of sudden death. It sometimes seems that more often than not patients with aortic stenosis are good athletes, highly motivated, and have a parent who is involved in coaching the patient, thereby making life difficult for the child's physicians. Patients who are asymptomatic (no palpitations, exercise-induced chest pain, or syncope) are encouraged to develop good exercise habits with mild to moderate amounts of aerobic activities; isometric exercise to maintain muscle tone is allowed in patients with moderate disease only to the extent that the patient may lift weights so long as it is still possible to hold a conversation without closing the glottis. Asymptomatic patients with mild disease (<30 mm Hg gradient and normal cardiac output) are encouraged to participate in all forms of organized athletic activity. Patients with moderate disease (30 to 60 mm Hg) are exercise-tested to evaluate ischemia and exercise-induced arrhythmias. Should these events occur, patients are allowed to participate only in activities of low intensity (e.g., golf, bowling). If there is no evidence of ventricular ectopy at rest and an exercise test is normal, patients are encouraged to participate in activities of low intensity, although they may be permitted activities of moderate intensity for isotonic demands (e.g., baseball, badminton, cross country running, tennis, volleyball) at the organized, competitive level. Patients with severe disease usually are under consideration for surgical or catheter intervention therapy, and only low-intensity activities at the noncompetitive level are allowed. Valvar aortic stenosis often is progressive, and serial evaluation to reassess severity is necessary.

Cyanotic patients who have not had an operation or who have had only a palliative procedure are encouraged to perform only mild forms of aerobic exercise at the noncompetitive level. Most patients within this group self-limit their activities because chronic hypoxemia predisposes them to symptoms with exercise. As more cardiac defects become repairable during infancy and early childhood, it is less common to have patients remaining cyanotic. Patients who are hypoxemic because obstructive pulmonary vascular disease precludes surgical correction are an exception to this trend. These patients are encouraged to do some walking, but they should not participate in organized competitive athletics. Even with bowling a low-weight bowling ball may be necessary.

Patients who have had repair of cyanotic congenital heart defects usually have improved exercise tolerance compared with that both measured and perceived preoperatively. Postoperative exercise tolerance, however, still is not normal. Formal exercise testing is helpful for evaluating the patient's objective level of exercise tolerance. These patients are excellent candidates for a postoperative cardiopulmonary rehabilitation program.

Patients with primary myocardial disease such as hypertrophic obstructive cardiomyopathy present difficult management decisions to the primary care physician and the pediatric cardiologist. Patients with severe hypertrophic obstructive cardiomyopathy, manifested by left ventricular wall thickness greater than 2.0 cm, significant left ventricular outflow obstruction at rest, family history of sudden death due to this disease, or ventricular ectopy should not participate in any organized competitive athletics. They should participate only in low-level noncompetitive activities.

Patients with Marfan syndrome may need to have their activity restricted. All such patients should have a cardiac evaluation with echocardiography. Those patients who have cardiovascular involvement, especially aortic root dilation, should be allowed to participate in organized competitive athletics only at the low-intensity level. They should completely avoid activities that put them at risk for sustaining acceleration–deceleration injuries that can result in aortic dissection (e.g., basketball). Those without cardiovascular involvement may participate in activities at the organized competitive athletic level that have isotonic dynamic and low isometric demands, such as baseball, running, tennis, and badminton.

Patients with a cardiac rhythm disturbance often have an otherwise normal heart. These individuals also need specific recommendations regarding daily exercise activities and competitive athletics. Virtually every such patient can participate in some form of exercise; not all are allowed to participate at the organized competitive level, however. The most frequent arrhythmia seen is supraventricular tachycardia (SVT). Patients who have SVT *without* the Wolff-Parkinson-White (WPW) syndrome, who are controlled on medication, and in whom the arrhythmia is not induced by exercise testing are allowed to participate in all types of organized competitive athletics. The physician must be aware that certain medications (e.g., β-blockers) interfere with exercise performance, and that patients may discontinue their medication if they perceive this interference, thereby increasing arrhythmia risk. Open and frank discussion of life style with the patient and the patient's family prior to beginning antiarrhythmic therapy may prevent this predicament.

Patients with WPW syndrome are at risk, albeit small, for sudden death. This tragedy may be due to the development of atrial fibrillation or flutter with a fast conducting bypass tract that in turn leads to ventricular fibrillation. Management within this patient population is changing rapidly. Patients with WPW syndrome who wish to participate in organized competitive athletics now can undergo radiofrequency ablation of their bypass tract (see Chapter 11).

Patients with ventricular arrhythmias must be grouped into those who are symptomatic, with syncope or near syncope, and those who are asymptomatic. Symptomatic patients, such as those who have long QT syndrome, may be allowed to participate in noncompetitive low-intensity activities. They should not, however, participate in organized competitive athletics. Asymptomatic patients, whose ventricular ectopy is suppressed during exercise testing, are allowed to participate at all levels of organized competitive athletics. Patients whose ectopy is either unchanged or exacerbated with exercise are treated and retested. If ectopy is controlled, these patients are allowed to participate in organized competitive athletics, provided compliance with medication can be documented.

Residual abnormalities may be present after surgical repair of a congenital cardiac defect. They include persistent right ventricular outflow obstruction, residual septal defects, and rhythm disturbances (supraventricular and ventricular tachyarrhythmias, as well as bradyarrhythmias with and without sinus mode dysfunction). Recommendations with regard to competitive athletics are complex in these patients. Control of an arrhythmia associated with exercise is essential. Patients with an excellent surgical repair (e.g., tetralogy of Fallot with no significant residual outflow gradient, no residual shunt, normal cardiac size on chest radiograph, and no significant arrhythmias at rest or with exercise) may participate in all forms of competitive athletics. Patients with moderate residual lesions, such as obstruction to ventricular outflow or a significant left-to-right shunt, are encouraged to participate in low-intensity activities. In the absence of ventricular ectopy, additional activities such as baseball, tennis, and volleyball are encouraged.

SEXUALITY

Most individuals with congenital cardiac malformations described in the Natural History Study married and had families at rates similar to those of the general population.[1] They also had the national average rate of marital longevity and divorce. Adolescents often are preoccupied with concerns regarding sexuality. Adolescence is commonly the time of sexual exploration; hence in addition to all the usual problems of adolescence, young people with heart malformations have other concerns. The practitioner may be asked by the patient for information regarding contraception, pregnancy, delivery, and risk to the offspring. If these concerns are not raised by the patient or parent, it is the physician's responsibility to initiate the discussion. This discussion of sexuality should be held with the patient without the presence of parents and should include whether the patient is heterosexual, bisexual, or lesbian/gay, as this information may direct further, specific counseling.

Contraceptive measures in most patients with congenital malformations of the heart are not different from those used by normal individuals. Abstinence from sexual intercourse should eliminate the possibility of pregnancy and substantially reduce the risk of sexually transmitted diseases. More young people now seem to be taking this approach. In a sexually active female patient, prevention of pregnancy usually is accomplished best by using low-estrogen birth control pills or barrier methods, such as a condom or diaphragm with spermicidal foam. An intrauterine device is not recommended because it introduces risk of bacteremia and therefore increases the risk of infective endocarditis. Higher-estrogen birth control pills can create a state of hypercoagulability, which could increase the risk of a cerebrovascular accident in cyanotic patients who have persistently high hemoglobin levels. The practitioner must counsel the patient that, although pregnancy may be prevented, the "pill" has no influence on exposure to sexually transmitted diseases. Barrier methods are somewhat less effective for preventing pregnancy, but they have few or no side effects regarding the patient's cardiac status.

Pregnancy planning is important for moderate- to high-risk female patients. Cardiac catheterization may be necessary to determine hemodynamics so the patient can be adequately advised about risks associated with pregnancy. Patients with artificial heart valves who require anticoagulation should be switched from sodium warfarin to heparin prior to conception to avoid the teratogenic effect of warfarin. Risk of teratogenic effect may apply also to certain antiarrhythmic medications. Patients who have supraventricular reentry tachycardias, such as WPW syndrome, and who require potentially teratogenic medication, may be treated by radiofrequency transcatheter ablation of the bypass tract before contemplating pregnancy.

Stringent precautions must be used in patients who have conditions that cannot be corrected and that present substantial risk of morbidity or mortality during pregnancy. For example, patients with Eisenmenger syndrome may develop a hypoxic crisis related to decreased pulmonary blood flow from which they may not recover. Indeed, patients with pulmonary vascular obstructive disease have approximately 50 per cent mortality when attempting to carry a pregnancy to term. Pregnancy termination also is associated with risk, so prevention is the best approach. Such patients who choose to be sexually active must consider surgical sterilization. Sterilization should be considered a permanent preventive procedure, as reversal is difficult and usually unsuccessful. Another option for long-term contraception is subcutaneous insertion of long-acting hormone-containing devices (Norplant). Such devices can be effective for up to 5 years, are removable, and seem to have no cardiovascular effects.

Other cardiac conditions in which risk of pregnancy is substantial are congestive cardiomyopathy and Marfan syndrome. A patient in low cardiac output state due to cardiomyopathy may not tolerate increased circulatory demands of the fetoplacental unit. Marfan syndrome and other conditions associated with cystic medionecrosis of the aorta involve the risk of aortic rupture. It might be argued that cardiomyopathy patients could become pregnant after cardiac transplantation. Risks to the fetus of immunosuppressive agents must be considered, however. Some patients with aortic cystic medionecrosis have had successful pregnancies after aortic root replacement. No patients have yet been reported to have successfully completed a pregnancy after heart–lung transplantation for Eisenmenger syndrome, but it may be possible in the future. Other potentially hazardous cardiac abnormalities could be treated operatively before pregnancy, lessening the chance of mortality and decreasing morbidity. They include severe mitral stenosis, severe hypertrophic obstructive cardiomyopathy, and aortic valvar stenosis. The patient who has had a Fontan procedure is at risk but usually not at the same level as those last mentioned.

Pregnancy management in most patients who have low-risk congenital malformations of the heart is little different from that necessary for the general population. Any complicated delivery requires antibiotic prophylaxis to minimize the possibility of bacterial endocarditis. It is usually given in the form of amoxicillin 3.0 gm PO followed 6 hours later by 1.5 gm PO[7] (see Chapter 15). If the patient's lesion is considered high risk, such as a prosthetic valve, treatment recommendation is intravenous or intramuscular ampicillin 50 mg/kg plus gentamicin 2.0 mg/kg 30 minutes before delivery, repeating these doses in 6 to 8 hours.

Delivery should take place where facilities, equipment, and personnel are available to manage these patients and their offspring. This point applies especially to those with high-risk pregnancies. Careful prelabor planning should include consideration of the anticipated type of delivery—vaginal or cesarean section. Patients with certain cardiac lesions (e.g., cystic medionecrosis of the aorta) may be afforded less risk if the second stage of labor can be avoided. These considerations must be discussed in detail by the patient, primary care physician, obstetrician, and cardiologist well before the estimated date of confinement.

Most women who have a congenital cardiac defect are concerned about their offspring's chance of having a similar malformation, and some studies have suggested that the overall risk is approximately 10 per cent.[8] There is risk for the offspring of an affected father as well. Fetal cardiac ultrasonography, performed at 18 to 24 weeks' gestation, usually is accurate and can reassure the mother that the fetal heart is normal.[9] The Natural History Study[1] showed that mothers with pulmonic stenosis and ventricular septal defect produced 1 malformation of the heart per 100 newborns, and those with aortic stenosis had a rate of 3 malformations per 100 births. Other studies have suggested that certain lesions in the mother are associated with a greater incidence of congenital heart lesions in newborns. It is especially the case with aortic valve stenosis and coarctation of the aorta.[10] Thus although fetal ultrasonographic cardiac screening of all pregnancies in mothers with congenital heart disease is probably desirable, screening those with left-sided outflow tract obstruction is especially useful. This topic is further discussed in Chapter 17.

Another concern of patients who underwent surgery during the early 1980s is possible exposure to human immunodeficiency virus (HIV)-contaminated blood products before testing for this virus was available. These patients had little risk of HIV exposure; but, if requested by the patient, antibody testing should be done.

DEVELOPMENTALLY RELATED PROBLEMS

More young people with congenital heart disease have developmental problems than do the general population. Examples include individuals with Down syndrome and Williams syndrome. These patients receive the same medical and surgical treatment as the developmentally normal population. Their self-care and that provided by others usually is helped by correction of their lesion, assuming that the treatment has been beneficial. It is much easier to care for a 20-year-old person with Down syndrome who has had a ventricular septal defect repaired

than for one who has Eisenmenger syndrome. Our present health care system should be able to provide for all, so there is little or no justification for not providing equal treatment to developmentally challenged patients. Ethical arguments are appropriate when lesions may not be correctable or can be treated only at high risk, but the same applies to the general population. The severity of the handicap is a valid argument at times, but this point must be carefully considered.

Advocacy for the handicapped adolescent and young adult often must be initiated by their health care provider in coordination with various community agencies and resources. Advocacy does not mean being sympathetic or feeling sorry for the person. It means helping them find ways to achieve as much independence as their physical condition and developmental abilities allow and improving understanding of their needs at the work place and in society.

CHOICE OF HEALTH CARE PROVIDER

The young adult, born with a congenital heart defect most likely was cared for by a family practitioner or pediatrician and a pediatric cardiologist. By their late teens or early twenties, however, many are dismissed from pediatric care resources. The patient may then gravitate from the care of a pediatric cardiologist to that of an internal medicine cardiologist, who may have had little training dealing with congenital heart lesions. The young adult often is not reevaluated for many years, despite previously having been evaluated annually.[1] Sporadic and incomplete care may be avoided by combining the expertise of both pediatric and internal medicine cardiology disciplines in a young adult cardiac clinic staffed with pediatric cardiologists and internal medicine cardiologists. Internal medicine should incorporate pediatric cardiologists into their cardiology educational training programs. Pediatric cardiologists should be willing to participate in the education of their internist colleagues and should attend conferences, clinics, and catheterizations on young adults who have congenital heart disease.

Pediatricians and pediatric cardiologists may continue responsibility for the care of the young adult with a congenital malformation of the heart until the patient feels more comfortable in other care resources, which may happen at age 18 or age 40. Accepting responsibility for care of the young adult infers more than just a continuing interest in one's patient. Pediatric physicians must be willing to learn about the needs and problems of this older population. Physicians who combine pediatric and internal medicine training may be ideally suited to provide care to this population.

Cardiology provider choice depends to some extent on the particular lesion. The internist-cardiologist may understand mitral valve prolapse and ventricular tachycardia better than the pediatric cardiologist, whereas the latter should have a better appreciation of tricuspid valve atresia following Fontan's repair. Combining the talents of each into a shared-care young adult cardiology clinic can enhance substantially the quality of patient care as well as physician satisfaction.

REFERENCES

1. Nadas AS, Miettinen OS, Rees JK, Weidman WH: Second Natural History Report of Congenital Heart Defects. Circulation(Suppl); 1993 (in press).

2. Allen HD, Gersony WM, Taubert KA: Insurability of the Adolescent and young adult with heart disease: based on the fifth conference on Insurability, Columbus, Ohio, October 1991. Circulation (in press).

3. Truesdell SC, Clark EB: Health insurance status in a cohort of children and young adults with congenital cardiac diagnoses [abstract]. Circulation 84:II-386, 1991.

4. Garson Jr A, Allen HD, Gersony WM, et al: Cost of congenital heart disease in children and adults: sources of variation assessed by multicenter study [abstract]. Circulation 84:II-385, 1991.

5. Talner NS, McCue Jr HM, Graham TP, et al: Guidelines for insurability of patient with congenital heart disease. Circulation 62: 1419A–1424A, 1980.

6. Mitchell JH, Maron BJ, Epstein SE: 16th Bethesda conference: cardiovascular abnormalities in the athlete: recommendations regarding eligibility for competition. J Am Coll Cardiol 6: 1185–1232, 1985.

7. Dajani AS, Bisno AL, Chung KJ, et al: Prevention of bacterial endocarditis: recommendations by the American Heart Association. JAMA 264: 2919–2922, 1990.

8. Rose V, Gold RJM, Lindsay G, Allen M: A possible increase in the incidence of congenital heart defects among the offspring of affected parents. J Am Coll Cardiol 6:376–382, 1985.

9. Wheller JJ, Reiss R, Allen HD: Clinical experience with fetal echocardiography. Am J Dis Child 144:49–53, 1989.

10. Boughman JA, Berg KA, Astemborski JA, et al: Familial risks of congenital heart defect assessed in a population-based epidemiologic study. Am J Med Genet 26:839–849, 1987.

INDEX

Note: Page numbers in *italics* refer to illustrations; numbers followed by t refer to tables.